Peritoneal Dialysis – State-of-the-Art 2012

IRRIV
International
Renal Research
Institute Vicenza

Contributions to Nephrology

Vol. 178

Series Editor

Claudio Ronco Vicenza

Peritoneal Dialysis – State-of-the-Art 2012

Volume Editors

Claudio Ronco Vicenza

Mitchell H. Rosner Charlottesville, Va.

Carlo Crepaldi Vicenza

28 figures, 2 in color, and 30 tables, 2012

KARGER

Basel · Freiburg · Paris · London · New York · New Delhi · Bangkok · Beijing · Tokyo · Kuala Lumpur · Singapore · Sydney

Contributions to Nephrology
(Founded 1975 by Geoffrey M. Berlyne)

Claudio Ronco
Department of Nephrology
Dialysis and Transplantation
International Renal Research Institute
San Bortolo Hospital
IT-36100 Vicenza

Mitchell H. Rosner
Division of Nephrology
University of Virginia Health System
Charlottesvile, VA 22908 (USA)

Carlo Crepaldi
Department of Nephrology
Dialysis & Transplantation
San Bortolo Hospital
IT-36100 Vicenza

Library of Congress Cataloging-in-Publication Data

Peritoneal dialysis : state-of-the-art 2012 / volume editors, Claudio Ronco, Mitchell H. Rosner, Carlo Crepaldi.
p. ; cm. -- (Contributions to nephrology, ISSN 0302-5144 ; v. 178)
Includes bibliographical references and indexes.
ISBN 978-3-318-02162-2 (hard cover : a k. paper) -- ISBN 978-3-318-02163-9 (e-ISBN)
I. Ronco, C. (Claudio), 1951- II. Rosner, Mitchell H. III. Crepaldi, Carlo. IV. Series: Contributions to nephrology, v. 178 ; 0302-5144.
[DNLM: 1. Peritoneal Dialysis. W1 CO778UN v.178 2012 / WJ 378]

617.4'61059--dc23

2012016243

Bibliographic Indices. This publication is listed in bibliographic services, including Current Contents® and Index Medicus.

Drug Dosage. The authors and the publisher have exerted every effort to ensure that drug selection and dosage set forth in this text are in accord with current recommendations and practice at the time of publication. However, in view of ongoing research, changes in government regulations, and the constant flow of information relating to drug therapy and drug reactions, the reader is urged to check the package insert for each drug for any change in indications and dosage and for added warnings and precautions. This is particularly important when the recommended agent is a new and/or infrequently employed drug.

www.karger.com
Printed in Germany on acid-free and non-aging paper (ISO 9706) by Bosch Druck, Ergolding
ISSN 0302–5144
e-ISSN 1662–2782
ISBN 978–3–318–02162–2
e-ISBN 978–3–318–02163–9

Contents

Preface

Thirty years ago, the first International Course on Peritoneal Dialysis took place in Vicenza, Italy, under the auspices of the International Society of Peritoneal Dialysis and under the guidance of Professor La Greca. Many courses were subsequently held in Vicenza always characterized by a common denominator: quality of the educational programme.

'The family is back.' That phrase is the one we always use to start the opening ceremony of the Vicenza International Course on Peritoneal Dialysis. There has been a special feeling and a particular environment in which the course has grown, making it clear why we call it 'the family'. In the early 1970s peritoneal dialysis (PD) was performed by repeated abdominal puncture using simple infusion sets and 2-liter bottles of PD solutions. The renal ward founded at San Bortolo Hospital in Vicenza by Giuseppe La Greca in 1970 had two rooms dedicated to PD since its beginnings. PD was performed intermittently, three times a week, and PD solution was delivered by gravity from the new 10-liter plastic containers. In those years, various schedules were prescribed, customized PD catheters were made in house and ultrafiltration was monitored by bed scales. When I joined the department's medical team in 1977, I was impressed by the enormous amount of experience that had matured in the group. I immediately understood how much could be learned in that environment and I decided to start my research in PD, where new developments were still very much needed. My first research work dealt with PD clearances at various dialysate flow

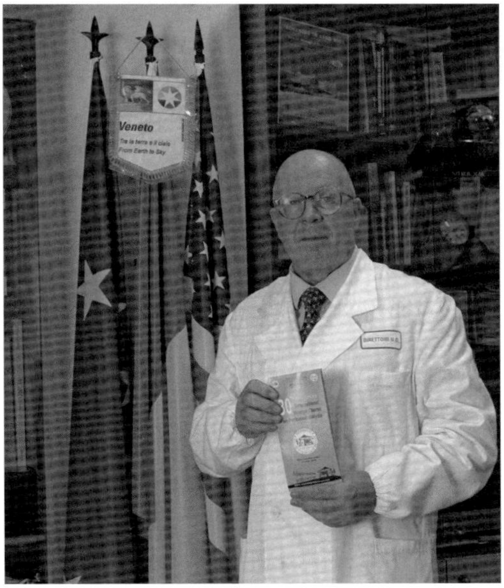

rates and dwell times. A few months later, the first paper that included my name among the members of the team was published. I still remember late evenings in the office of Professor LaGreca, all of us struggling with the difficult undertaking of writing in English. A few months later, continuous ambulatory peritoneal dialysis (CAPD) appeared on the scene and interest in PD skyrocketed. In those days the idea matured to write a book on PD: The 'yellow book' was the ideal academic completion of a huge body of clinical work. At the same time we decided to organize the first international course on PD in Vicenza.

We then started planning topics and speakers for the program. The first telephone calls overseas to invite Popovich, Moncrief, Nolph, and other experts in the field were difficult. Nobody knew who we were or where Vicenza was, but in the end we gathered a series of positive answers and a general consensus. The first Vicenza International Course on Peritoneal Dialysis was announced in 1981. As a logo for the course, we decided to use one of the most important architectural jewels of Vicenza: the Villa Capra detta 'la Rotonda' di Andrea Palladio. We felt that this logo gave a local trademark to the course, while at the same time being internationally recognizable. With the years, this has become the logo of our department. The congress center, located at the Ente Fiera of Vicenza, was just a big room without amenities or services. We were kept very busy preparing the screen and the audiovisuals, all the signage (including those pointing the way to the restrooms), and the congress kits. For the first course, we prepared picture-ID badges in advance, and all delegates were immediately recognized and welcomed when they arrived at the registration desk. The opening ceremony was held at the Teatro Olimpico, another masterpiece by Andrea Palladio. These appealing special events and the quality of the scientific program made the first International course a real success. The most important experts in the field gathered in Vicenza in 1982, and the faculty of the course included the top experts of the day in PD. Fred Boen, Lazaro Gotloib, Robert Popovich, Jack Moncrief, Charles Mion, Karl Nolph, Steven Vas and Jack Maher were just a few names of the friends who honored the Vicenza course with their presence. The Course became a mixture of high scientific quality and cheerful Mediterranean environment. The scientific programs of the Vicenza Course have always been up to date. At later courses, the most important topics of the moment were always included in the program. Main themes have been the kinetics of ultrafiltration, the reduction of peritonitis, the effects of diabetes and metabolism, and new catheters for chronic PD. Morphological modifications of the peritoneal membrane and the role of the immune response to bacterial invasion of the peritoneal cavity were also discussed. In 1988, the first industry panel was organized including companies interested in PD such as Bieffe, Braun, Fresenius, Pierrel, Sifra and Baxter. The initial experience of PD registries in various regions of the world was reported by Nolph and Oreopoulos. The important issue of comparing PD outcomes with those of hemodialysis was also debated. In 1991, the course focused on the prescription and delivery of PD and on new criteria to assess the adequacy of therapy. New trends in PD solutions were presented at following meetings and they are even discussed in this latest edition. Cytokine production by peritoneal macrophages and the clinical application of erythropoietin were presented by Jörres, Gahl and Winchester in subsequent editions. The optimization of the Y-set for CAPD was described by Buoncristiani in 1994. Until 1991, the course proceedings were always published in time for the meeting, so that delegates always had the book in their course bag. The books were published by Wichtig Editore as standalone publications, and the number of literature citations for these books were increasing progressively. In 1994, we decided to continue the tradition of timely publication of the proceedings, but the papers were collected in a special issue of *Peritoneal Dialysis International*. Dr. LaGreca was president of the International Society of Peritoneal Dialysis at the time, and we felt it important to publish the proceedings of our course in the official journal of the society. In the 1994 proceedings, specific papers were dedicated to new osmotic agents and new PD solutions. In 1997, the interest in new PD solutions continued, and new, vital issues such as automated PD, the importance of residual renal function, and the importance of computers and the Internet in the management of PD programs were discussed. Another important topic first discussed at the Vicenza Course was the integration of PD with hemodialysis and transplantation in active uremia treatment. Subsequent editions were dedicated to the most actual topics of PD and the programs can be found at the web site www.vicenzanephrocourses.com or in the index of the several books containing the proceedings and published by Karger in the book series *Contributions to Nephrology*. In 1991, the International Vicenza Award was instituted and given to a distinguished scientist in the field of PD. The late John F. Maher was the first winner. Subsequent winners were Karl D. Nolph and Dimitri Oreopoulos, Ram Gokal and Lazaro Gotloib, and Jonas Bergstrom. As we gather today, we are celebrating 30 years of science and education in the field of PD. The Vicenza International Course has indeed represented a cornerstone in the education and practice of PD. The design of the course itself is unchanged and will remain so. We are indebted to all the people who have made possible the progressive growth and the remarkable success of the course. Our audience has expanded, and we now have delegates from around the world, including Africa and Asia. We hope that our educational effort has been useful to many people and that it will continue to be useful to coming generations of physicians and nurses. A special thanks to Anna Saccardo, Marta Scabardi, Alessandra Brando and Ilaria Balbo who have organized the logistics and all the details of the Vicenza courses in the past and present editions. A special thanks goes to Karger publishing house for the usual outstanding quality of the publication. The 30th Annual International Vicenza Course has yet another exceptional group of speakers and we are excited that this special issue of *Contributions to Nephrology* is ready to guide attendees through the event and serve as a valuable tool for the future. We hope that the readers will enjoy the book and will consider it a companion for their daily clinical practice as well as for research.

Claudio Ronco, Vicenza

The International Vicenza Course on Peritoneal Dialysis – 30 Year Anniversary

From 1975–1982, there were many important developments and events that had a very significant impact on the growth and advancement of peritoneal dialysis(PD) as a renal replacement therapy. In 1975, Drs. Moncrief and Popovich placed their first patient on continuous ambulatory peritoneal dialysis (CAPD). In 1977, the University of Missouri began a collaboration with with Drs. Moncrief and Popovich to do clinical studies in patients on CAPD funded by NIH. This collaboration led to the NIH CAPD Registry which operated from 1981–1988 before being integrated with the United States Renal Data System. In 1978, Dr. Trevino-Becerrra organized and chaired the first International PD Congress in Chapala, Mexico. At this congress in Mexico, the decision for subsequent conferences in other areas of the world gave birth to the ISPD. The second congress was held in Berlin in 1981, organized by Drs. Kessel and Gahl. In 1981, in order to promote participation in the NIH CAPD Registry, the University of Missouri organized a CAPD Conference which was held in Kansas City, Mo.; this became a yearly event and grew into the International PD Conference and eventually the International Annual Dialysis Conference (ADC); the 32nd ADC was held in San Antonio, Tex., in February 2012.

In 1982, the Department of Nephrology at S. BortolamiusHospital in Vicenza, Italy, under the direction of Dr. La Greca, organized the first International Vicenza Course on Peritoneal Dialysis (IVC). Dr. Ronco served as General Secretary of the IVC from 1982 until he became IVC Director in 2001 when Dr. La Greca retired. This course has been presented every three years and this summer will celebrate its 30th anniversary.

Thus, the IVC now joins the ADC and ISPD as a family of meetings that have worked to promote education, research and the best clinical practices in PD therapy. These meetings have exhibited marvelous collaborations during these 30 or more years. Meeting planners and speakers overlap extensively. Each meeting promotes the other two meetings. Many have had the privilege of serving and/or being recognized by several of these meetings. For example, the late Jack Maher, MDwas the first President of ISPD, the recipient of the first International Vicenza Award at the fourth IVC in 1991 and the winner of the Lifetime Achievement Award in PD at the ADC in 1993. I was honored to be the 3rdpresident of ISPD, have chaired the ADC for 32 years and was awarded the second International Vicenza Award at the IVC in 1994. Claudio Ronco, current chair of the IVC, was awarded the ADC Lifetime Achievement Award in PD at the 32nd ADC this year.

Those who have been involved in all three meetings over many years have been welcomed at the IVC by Dr. Ronco as 'the family'. This reflects the spirit of cooperation and comradeship among those who have had the common goal of making PD a better therapy over many decades. The spirit of cooperation among those involved in these three meetings serves as a role model for other specialty areas.

The topics and speakers at the IVC have a tradition of excellence. The publication of the IVC proceedings have often been accomplished ahead of the meeting dates and have been valuable additions to the PD literature.

The IVC has experienced remarkable success in exposing those of us who attend to Italian history and culture. Touring the amazing architectural accomplishments in the city of Vicenza, especially those of Palladio are an extra benefit of attending the IVC. Dinners and receptions are hosted in charming villas. Italian hospitality is legendary.

Dr. ZbylutTwardowski (Columbia, Mo.) summarizes all of the above very well:

'I participated twice at the International Courses on Peritoneal Dialysis organized by St. Bortolo Hospital in Vicenza. The first time it was during the 5th Course in May 24–25, 1994, organized by Prof. Giuseppe La Greca. The meeting was held in the Convention Hall of the BancoAmbrosiano Veneto. The second time I participated on the 15th International Vicenza Course on Peritoneal Dialysis, organized by Prof. Claudio Ronco from May 30 to June 01, 2006, in the Congress Center EnteFiera in Vicenza. The courses were very well organized with important presentations of the best PD experts. In the evening after the course in 2006 we had an impressive Gala Dinner in Villa Imperiali Lampertico.

In addition to valuable presentations I could visit several places of interest designed by famous Andrea Palladio including Villa Capra detta'la Rotonda', Basilica Palladiana, TeatroOlimpico and other places like Villa Trissino where Palladio worked as a mason. It is worth mentioning that the main building of the University of Virginia was named The Rotunda by Thomas Jefferson in honor of Andrea Palladio'.

Dr. Jack Moncrief (Austin, Tex.) also shares his thoughts:

'Thank you for the opportunity to write about the great conferences held in Vicenza. I attended the very first and many subsequent meetings and found them all educational, very well organized and great fun for the participants. The conference was instrumental in helping initiate and demonstrate the value of the transformation of peritoneal dialysis due to the 'long dwell' concept developed by Dr. Robert Popovichand myself here in Austin, Tex. Your conference was responsible for the early and rapid adoption of the CAPD technique by the Italian nephrology community. This interest and utilization has proved correct as there is now a major shift taking place in many countries toward wider use of peritoneal dialysis as an alternative to 'center' hemodialysis.

The nephrology community has recognized your contribution by both the support of the conference and by the many awards you have received, including the recent 'Lifetime Achievement in PD' award at the 'Annual Dialysis Conference' in San Antonio, Tex. This early interest stimulated by the Vicenza conference was directly responsible for the reduction in episodes of peritonitis in PD by the 'drain before fill' concept in which you participated. This concept has now become standard practice throughout the world. Thanks for the opportunity to come to Vicenza and to Italy for so many good reasons'.

Dr. Bengt Lindholm (Stockholm, Sweden had the following to say:

'I feel honored to be given this opportunity to express my appreciation of this important anniversary. Since the first International Course on Peritoneal Dialysis in Vicenza in 1982, and still going strong for the 30 years thereafter, the Vicenza courses have provided a great educational opportunity for clinicians and researchers wanting to learn more about peritoneal dialysis. The courses which put Vicenza on the map of important nephrology centers in the world have been an ideal platform also for in-depth scientific and clinical updates and discussions among experts dedicated to peritoneal dialysis.

With Giuseppe La Greca as President during the early years, and always with Claudio Ronco as the primus motor, the courses (and the proceedings) have been of great importance and truly conducive to the acceptance, dissemination and development of the new therapy not least during the sensitive infant period of CAPD. The personal, wonderful warm atmosphere of the conferences, and the excellent opportunities for discussions during the social programs, have contributed very much to its success.

The nephrology community is indebted to the organizers for their visions, endurance and very hard work for the benefit of the patients. I salute, congratulate and thank Claudio Ronco and his team for this achievement!'

Congratulations to the Vicenza Nephrology Group for the important contributions of the IVC over the past 30 years.

Karl D. Nolph, MD
Curators's Emeritus Professor of
Internal Medicine
University of Missouri School of Medicine,
Columbia, Mo.

Ronco C, Rosner MH, Crepaldi C (eds): Peritoneal Dialysis – State-of-the-Art 2012.
Contrib Nephrol. Basel, Karger, 2012, vol 178, pp 1–5

Twenty Years of Bicarbonate Solutions

Mariano Feriani

Department of Nephrology and Dialysis, dell'Angelo Hospital and S.S. Giovanni e Paolo Hospital, Mestre and Venice, Venice, Italy

Abstract

For many years, lactate has been used successfully as a buffer in peritoneal dialysis solutions although its effectiveness in the correction of uremic acidosis and its biocompatibility on peritoneal resident cells have been questioned. In addition, some investigators have suggested other potential adverse metabolic effects resulting from the unphysiologically high lactate flux into the body during CAPD. These potential problems associated with lactate-containing CAPD solution prompted the search for alternative buffer-containing solutions. Bicarbonate, the physiological buffer, was considered when the problem of calcium and magnesium carbonate solubility was solved by the use of a two-compartment bag system allowing the mixing of bicarbonate and divalent cations immediately before infusion. The long-term tolerance, safety, efficacy and therapeutic value of a bicarbonate-buffered peritoneal dialysis solution have been evaluated for about 15 years. RCT studies demonstrated a benefit for acid base improvement, while observational reports showed other clinical effects such as a preservation of residual renal function, less inflammatory effect and peritonitis prevention. In addition, there is a consensus that local biocompatibility is improved. Therefore, as bicarbonate is the physiological buffer of the body, it should become the solution of choice in PD patients.

In end-stage renal failure patients the buffer capacity is restored by providing a buffer source in the dialysis fluid. In peritoneal dialysis the buffer is included in the fresh dialysis solution daily infused in the peritoneal cavity.

Bicarbonate was initially used by Boen [1] in peritoneal dialysis fluid, but it was soon replaced by lactate when it was found that calcium carbonate precipitated and the solution became alkaline during autoclaving.

Subsequently, acetate and lactate were introduced as buffer substance in peritoneal dialysis fluid. Despite acetate has been proved to be effective in correcting uremic metabolic acidosis both in CAPD and in intermittent treatment [2], it was quickly abandoned because it seemed to produce vasodilation and alterations of the peritoneal membrane leading to hyperpermeability, loss of ultrafiltration and possibly development of sclerosing peritonitis [3, 4].

Lactate is now the most commonly used buffer and no major clinical adverse events related to its use have been reported in PD patients since the introduction of peritoneal dialysis in clinical practice. However, in the last decade, several investigations have pointed out that the standard lactate buffered PD solution presents some problems:

a potential metabolic side effects,
b biocompatibility,
c not full correction of metabolic acidosis.

Chemical Principle of the Bicarbonate Solution

The undesired effects ascribed to lactate-containing solutions have prompted a search for alternative buffering agents.

Bicarbonate, the physiological buffer, was proposed again in 1985 [5].

The key idea for avoiding the chemical precipitation was the separation of the calcium and magnesium from bicarbonate by a two-compartment bag system, which allows the mixing of bicarbonate and divalent cations only just before the use [6].

The alkaline compartment contains only sodium bicarbonate and the pH is rather high (pH 7.80–8.0), while the acidic part contains all the other electrolytes and glucose, but also includes a small amount of an acid. At the beginning this was the acetic acid, similarly to the bicarbonate dialysate used in hemodialysis, afterwards it was replaced by the metabolically inert hydrochloride acid. The pH of the acid compartment is very low (pH 2.5–3) thus avoiding the formation of the glucose degradation products (GDPs) deriving from the glucose sterilization. This principle of the two-compartment bag is now exploited by all the new biocompatible solutions with a low GDPs content.

When the two compartments are mixed, the hydrochloride acid reacts with the sodium bicarbonate generating carbon dioxide and water and adjusting the pH of the final solution to the physiological value (7.40). Since carbon dioxide is a gas it possesses a certain pressure (pCO_2) and consequently tends to evaporate from the bag. The pH increases according to the CO_2 content decrease and when the solubility product of the calcium carbonate is reached, this molecule precipitates. It was theoretically and empirically demonstrated that the final solution remains stable (i.e. without precipitate) for more than 24 h, which is much more than its use both in CAPD than in APD.

Early Studies with the Bicarbonate Solution

After several in vitro studies and in an animal model, a first acute study was performed in 1985 in patients with a homemade solution containing 35 mmol/l of bicarbonate and 5 mmol/l of acetate [7]. A total of 45 exchanges were performed in 4 patients, 1 of them being treated for a week. No side effects were recorded and in the patient treated for a longer period a detectable increase in blood bicarbonate was demonstrated.

Some months later, another patient was treated for 2 months until she was transplanted and, again, no side effects were registered. In this patient a solution with a reduced content of acetate (2 mmol/l) was used [not published].

The first pilot study with an industrially made bag was performed after about 10 years from the beginning of the bicarbonate history [8]. The most important innovation was the substitution of the acetate with the inert hydrochloride avid.

Six patients treated for 4 weeks with a 34-mmol/l bicarbonate CAPD solution demonstrated that the solution was safe and well tolerated, did not affect dialytic adequacy and increased serum bicarbonate levels.

In the meantime, other proposals for producing a stable bicarbonate CAPD solution suitable for clinical use were published.

Yatzidis [9] proposed a bicarbonate-based PD solution in a single compartment where bicarbonate (30 mmol/l) is stabilized by the addition of a dipeptide, glycylglycine (10 mmol/l). This solution has been shown to be stable after 18 months in storage and has been tested in rabbits for up to 25 days with no pathological findings in the peritoneum. About 80% of glycylglycine was absorbed. In humans, this substance is enzymatically degraded to glycine which, in turn, is metabolized to other nonessential amino acids.

The first clinical acute study demonstrated that a glycylglycine-bicarbonate solution was well tolerated by patients and significantly increased net ultrafiltration as compared to a standard lactate solution [10]. In addition, since the solution must be cold sterilized by filtration in order to avoid glucose caramelization, the concentration of glucose by-products was reduced considerably [11].

A mixture of several buffers in the same solution was proposed by Veech [12] on theoretical grounds and was later investigated both in vitro and in an animal model [13].

Studies with the Modern Bicarbonate Solution

From these studies, a solution suitable for clinical practice, containing a mixture of bicarbonate (25 mmol/l) and lactate (15 mmol/l), was prepared. This solution was compared with a conventional solution containing 40 mmol/l of lactate and with a pure bicarbonate solution (38 mmol/l) in a randomized multicenter study involving 45 patients [14]. There was no difference in plasma bicarbonate levels, irrespective of the dialysis solution used and it could be concluded that the lactate/bicarbonate solution is as effective as lactate solution in treating uremic acidosis. This solution was able to reduce the infusion pain experienced by some patients with the lactate solution [15].

The original bicarbonate solution called 'pure bicarbonate' (Bicavera®) was tested in a randomized multicenter long-term study [16]. The trial was designed to evaluate the long-term tolerance, safety, efficacy and therapeutic value of a bicarbonate-buffered peritoneal dialysis solution versus a conventional lactate-buffered peritoneal dialysis solution for CAPD patients. A total of 69 patients from 14 centers completed the 6-month study period (36 patients in the bicarbonate group and 33 in the lactate group). Twenty-seven patients treated with the bicarbonate solution were followed for more than 6 months (15 for more than 1 year).

At baseline evaluation, a wide range of patient's acid base status was recorded: 9.23% of patients were alkalotic, 12.3% had a normal acid base status and 78.46% were acidotic. During the study, despite that the acid base status of the two groups of patients did not change significantly, on the whole, plasma bicarbonate concentrations of acidotic patients in the bicarbonate group tended to increase and in patients with alkalosis there was a tendency to decrease. On the contrary, in the lactate group, no substantial changes of distribution values were recorded. The small fraction of patients with metabolic alkalosis or normal acid base status did not allow a statistical evaluation.

Patients with metabolic acidosis in the bicarbonate group (25 patients) significantly improved their acid base status during the 6-month study and even the mean increase in arterial plasma bicarbonate was small (about 2 mmol/l). On the contrary, lactate patients with acidosis at baseline (26 patients) did not show any significant changes.

A qualitative analysis performed in the 27 patients treated for more than 6 months with the bicarbonate solution showed that 62.9% (17 patients) had an improved acid base status during the bicarbonate treatment (improvement was defined as a change in arterial plasma bicarbonate towards the normal range 23.5–26.1 mmol/l). In 3 patients (11.1%), a worsening of plasma bicarbonate was recorded during the study, while in 7 patients (26%) plasma bicarbonate did not change or its fluctuation was inside the normal range.

Despite lactate- and bicarbonate-buffered CAPD solutions providing the same amount of buffer in the fresh dialysis solution (35 and 34 mmol/l, respectively), this study suggested that the bicarbonate solution has a beneficial effect on patients with metabolic alkalosis and severe acidosis.

In addition, a significant increase in normalized protein catabolic rate was recorded in the bicarbonate group and also BUN slightly, but not significantly, increased even though no changes in urea nitrogen clearance were registered. Despite the daily protein intake not being assessed during the study, this effect is generally attributed to an increase of diet protein intake. Therefore, a nutritional improvement in the bicarbonate group could be suggested.

In this long-term study involving a large number of patients, use of the bicarbonate-buffered solution was not associated with any adverse event related to the solution, and dialysate protein loss did not increased as recorded in older studies. The subjective patient well-being was improved mainly because of a reduction of abdominal pain induced by the standard lactate solution.

Despite the 34 mmol/l bicarbonate solution being more effective than the conventional 35 mmol/l lactate solution in the acid base correction, an alternative formulation with a higher bicarbonate concentration (39 mmol/l) was proposed in order to extend the percentage of the CAPD population with a normal acid base status [17].

An interventional study in a large population was performed [18] with the aim to normalize the acid base status of CAPD patients by using two bicarbonate concentrations in the dialysis fluid. Patients with normal acid base status at baseline (19 patients) used the low bicarbonate solution (34 mmol/l) during the study, while patients with metabolic acidosis (42 patients) used the high bicarbonate solution (39 mmol/l). During the study, the use of the two solutions was modulated according to the blood bicarbonate levels of patients. After 6 months, the percentage of patients with normal acid base status rose from 27.6% to 63.9% at baseline and the potential benefit on nutrition, already recorded in the previous randomized study, was confirmed. Since factors affecting acid base homeostasis are intrinsic characteristics of the individual patient (ultrafiltration, metabolic acid production, etc.), it is not surprising that only a certain modulation of buffer infusion may ensure a good correction in a large percentage of patients.

A more recent long-term (3 years) clinical study with Bicavera® in 100 patients demonstrated further beneficial clinical effects of this solution in comparison with the standard lactate solution including a significant reduction of peritonitis, less inflammation, a significant decrease in the residual renal function decline, and a reduced mortality [19].

Since bicarbonate solution is a low GDPs fluid, local biocompatibility effects are expected. After a thorough in vitro evaluation [20], an in vivo analysis was performed by Weiss et al. [21] in a cross-over study in 53 patients. In the overnight effluent, the CA125 was higher and the hyaluronic acid was lower in the bicarbonate solution as compared with the standard lactate solution. TNF-α and TGF-β_1 were also higher in the effluent of the bicarbonate solution, while no differences in IL-6, VEGF and IFN-γ were detected.

Conclusions

All these studies demonstrated that the bicarbonate-buffered CAPD solution is safe, well tolerated and does not present any, even potential, side effects. In addition, some beneficial effects have been demonstrated (improvement of the acidosis correction) or suggested (preservation of residual renal function, better response to peritonitis, decreased inflammation, improvement of the nutritional status). Furthermore, there is evidence that the bicarbonate PD solution, bicarbonate being the physiological buffer of the body and the solution with low GDPs and physiological pH, is more biocompatible in terms of local and systemic effects than the conventional lactate-buffered solution. Thus, it seems reasonable to consider the bicarbonate-buffered solution the standard instead of the alternative solution and it might entirely substitute lactate as a buffer in peritoneal dialysis fluid.

References

1 Boen TS: Kinetic of peritoneal dialysis. A comparison with the artificial kidney. Medicine 1961;40:243–287.
2 La Greca G, Biasioli S, Chiaramonte S, et al: Acid base balance on peritoneal dialysis. Clin Nephrol 1981;16:1–7.
3 Faller B, Marichal JF: Loss of ultrafiltration in CAPD a role for acetate. Perit Dial Bull 1984;4:10–13.
4 Slingeneyer A, Mion C, Mourad G, Canaud B, Faller B, Béraud JJ: Progressive sclerosing peritonitis. A late and severe complication of maintenance peritoneal dialysis. Trans Am Soc Artif Intern Organs 1983;29:633–636.
5 Feriani M, Biasioli S, Borin D, et al: Bicarbonate solutions for peritoneal dialysis: a reality. Int J Artif Organs 1985;8:57–58.

6 Feriani M, Reinhardt B, La Greca G: $CaCO_3$ precipitation in oversatured bicarbonate containing CAPD solution; in La Greca G, Ronco C, Feriani M, Chiaramonte S, Conz P (eds): Peritoneal Dialysis – Proceedings of the 4th International Course on Peritoneal Dialysis. Milano, Wichtig editore, 1991, pp 145–150.
7 Feriani M, Biasioli S, Borin D, et al: Bicarbonate buffer for CAPD solution. Trans Am Soc Artif Intern Organs 1985;31:668–672.
8 Feriani M, Dissegna D, La Greca G, Passlick-Deetjan J: Short term clinical study with bicarbonate-containing peritoneal dialysis solution. Perit Dial Int 1993;13:296–301.
9 Yatzidis H: A new stable bicarbonate dialysis solution for peritoneal dialysis: preliminary report. Perit Dial Int 1991;11:224–227.
10 Yatzidis H: Enhanced ultrafiltration in rabbits with bicarbonate glycylglycine peritoneal dialysis solution. Perit Dial Int 1993;13:302–306.
11 Slingeneyer A, Faller B, Michel C, Przbylski C, Rolland R, Mion C: Increased ultrafiltration capacity using a new bicarbonate CAPD solution (abstract). Perit Dial Int 1993;13(suppl 1):S57.
12 Veech RL: The untoward effects of the anions in dialysis fluids. Kidney Int 1988;34:587–597.
13 Schambye HT, Flesner P, Pedersen RB, et al: Bicarbonate versus lactate-based CAPD fluids: a biocompatibility study in rabbits. Perit Dial Int 1992;12:281–286.
14 Coles GA, Gokal R, Ogg C, et al: A randomized controlled trial of a bicarbonate and a bicarbonate/lactate containing dialysis solution in CAPD. Perit Dial Int 1997;17:48–54
15 Mactier RA, Sprosen TS, Gokal R, et al: Bicarbonate and bicarbonate/lactate peritoneal dialysis solutions for the treatment of infusion pain. Kidney Int 1998;53:1061–1068.
16 Feriani M, Kirchgessner J, La Greca G, Passlick-Deetjen J, Bicarbonate CAPD Cooperative Group: Randomized long-term evaluation of bicarbonate-buffered CAPD solution. Kidney Int 1998;54:1731–1738.
17 Feriani M, Carobi C, La Greca G, Buoncristiani U, Passlick-Deetjen J: Clinical experience with a 39 mmol/l bicarbonate-buffered peritoneal dialysis solution. Perit Dial Int 1997;17:17–21.
18 Feriani M, Passlick-Deetjen J, Jaeckle-Meyer I, La Greca G, Study Group: Individualized bicarbonate concentrations in the peritoneal dialysis fluid to optimize acid-base status in CAPD patients. Nephrol Dial Transplant 2004;19:195–202.
19 Montenegro J, Saracho R, Gallardo I, Martinez I, Munoz R, Quintanilla L: Use of pure bicarbonate-buffered peritoneal dialysis fluid reduces the incidence of CAPD peritonitis. Nephrol Dial Transplant 2007;22:1703–1708.
20 Topley N, Kaur D, Petersen MM, Passlick-Deetjen J, Coles GA, Williams JD: Biocompatibility of bicarbonate buffered peritoneal dialysis fluids: influence on mesothelial cell and neutrophil function. Kidney Int 1996;49:1447–1456.
21 Weiss L, Stegmayr B, Malmsten G, et al: Biocompatibility and tolerability of a purely bicarbonate-buffered peritoneal dialysis solution. Perit Dial Int 2009;29:647–655.

Dr. Mariano Feriani
Director of the Unità Operativa di Nefrologia e Dialisi
Ospedale dell'Angelo Mestre e S.S. Giovanni e Paolo
Mestre e Venezia
IT–30174 Venice (Italy)
Tel. +39 041 965 7383, E-Mail mferiani@goldnet.it

Ronco C, Rosner MH, Crepaldi C (eds): Peritoneal Dialysis – State-of-the-Art 2012.
Contrib Nephrol. Basel, Karger, 2012, vol 178, pp 6–10

Peritoneal Dialysis Solution and Nutrition

Christian Verger

RDPLF, Pontoise, France

Abstract

20–70% of peritoneal dialysis patients have some signs of malnutrition. Anorexia, protein and amino acid losses in dialysate, advanced age of elderly patients, inflammation and cardiac failure are among the main causes. Modern dialysis solutions aim to reduce these causes, but none of them is without side effects: glucose is relatively safe and brings additional energy but induces anorexia and lipid abnormalities, amino acids compensate dialysate losses but may increase uremia and acidosis, icodextrin helps control hyperhydration and chronic heart failure and minimizes glucose side effects, but may sometimes cause inflammation, and poly chamber bags allow the replacement of lactate by bicarbonate and are more biocompatible, decrease GDP, induce less inflammation and have a better effect on nutritional status. However, it appears that the management of nutrition with the different solutions available nowadays necessitates various combinations of solutions adapted to different patient profiles and there is not actually a single universal solution to minimize malnutrition in peritoneal dialysis patients.

Whether on hemodialysis or on peritoneal dialysis (PD), malnutrition is a frequent complication which is diagnosed in 20–70% of patients, depending upon the way it is evaluated, the selection of the patients and the duration on chronic renal replacement therapy. In France, in the French Language Peritoneal Dialysis Registry (RDPLF) (http://www.rdplf.org), 1.7% of transfers to hemodialysis are due to malnutrition and 3.2% of deaths are due to malnutrition. However, the percentage of malnourished patients maintained on dialysis is obviously higher. Various approaches have been recommended to cope with the frequent malnutrition of dialysis patients. Among them is the research for PD solutions. This paper is a summary of the influence of dialysis solutions on nutritional fate of PD patients.

Preliminary Known Context

Age

Aging is associated with a progressive decrease of muscle mass (fig. 1) and with a different evolution in males and females. Males start with greater muscle mass than females which decreases progressively during their life; females start at a lower level, but remain quite stable until the age of 60 years, then decreases rapidly. In the oldest, muscle mass is identical in both groups.

Dose of Dialysis

It is well known that dialysis adequacy is an important factor to prevent denutrition; however,

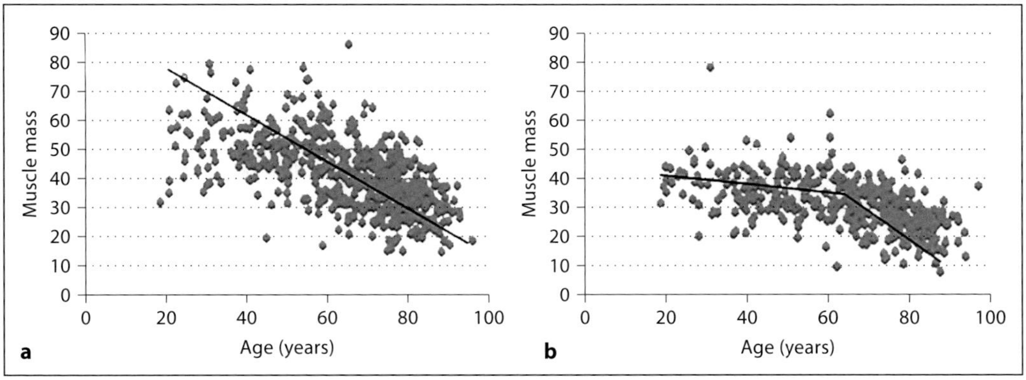

Fig. 1. Evolution of muscle mass estimated by creatinine generation with age in (**a**) males (n = 578) and (**b**) females (n = 421). C. Verger – data from the RDPLF.

Table 1. Patients who lose muscle mass and have poorer survival, start DP with a lower initial muscle mass (estimated by creatinine generation), a lower protein intake, but receive same dose of dialysis and lose the same amount of protein in dialysate [data from RDPLF]

	Loss of muscle mass >1 kg during first 2 years	Stable or increased muscle mass during first 2 years
Initial muscle mass, kg	35.11±11.49	42.04±11.39
Initial body weight, kg	67.8±13.3	71.0±15.5
Dietary protein intake/ideal body weight, g/kg	1.09±0.36	1.17±0.37
Dietary caloric intake/ideal body weight, cal/kg	29.21±8.3	30.13±7.9
Daily dialysate protein losses, g/24 h	6.9±4.9	6.8±3.2
Total volume drained, liters	11.22±5.07	11.64±4.45

increasing or maintaining a stable volume of dialysate may sometimes have deleterious effect on frail patients.

Table 1 was obtained from the RDPLF data base in two groups of patients; those who lost 1 kg of estimated muscle mass during the first 2 years, and those who are stable or increase their muscle mass. Those who lost their muscle mass were the ones who already started with the lowest muscle mass, whereas they were receiving the same amount of dialysis and losing the same amount of protein per day in the dialysate: the protein losses/protein reserves ratio had a trend to be higher, increasing the risk of malnutrition if not compensated.

Other factors that impact the nutritional status are well known and a nonlimitating list includes inflammation, acidosis, glucose load, chronic cardiac failure, etc.

Effect of Dialysis Solution on Nutritional Status

Glucose-Containing Solutions

The most use osmotic agent has been and remains glucose in a lactate-buffered solution. These conventional solutions, in addition to their high glucose concentration, are acidic. The glucose absorbed can lead to hyperglycemia and induces hyperinsulinemia [1]. The amount of glucose intake through the peritoneum is increased in hyperpermeable patients or those who necessitate hypertonic solutions to manage their hydration status; this higher glucose exposure through PD fluid is associated with an increase in total fat mass and increased fat accumulation [2]. In addition, in susceptible subjects, an induced hyperglycemic status can directly suppress appetite [3, 4]. Eventually, despite higher ultrafiltration, it has been demonstrated that the use of 3.86% glucose solutions may be associated with some cardiac abnormalities, compared to nonglucose solutions [5].

However, glucose is far from having disadvantages on nutritional status. Many patients have insufficient caloric intake and the glucose absorbed is therefore an additional source of energy. In the data base of RDPLF, the average caloric intake is 25 kcal/ideal body weight: when glucose absorption from the dialysate is taken in account it is 28 (in this study patients receiving AA dialysate and Icodextrin were included).

Glucose Polymer (Icodextrin) PD Solution

Icodextrin has been designed to maintain sustained ultrafiltration due to its high molecular weight [6]. Icodextrin, due to its larger molecular size, is less absorbed (mainly through the lymphatics) and is not metabolized locally during a dwell. It is metabolized in maltose not used by the human organism, so it acts as glucose sparing and prevents hyperglycemia and hyperinsulinemia. In addition to its interest in ultrafiltration during long dwell, it is particularly useful in diabetic patients to minimize insulin requirement and weight gain. In diabetics, an improvement of the HbA1c and a better lipid profile has been shown [7, 8].

However, intolerance to icodextrin can sometimes be observed in some patients with an inflammatory response and may be a source of concern [9], but other studies are conflicting and, on the other hand, showed a significant drop of inflammatory markers with icodextrin compared to standard solution, associated with an improvement of the nutritional status [10].

Amino Acid-Containing Solutions (AA Solutions)

Nutrients are lost into the dialysate. As an example, amino acid losses into dialysate can average 4–8 g/day in PD [11].

AA-containing PD solution as a means to replace the protein loss has been proposed since early 1980. Use of an AA solution can minimize the undesirable effects of glucose solution. It is most effective when associated with a glucose solution which acts as an additional caloric intake to synthetize proteins from the amino acids absorbed [11].

With PD, losses rise much higher during episodes of peritonitis [12]. Max Dratwa [Bruxelles, pers. commun.] demonstrated that use of AA solutions during peritonitis prevented an important drop in albumin and accelerated recovery of pre-peritonitis albumin levels.

The amino acid solution used in a modern solution is a 1.1% solution of a combination of essential amino acids and some nonessential amino acids. The pH of this solution is 6.7 and osmolality is 365 mosm/kg. In various studies, this solution has been shown to improve the nutritional status of dialysis patients [13]. However, due to its low pH, and in cases of insufficient caloric intake this solution has some side effects such as worsening of acidosis and a rise in urea. Amino acid dialysate may also lead to metabolic acidosis which is primarily due to the hydrogen ion contained in cationic amino acids (such as lysine) [14]. So, recommendations have been proposed when prescribing amino acid peritoneal dialysis solutions [15]: they are indicated for use only in malnourished or diabetic patients and/or during peritonitis, or in patients with recurrent peritonitis. No more than one exchange per day of AA solution should be prescribed, seldom 2, but in all cases blood urea and bicarbonate status should be closely monitored [16]. Sufficient concurrent alternative caloric intake should be guaranteed.

Dialysis Solution to Prevent Acidosis

As ESRD patients are unable to excrete the daily acid load, they have a strong trend to be in metabolic acidosis. Until recently, PD solutions used lactate as a buffer, which converts to bicarbonate in the liver and corrects the acidosis. However, lactate is not fully biocompatible and may cause adverse metabolic effects [17]. To conterbalance these side effects new solutions have been designed to use bicarbonate instead of lactate as a buffer. To avoid calcium precipitation, dialysis bags are divided in a two-chambered system separating bicarbonate and calcium. This allows the use of bicarbonate near physiologic pH. As glucose is separated, it can be sterilized at a lower pH which prevents caramelization and the release of GDP, the source of inflammation and secondary malnutrition. When the two chambers are mixed at the time of exchange, the dialysate has a more physiological pH and is more biocompatible.

Dialysis Solution to Prevent Inflammation-Induced Malnutrition

Inflammation is part of the MIA syndrome and probably its trigger. In this case both protein and caloric intake increase is ineffective as long as inflammation is present. There have been numerous papers showing that neutral pH, low GDP and more biocompatible solutions are associated with lower inflammatory markers and better nutritional status. This suggests that a modern PD program should favor these new types of solutions [18–20].

In conclusion, there is no unique PD solution that allows to correct all the consequences of end-stage renal failure, inflammation, protein starvation, cardiac failure, etc., but knowledge of the characteristics of each solution should allow one to make the adequate choice to improve or at least stabilize the nutritional status of PD patients. Most modern biocompatible solution have characteristics which are effective in reaching, at least partly, this aim. The physician must continue to keep an open mind to sometimes prescribe a nonstandard regimen of dialysis solution, taking into account that each patient has his owns characteristics. There are several ongoing lines of research which are testing the possibility of mixtures of solutions in pluricompartmental bags, each solution being supposed to compensate the disadvantage of the other.

References

1 Fernstrom A, Hylander B, Moritz A, Jacobson H, Rossner S: Increase in intra-abdominal fat in patients treated with continuous ambulatory peritoneal dialysis. Perit Dial Int 1998;18:166–171.

2 Fernstrom A, Hylander B, Moritz A, Jacobson H, Rossner S: Increase in intra-abdominal fat in patients treated with continuous ambulatory peritoneal dialysis. Perit Dial Int 1998;18:166–171.

3 Bouma SF, Dwyer JT: Glucose absorption and weight change in 18 months of continuous ambulatory peritoneal dialysis. J Am Diet Assoc 1984;84:194.

4 Aguirre Galindo BA, Prieto Fierro JG, Cano P, et al: Effect of polymeric diets in patients on continuous ambulatory peritoneal dialysis. Perit Dial Int 2003;23:434.

5 Selby NM, Fonsesca S, Hulme H, Fluck RJ, Tall MW, McIntyre CW: Hypertonic glucose based peritoneal dialysis is associated with higher blood pressure and adverse hemodynamics as compared with icodextrin. Nephrol Dial Transplant 2005;20:1848–1853.

6 Mistry CD, Gokal R, Peers E: A randomized multicenter clinical trial comparing isosmolar icodextrin with hyperosmolar glucose solutions in CAPD. MIDAS study group. Multicenter investigation of icodextrin in ambulatory peritoneal dialysis. Kidney Int 1994;46:496–503.

7 Babazono T, Nakamoto H, Kasai K, Kuriyama S, Sugimoto T, Nakayama M, Hamada C, Furuya R, Hasegawa H, Kasahara M, Moriishi M, Tomo T, Miyazaki M, Sato M, Yorioka N, Kawaguchi Y, Japanese Extraneal Collaborated Study Group: Effects of icodextrin on glycemic and lipid profiles in diabetic patients undergoing peritoneal dialysis. Am J Nephrol 2007;27:409–415.

8 Bredie SJ, Bosch FH, Demacker PN, Stalenhoef AF, van Leusen R: Effects of peritoneal dialysis with an overnight icodextrin dwell on parameters of glucose and lipid metabolism. Perit Dial Int 2001;21:275–281.

9 Martikainen TA, Teppo AM, Grönhagen-Riska C, Ekstrand AV: Glucose-free dialysis solutions: inductors of inflammation or preservers of peritoneal membrane? Perit Dial Int 2005;25:453–460.
10 Lin W, Chen YC, Wu MS, Hsu HJ, Sun CY, Lin YK, Wu IW: Icodextrin dialysate improves nutritional and inflammatory profiles in peritoneal dialysis patients. Ren Fail 2009;31:98–105.
11 Blumenkrantz MJ, Gahl GM, Kopple JD, et al: Protein losses during peritoneal dialysis. Kidney Int 1981;19:593.
12 Tjiong HL, Rietveld T, Wattimena JL, van den Berg JW, Kahriman D, van der Steen J, Hop WC, Swart R, Fieren MW: Peritoneal dialysis with solutions containing amino acids plus glucose promotes protein synthesis during oral feeding. Clin J Am Soc Nephrol 2007;2:74–80.
13 Ohkawa S, Kaizu Y, Odamaki M, et al: Optimum dietary protein requirement in nondiabetic maintenance hemodialysis patients. Am J Kidney Dis 2004;43:454.
14 Tjiong HL, van den Berg JW, Wattimena JL, et al: Dialysate as food: combined amino acid and glucose dialysate improves protein anabolism in renal failure patients on automated peritoneal dialysis. J Am Soc Nephrol 2005;16:1486.
15 Dialysis Outcomes Quality Initiative Guidelines: Clinical practice guidelines for nutrition in chronic renal failure. Guideline 15. Am J Kidney Dis 2000;35(suppl 2):S40.
16 European Best Practice Guidelines for peritoneal dialysis. Nephrol Dial Transplant 2005;20(suppl 9):3.
17 Veech RL: The untoward effect of the anions of dialysis fluids. Kidney Int 1988;34:587–597.
18 Williams JD, Topley N, Craig KJ, Mackenzie RK, Pischetsrieder M, Lage C, Passlick-Deetjen J: The Euro-Balance Trial: the effect of a new biocompatible peritoneal dialysis fluid (balance) on the peritoneal membrane. Kidney Int 2004;66:408–418.
19 Szeto CC, Chow KM, Lam CW, Leung CB, Kwan BC, Chung KY, Law MC, Li PK: Clinical biocompatibility of a neutral peritoneal dialysis solution with minimal glucose-degradation products – a 1-year randomized control trial. Nephrol Dial Transplant 2007;22:552–559.
20 Schambye HT, Flesner P, Pedersen RB, Hardt-Madsen M, Chemnitz J, Christensen HK, Detmer A: Bicarbonate-versus lactate-based CAPD fluids: a biocompatibility study in rabbits. Perit Dial Int 1992;12:281–286.

Dr. Christian Verger
Registre de Dialyse Péritonéale de Langue Française (RDPLF)
30, rue Séré Depoin
FR–95300 Pontoise (France)
Tel. +33 608765991, E-Mail c.verger@wanadoo.fr

Ronco C, Rosner MH, Crepaldi C (eds): Peritoneal Dialysis – State-of-the-Art 2012.
Contrib Nephrol. Basel, Karger, 2012, vol 178, pp 11–15

Alternative Dialysis Strategies with Icodextrin

Sarah E. Panzer · Isaac Teitelbaum

Division of Renal Diseases and Hypertension, University of Colorado, Aurora, Colo., USA

Abstract

Proper volume management continues to be a major challenge in patients requiring renal replacement therapy. In patients performing peritoneal dialysis the introduction of icodextrin represented a major advance in this effort. Recent studies have demonstrated a potential role for the use of novel dialysis strategies employing icodextrin to further enhance ultrafiltration and to improve cardiac indices in patients with ultrafiltration failure. These alternative strategies include the use of icodextrin in non-traditional patient populations (low transporters), the simultaneous use of glucose-based and icodextrin solutions in combination, and the use of icodextrin twice daily rather than for just a single dwell. This paper will briefly review the current status of these alternative dialysis strategies with icodextrin. In addition, the potential role for icodextrin to decrease postoperative adhesions will be discussed as well.

One of the major challenges in the treatment of dialysis patients is failure to achieve appropriate ultrafiltration (UF). UF failure is a common cause of technique failure and may necessitate a change of modality to hemodialysis. Additionally, cardiac mortality is high in this population and there are concerns that volume overload, hypertension, and heart failure related to poor UF may worsen cardiac outcomes in these patients.

Standard glucose-based peritoneal dialysis (PD) solutions contain high concentrations of glucose, lactate, and glucose degradation products. Over time, these compounds cause damage to the peritoneal membrane [1]. There is also concern regarding the direct toxicity of hypertonic glucose solutions on the peritoneal membrane. In addition, the use of hyperosmolar glucose solutions results in systemic absorption of a glucose load. This can lead to hyperglycemia, insulin resistance, metabolic derangements, dyslipidemia, concern for worsened outcomes in diabetic patients, and potential negative impact on mortality [2].

The introduction of icodextrin, a solution containing large polymers from a digestion of cornstarch resulting in molecules of varying size between 13 and 19 kDa, represented a major advance in PD therapy. Icodextrin generates UF through colloidal osmotic pressure, is iso-osmotic, and does not activate peritoneal capillary aquaporins. Thus, icodextrin has the benefit of sodium and water removal via fluid movement through small and large pores resulting in both water and sodium clearance. Icodextrin has a unique UF curve that is sustained over 12–14 h; it is currently recommended for increasing UF in long dwell only.

Icodextrin is felt to be more biocompatible because the solution is iso-osmolar, it contains no glucose, and has much lower levels of glucose degradation products. Icodextrin is not absorbed across the peritoneal membrane due to its large size. Rather, it is absorbed by lymphatics and within the circulation is degraded by serum amylase to maltose. Maltose then enters cells and is converted by maltase to glucose. The effect of these maltose degradation products needs further investigation. Clinicians are now aware of potential toxicities related to glucose containing solutions and trying to utilize glucose-sparing techniques. Thus, there are potential advantages to increasing the use of icodextrin in lieu of glucose. In this article, we will briefly review the status of nonconventional or alternative uses of icodextrin.

Use of Icodextrin in Low Transporters

Identification of peritoneal membrane characteristics is of utmost importance in prescribing adequate PD therapy. Peritoneal transport characteristics are an independent predictor of patient and technique survival [3]. Though initially intended for use in rapid transporters only, recent data suggest that icodextrin's effects may be somewhat independent of peritoneal membrane characteristics [4]. A 4-week randomized double-blind trial of just over 200 CAPD patients in Asia compared the use of 7.5% icodextrin to that of 2.5% glucose during a long nighttime dwell. Peritoneal creatinine clearance and UF were significantly higher in the icodextrin-treated group. The increase in UF was more pronounced in higher transporters, but was significantly increased in high, high-average, and even low-average transporters. Low transporters did not demonstrate increased UF with icodextrin. Compared to the glucose-based solution, 7.5% icodextrin significantly improved both UF and small solute clearance, even in low-average transport patients [4].

Use of Icodextrin in Combination with Glucose-Based Dialysate

High glucose solutions provide rapid UF but as the osmotic gradient lessens the UF effect diminishes and the patient is subject to systemic glucose absorption. In an effort to decrease the glucose load while maintaining UF, researchers have investigated alternative dialysis strategies. Computer simulations involving mathematical modeling of peritoneal membrane physiology based on the three-pore model suggested that a dialysis solution composed of a combination of 1.36% glucose and 7.5% icodextrin would offer an improved UF profile [5]. In a very small exploratory study, this combination fluid of 1.36% glucose and 7.5% icodextrin showed a biphasic UF profile with an initial steep increase in UF with subsequent maintenance of a plateau over seven hours. This combination fluid allows for both crystalloid and colloid osmosis to take place during the same exchange, which is reflected in the biphasic UF profile. Preliminary studies demonstrated that the combined 1.36% glucose/7.5% icodextrin solution provided improved UF compared to either icodextrin or glucose alone with increased water and sodium removal sustained over a longer period of time. This combination solution provided a similar degree of UF as high glucose solutions (3.86% was used in this study) but avoided the high glucose concentrations [5, 6].

Subsequent studies using a combination of 2.6% glucose and 6.8% icodextrin for the long dwell in rapid transporters demonstrated a twofold increase in UF and a threefold increase in sodium removal [7, 8]. In the second of these two studies, patients were maintained on the 2.6% glucose/6.8% icodextrin combination fluid for 4 months. These patients exhibited a higher 24-hour UF and peritoneal sodium removal compared to control groups. Thus, this therapy might be particularly helpful in anuric patients with UF failure. It must be noted, however, that due to small numbers of patients and significant scatter of the data statistical significance could be achieved only when examining percent changes; there were no significant changes in absolute values for peritoneal UF or sodium removal. Furthermore, in those patients who had residual kidney function there was a trend toward lower urine volume over the four months of treatment [8]. Though it did not achieve statistical significance, this trend toward lower urine output with enhanced UF and sodium removal does raise concern about possible loss of residual renal function. Finally, in contrast to conventional PD fluid which has a sodium concentration of 132 mEq/l, the sodium concentration of the bimodal fluid was only 121 mEq/l. One wonders, therefore, how much of the beneficial effect of the bimodal fluid, particularly on sodium removal, was due not to the addition of icodextrin but rather to the lower sodium concentration. Additional careful study of these issues is necessary before one may advocate the widespread use of bimodal solutions.

Twice-Daily Icodextrin

As outlined earlier, icodextrin is currently recommended for use once daily during long dwell in patients with poor UF. Some studies suggest that the UF obtained with icodextrin is variable and may not increase further after ten hours. Accordingly, attention has been given to the possibility of using icodextrin for two exchanges daily. In one recent study, 9 patients on long-term PD with UF failure (weight gain and edema) were treated with two icodextrin exchanges of 8 h each for a period of 6 months. In patients on CAPD the icodextrin exchanges were separated by exchanges in which glucose-based solutions were used; in patients on APD the two icodextrin exchanges were performed consecutively in lieu of a single long day dwell. Within 2 months, body weight was significantly reduced in the majority of patients; this was maintained for the duration of the study. Patients also demonstrated a reduction in mean blood pressure and a modest decline in serum sodium levels. Of the 3 patients who had residual renal function, mean creatinine clearance remained stable in 2 [9].

Similar results were obtained in another recent study. Eight PD patients were switched from once daily to twice daily icodextrin for 8 h each. All but 1 patient was either a high or high-average transporter. This study demonstrated a significant increase in UF in all patients within the first week, which was maintained over 6 months. Residual urine output remained unchanged and was not significantly different at 6 months [10].

This study also reported on the effect of twice daily use of icodextrin on the levels of icodextrin metabolites. Icodextrin is gradually absorbed by lymphatics and is then metabolized systemically by serum amylase to produce maltose and other small multimers thereof. There are some concerns that using increased exchanges of icodextrin could result in accumulation of maltose metabolites. Icodextrin metabolites (maltose, maltotriose, or total metabolites) were measured in 6 patients prior to the study and again at 6 months and found to not be significantly different. Nevertheless, there was a small but statistically significant decrease in the serum sodium concentration [10] presumably reflecting the presence of osmotically active icodextrin metabolites.

Cardiac Outcomes with Twice-Daily Icodextrin

A recent study analyzed left ventricular hypertrophy in 34 PD patients with high or high-average membrane permeability and UF failure receiving treatment with icodextrin. UF failure was defined as less than 400 ml of UF after a 4-hour exchange of 2,000 ml of a 3.86% glucose dialysis solution. Patients were then randomly divided into two groups: either a single 12-hour dwell with icodextrin (with three other glucose-based exchanges of 4 h each) or two daily 9-hour dwells with icodextrin (with two other glucose-based exchanges of 3 h each). After 3 months, patients in the twice daily icodextrin group had a significant reduction in mean body weight, increase in UF volume, and decreased average systolic BP. Left ventricular mass index determined by echocardiography was significantly lower compared to baseline but was not different between the two groups at 3 months. There was no significant difference in serum sodium levels, weekly Kt/V, urine volume, and no significant increase in total icodextrin metabolite levels [11].

Brain natriuretic peptide (BNP) is elevated in left ventricular dysfunction and increased with ventricular volume expansion. It is also present at increased levels in patients with decreased kidney function. Left ventricular mass index (LVMI) has been shown to correlate with BNP levels and may be a prognostic indicator for survival. A recent study followed 28 PD patients with UF failure for 8 weeks randomized to treatment with either 7.5% icodextrin twice daily for 9 h or 7.5% icodextrin once daily for 12 h per the protocols described above. UF failure was defined as less than 400 ml of UF after an exchange of 2,000 ml of 3.86% glucose for 4 h. All patients were high or high-average transporters. GFR, Kt/V, and urine volume were not significantly different between groups. At 8 weeks of treatment there was a significant reduction in body weight, mean LVMI, heart rate, blood pressure, and BNP and an increase in ejection fraction and UF compared to baseline in the twice-daily icodextrin group. In contrast, the once-daily icodextrin group did not have a significant change compared to their baseline in body weight or blood pressure. While, the patients in the once-daily icodextrin group did experience significant changes compared to their baseline in mean LVMI, heart rate, ejection fraction, and BNP these changes were all significantly larger ($p < 0.05$ for each) in the twice-daily icodextrin patients compared to those treated with icodextrin only once daily [12].

Left ventricular hypertrophy and cardiovascular mortality are common in the dialysis population. The current studies link UF achieved with icodextrin to changes in left ventricular hypertrophy, BNP levels, and LVMI. The observation that left ventricular hypertrophy was reduced compared to baseline but was not significantly different between the two treatment groups suggests that longer duration studies are needed to determine effects of treatment with icodextrin on cardiac remodeling. Thus, further studies are required to determine if volume management with increased icodextrin usage will favorably impact long-term cardiovascular mortality in PD patients.

Surgical Indications for the Use of Icodextrin: Reduction of Adhesions

Though not specifically related to its use for PD, it is interesting to note that studies in the surgical literature suggest a role for icodextrin to lessen postoperative peritoneal scarring and adhesions. Following laparotomy there is a high risk of the development of intraperitoneal adhesions, which is associated with significant morbidity and mortality. Surgical damage to the peritoneal membrane results in an inflammatory response with release of cytokines, activation of the coagulation cascade, and thrombin formation. Early fibrinolysis (within 5 days) encourages healing of the peritoneum without adhesions. However, if fibrinolysis does not occur within five to seven days of injury, temporary fibrin matrix persists and organizes leading to adhesion formation. A 4% icodextrin solution instilled following surgery decreases adhesion formation through temporary separation of peritoneal surfaces by hydroflotation with a fluid reservoir kept in place for 3–4 days following surgery [13].

Studies of patients undergoing adhesiolysis surgery randomized to 4% icodextrin or lactated Ringer's solution instillation prior to closure have demonstrated a significant reduction in adhesions on second-look surgery [14]. Other studies have demonstrated a trend towards reduced adhesion formation on second-look surgery after treatment with 4% icodextrin [15, 16]. A recent study of patients undergoing adhesiolysis for adhesive bowel obstruction was randomized to treatment with 4% icodextrin or traditional treatment. A significantly lower small bowel obstruction rate was found in the icodextrin-treated group after follow-up for an average of 41 months. There was no significant difference in the need for laparotomy for small bowel obstruction recurrence or change in adhesion severity score [17]. In the US, a 4% icodextrin solution is approved by the FDA for reducing adhesions in gynecologic laparoscopic surgery. In Europe, 4% icodextrin is approved as an adhesion reduction agent for laparoscopy and laparotomy.

Conclusion

UF failure represents a major problem in the PD population. Icodextrin enhances UF and sodium removal and recent studies suggest a role for icodextrin in controlling volume status and LVMI. Current research demonstrates a potential role for alternative strategies utilizing bimodal solutions of glucose plus icodextrin or twice-daily icodextrin in PD patients. However, there are also several limitations including cost, possibility of loss of residual renal function, and unknown long-term effect of accumulation of icodextrin breakdown products. Future long-term studies are needed to assess whether these alternative uses of icodextrin will impact cardiac death.

References

1 Williams JD, Craig KJ, Topley N, Von Ruhland C, Fallon M, Newman GR, Mackenzie RK, Williams GT: Morphologic changes in the peritoneal membrane of patients with renal disease. JASN 2002;13:470–479.
2 Duong U, Mehrotra R, Molnar MZ, Noori N, Kovesdy CP, Nissenson AR, Kalantar-Zadeh K: Glycemic control and survival in peritoneal dialysis patients with diabetes mellitus. CJASN 2011;6:1041–1048.
3 Rumpsfeld M, McDonald SP, Johnson DW: Higher peritoneal transport status is associated with higher mortality and technique failure in the Australian and New Zealand peritoneal dialysis patient populations. JASN 2006;17:271–278.
4 Lin A, Qian J, Li X, Yu X, Liu W, Sun Y, Chen N, Mei C: Randomized controlled trial of icodextrin versus glucose containing peritoneal dialysis fluid. CJASN 2009;4:1799–1804.
5 Jenkins S, Wilkie M: An exploratory study of a novel peritoneal combination dialysate (1.36% glucose/7.5% icodextrin), demonstrating improved ultrafiltration compared to either component studied alone. Perit Dial Int 2003;23:475–480.
6 Dallas F, Jenkins SB, Wilkie ME: Enhanced ultrafiltration using 7.5% icodextrin/1.36% glucose combination dialysate: a pilot study. Perit Dial International 2004;24:542–546.
7 Freida P, Galach M, Divino Filho JC, Werynski A, Lindholm B: Combination of crystalloid (glucose) and colloid (icodextrin) osmotic agents markedly enhances peritoneal fluid and solute transport during the long PD dwell. Perit Dial Int 2007;27:267–276.
8 Freida P, Issad B, Dratwa M, Lobbedez T, Wu L, Leypoldt J, Divino-Filho JC: A combined crystalloid and colloid PD solution as a glucose-sparing strategy for volume control in high-transport APD patients: a prospective multicenter study. Perit Dial Int 2009;29:433–442.
9 Dousdampanis P, Trigka K, Chu M, Khan S, Venturoli D, Oreopoulos DG, Bargman JM: Two icodextrin exchanges per day in peritoneal dialysis patients with ultrafiltration failure: one center's experience and review of the literature. Int Urol Nephrol 2011;43:203–209.
10 Ballout A, Garcia-Lopez E, Struyven J, Marechal C, Goffin E: Double-dose icodextrin to increase ultrafiltration in PD patients with inadequate ultrafiltration. Perit Dial Int 2011;31:91–94.
11 Sav T, Oymak O, Inanc MT, Dogan A, Tokgoz B, Utas C: Effects of twice-daily icodextrin administration on blood pressure and left ventricular mass in patients on continuous ambulatory peritoneal dialysis. Perit Dial Int 2009;29:443–449.
12 Sav T, Inanc MT, Dogan A, Oymak O, Utas C: Two daytime icodextrin exchanges decrease brain natriuretic peptide levels and improve cardiac function in continuous ambulatory peritoneal dialysis patients. Nephrology 2010;15:307–312.
13 Schnuriger B, Barmparas G, Branco BC, Lustenberger T, Inaba K, Demetriades D: Prevention of postoperative peritoneal adhesions: a review of the literature. Am J Surg 2011;201:111–121.
14 Brown CB, Luciano AA, Martin D, Peers E, Scrimgeour A, diZerega GS: Adept (icodextrin 4% solution) reduces adhesions after laparoscopic surgery for adhesiolysis: a double-blind, randomized, controlled study. Fertil Steril 2007;88:1413–1426.
15 Kossi J, Gronlund S, Uotila-Nieminen M, Crowe A, Knight A, Keranen U: The effect of 4% icodextrin solution on adhesiolysis surgery time at the Hartmann's reversal: a pilot, multi-centre, randomized control trial vs. lactated Ringer's solution. Colorectal Dis 2009;11:168–172.
16 Trew G, Pistofidis G, Pados G, Lower A, Mettler L, Wallwiener D, Korell M, Pouly JL, Coccia ME, Audebert A, Nappi C, Schmidt E, McVeigh E, Landi S, Degueldre M, Konincxk P, Rimbach S, Chapron C, Dallay D, Roemer T, McConnachie A, Ford I, Crowe A, Knight A, diZerega G, DeWilde R: Gynaecological endoscopic evaluation of 4% icodextrin solution: a European, multicentre, double-blind, randomized study of the efficacy and safety in the reduction of de novo adhesions after laparoscopic gynaecological surgery. Hum Reprod 2011;26:2015–2027.
17 Catena F, Ansaloni L, Di Saverio S, Pinna AD, POPA Study: Prevention of postoperative abdominal adhesions by icodextrin 4% solution after laparotomy for adhesive small bowel obstruction. A prospective randomized controlled trial. J Gastrointest Surg 2012;16:382–388.

Isaac Teitelbaum, MD
Division of Renal Diseases and Hypertension, University of Colorado School of Medicine
12605 E. 16th Avenue, F774
Aurora, CO 80045 (USA)
Tel. +1 720 848 7601, E-Mail isaac.teitelbaum@ucdenver.edu

Ronco C, Rosner MH, Crepaldi C (eds): Peritoneal Dialysis – State-of-the-Art 2012.
Contrib Nephrol. Basel, Karger, 2012, vol 178, pp 16–22

Are Current Peritoneal Dialysis Solutions Adequate for Pediatric Use?

Enrico Eugenio Verrina[a] · Rossella Cannavò[a] · Betti Schaefer[b] · Claus Peter Schmitt[b]

[a]Dialysis Unit, G. Gaslini Children Hospital, Genoa, Italy; [b]Division of Pediatric Nephrology, Center for Pediatric and Adolescent Medicine, Heidelberg, Germany

Abstract

Peritoneal dialysis (PD) is the treatment modality of choice in pediatric CKD5D patients awaiting renal transplantation. Facing many decades of renal replacement therapy long term preservation of peritoneal membrane function is of particular importance in this patient group. Whereas conventional PD fluids induce severe morphological and functional alterations of the peritoneal membrane within a few years, reduction of glucose degradation product content by multichamber systems, replacement of glucose by icodextrin and amino acids, and of lactate by bicarbonate at a neutral to physiological pH are expected to preserve peritoneal membrane integrity. Based on numerous in vitro, experimental and clinical studies, the European Pediatric Dialysis Working Group recommended the use of low glucose degradation product solutions whenever possible. Icodextrin is considered a useful option, in particular in children with sodium and water overload, even though infants may absorb higher amounts of icodextrin and achieve less ultrafiltration. The concept of amino acid-based PD fluids is intriguing, but pediatric benefits are insufficiently described and cannot replace tube feeding in malnourished children. Bicarbonate-based PD fluids better control metabolic acidosis and have been recommended in children with acute kidney injury and impaired lactate metabolism. This review discusses the scientific evidence and potential advantages of PD solutions with an improved biocompatibility profile, with a particular focus on pediatric studies.

Peritoneal dialysis (PD) remains the dialysis modality of choice for pediatric patients awaiting kidney transplantation. In growing children, adequate metabolic control and acid-base balance maintenance are even more important than in adults [1]. Furthermore, the preservation of peritoneal membrane (PM) integrity and function is of major importance in view of renal replacement therapy required for many decades. Deleterious effects of conventional PD solutions have been long debated, and a series of studies raised major clinical concerns regarding the prolonged exposure of the peritoneal membrane to standard PD solutions with high glucose and lactate concentrations, low pH, high osmolarity, and high levels of glucose degradation products (GDP). These concerns are substantiated by adult peritoneal biopsy data [2] and pediatric data on deterioration of PD membrane transport function with time even in the absence of peritonitis episodes [3]. The pH of acidic PD solutions is equilibrated within 1–2 h of dwell time and GDP are rapidly absorbed [4, 5]. In automated PD (APD), the modality usually prescribed in pediatric patients, the PD solution is frequently exchanged over the course of a dialysis session. Oligoanuric infants may even require exchanges every 45–60 min to achieve adequate ultrafiltration (UF). Such treatment regimens further increase the significance of PD fluid biocompatibility. In addition, the progressive decline of residual renal function, a major determinant of PD treatment outcome, is exacerbated by the metabolic and cardiovascular burden related to the PD-associated glucose load, GDP accumulation and oxidative stress [6, 7].

This review discusses the evidence and expected advantages of so called biocompatible PD solutions with a focus on the pediatric studies, which have been recently published on this issue.

Choice of PD Solution Type in Children

Osmotic Agents

Glucose

The most widely employed osmotic agent in the clinical setting is still glucose at supraphysiological concentrations (1,360–4,250 mg/dl). The absorption of large amounts of glucose aggravates uremic anorexia, hyperglycemia, dyslipidemia, and insulin resistance as well as the increased oxidative stress associated with renal failure. Moreover, long-term exposure to high concentrations of glucose and GDP induces structural alterations of the peritoneal membrane, such as submesothelial thickening, fibrosis and vascular proliferation, and substantial functional impairment [3]. Reduced GDP formation has been achieved by the separation of glucose at a very low pH from the other fluid constituents in double and triple chamber bag systems. A prospective short-term randomized cross-over trial in children demonstrated similar solute transport and ultrafiltration capacity with multichamber compared with conventional PD solution [4]. A subsequent 3 months' cross-over trial in children reconfirmed these findings and suggested a better correction of metabolic acidosis with pure bicarbonate-based PD fluid. In addition, plasma advanced glycation end-product levels significantly declined within 4 weeks of switching from conventional to low GDP solution [5].

According to the recommendation given by the European Pediatric Dialysis Working Group [8], conventional, single-chamber PD solutions should be replaced by low GDP multichamber solutions. In contrast to adult nephrologists [9], pediatricians generally consider these solutions as the standard of care for children on PD. Unfortunately, in some settings the adoption of these PD solutions may still be limited due to cost constraints.

Of note, the GDP concentrations differ substantially between the currently available multichamber solutions. Compared to single chamber PD fluids some manufactures achieved a 50% reduction in GDP, others by more than 90% [10]. Even though the clinical impact of these differences has not yet been delineated, a clinical impact is likely to exist. The amount of the well-characterized GDP 3-deoxyglucosone absorbed during a 4-hour dwell is reduced by 80% when a glucose based PD solution with the lowest GDP concentrations instead of a single-chamber fluid is used [5]. This difference is less than 50% when a multichamber PD fluid with still high GDP concentrations is administered. For the latter even no difference in 3,4-dideoxyglucosone-3-ene concentrations exists compared to single chamber solutions. The relative amount of GDP absorbed during a PD dwell is similar with different PD fluids [5].

Icodextrin

Similar to adult patients, children achieve sustained UF with 7.5% icodextrin solution during a prolonged dwell, and an increase in solute removal. Since the icodextrin induced colloid osmosis is exerted via the small pores of the peritoneal membrane and not via aquaporine 1, free water transport and sodium sieving do not occur and thus sodium removal is higher than with respective glucose-based solutions. Side effects comprise mild to moderate skin rash and exfoliative dermatitis (in up to 10% of treated patients), which usually resolve without any sequelae after icodextrin discontinuation [11–13]. In a group of 9 children, Rusthoven et al. [14] demonstrated that during a 4-hour dwell 3.86% glucose solution

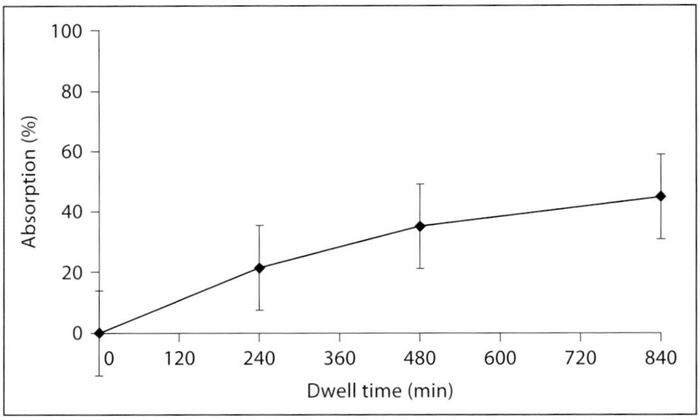

Fig. 1. Icodextrin absorption rate along a daytime 14-hour dwell with 600 ml/m^2 body surface area of 7.5% icodextrin solution in 7 children with a median age of 9.2 years (range 2.7–13.4 years).

induces a rapid increase in intraperitoneal pressure (IPP), closely related to transcapillary UF rate and inversely related to BSA, while icodextrin induces a slow but sustained UF, which is not associated with an increase in IPP within 4 h. Of note, a positive correlation between age and net UF was reported in a small group of patients, with an even negative UF in infants characterized as high transporters on peritoneal equilibration test, presumably due to faster icodextrin absorption [15]. In pediatric patients icodextrin absorption, which occurs via convective pathways such as peritoneal lymphatics, was reported to be 40–45% within 12–14 h [13]. In 7 children with an age range of 2.7–13.4 years the mean caloric load associated with a daytime dwell of 600 ml/m^2 BSA of 7.5% icodextrin solution corresponded to 3.4 ± 1.3% of the recommended age adapted daily allowance of energy. The icodextrin absorption curve (fig. 1) almost linearly increased with dwell time [13] which would be consistent with the disappearance of icodextrin from the peritoneal cavity independent of the molecular size and the concentration gradient via the lymphatic system at a constant rate. Icodextrin is metabolized by amylase to maltose and a number of oligosaccharides, which usually reach a steady-state concentration within 2 weeks from the start of treatment, and return back to zero 1–2 weeks after the discontinuation of icodextrin [11]. Serum osmolality increases by 5 mmol/l, but clinical side effects of icodextrin metabolite accumulation during chronic PD have not yet been delineated.

In vitro and ex vivo studies have shown increased biocompatibility of icodextrin solution compared to single chamber glucose-based solutions, possibly due to its iso-osmolar property, lack of glucose, and lower GDP content. However, icodextrin may inhibit the physiological mesothelial cell repopulation process and induce connective tissue formation [16]. Moreover, icodextrin solution has a high concentration of lactate (40 mmol/l) and a low pH. Long-term results of randomized controlled studies on the effect of icodextrin PD fluid on peritoneal membrane function and integrity in pediatric patients are not yet available.

According to the European pediatric PD recommendations [8], icodextrin solution is a useful option, in particular in children with sodium and water overload. It may help to maintain patients on PD despite the presence of a high peritoneal membrane transport function. Icodextrin is recommended for one daily dwell only. Twice daily administration cannot be advised in children since the metabolic impact of the additional icodextrin and oligosaccharide load is unknown.

Amino Acids

Osmotically, a 1.1% amino acid-based PD solution is as efficient as a 1.36% glucose-based solution. It compensates for dialytic amino acid losses and provides a phosphate-free amino acid supply. In addition, use of amino acid-based solutions was expected to improve PD biocompatibility thanks to the lack of glucose and GDP and the only slightly acidic pH of 6.2–6.7. However, the results of experimental studies did not univocally confirm this expectation, unless the buffer lactate was replaced by bicarbonate [17].

In children on CAPD the use of amino acid solution in a single long dwell yielded conflicting results regarding the nutritional impact and was associated with increases in blood urea nitrogen and metabolic acidosis [18]. On the other hand, combined intraperitoneal infusion of amino acid and glucose during a nocturnal APD session in children promoted amino acid utilization for protein synthesis and improved some anthropometric indices [19]. Up to now, there is not sufficient clinical evidence regarding a positive nutritional effect of dialytic amino acid supplementation. Thus, amino acid-containing PD solutions cannot replace the enteral nutrition via nasogastric tubes or percutaneous endoscopic gastrostomies in malnourished children on PD [8].

Combination Therapies

A triple combination of low GDPs, multichamber PD solutions with icodextrin- and amino acid-based PD fluids has been reported to be safe and effective in some observational studies in adult patients [20]. Recently, PD solutions containing a combination of both crystalloid (glucose) and colloid osmotic agents (icodextrin) have been employed to increase sodium removal and ultrafiltration, especially in anuric adult patients on APD. Results are controversial [21, 22]; pediatric experience on 'bimodal' PD solutions does not exist.

Buffers

Lactate

Lactate has long been the standard buffer traditionally applied in PD solutions. However, a body of literature shows that the use of acidic (pH 5.5–6.5) lactate-buffered PD solutions is associated with a series of clinical, metabolic and biocompatibility drawbacks, such as inflow pain and local release of growth factors that stimulate fibrogenic processes and neoangiogenesis. Thus, high concentrations of lactate buffer at an acid pH impair peritoneal membrane transport function. Even at neutral pH, lactate-based PD fluid has been associated with toxicity with regard to mesothelial cell viability and function [23, 24], and with reduced ultrafiltration [25]. A multicenter randomized controlled trial comparing two neutral pH, low GDP PD solutions differing only with respect to lactate or bicarbonate buffer in children is underway.

Metabolic acidosis of patients with acute kidney injury (AKI) associated with shock, lactic acidosis or multi-organ failure is inadequately corrected by lactate-based PD solutions. Close monitoring of blood lactate levels is recommended in children with impaired liver function, e.g. due to sepsis or inborn errors of metabolism, and in newborns. Lactate-based PD fluids should be avoided [8].

Bicarbonate

Both in adult and pediatric patients, experimental and clinical studies showed that the use of low GDP bicarbonate-buffered PD solutions is associated with improved biocompatibility, reduced capillary recruitment [26] and better correction of acidosis [27], and a lower incidence of infusion pain as compared to conventional lactate-buffered solutions. Overcorrection of metabolic acidosis, which may occur with frequent cycles on an APD regimen, is rare when using a 34- or 35-mmol/l bicarbonate solution (fig. 2) [27]. Recently, a higher free water transport was observed in 28 pediatric patients using a 25-mmol bicarbonate and 10–15 mmol lactate-containing, neutral pH, low GDP solution compared to 37 pediatric patients using a conventional purely lactate-based, low pH, high GDP solution [28].

According to pediatric recommendations [8], acidic PD solutions should be avoided. Bicarbonate-based PD solutions are recommended in children with AKI and should

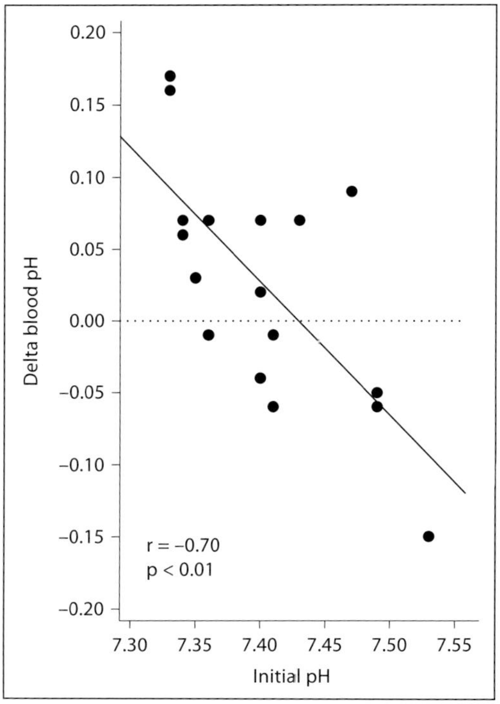

Fig. 2. Inverse association of changes in blood pH during PD with 34 mmol bicarbonate-based double-chamber PD fluid (BPDF). The x-axis gives the blood pH at time of switching from single chamber, 35 mmol lactate PDF to BPDF, and the y-axis the respective difference after 3 months of APD with BPDF. Children with a low pH had an increased, while those with a high pH a decreased blood pH; overcorrection was not observed. Modified with permission from Haas et al. [27].

generally be preferred to single-chamber lactate-based PD solutions in children on chronic PD.

Sodium

Since most of the commercially available PD solutions contain sodium at concentrations only slightly below those in plasma (132–134 mmol/l), dialytic sodium removal via diffusion is low and relatively less important than the convective sodium transport via transcapillary UF. In infants, higher dialysate sodium concentrations (137–138 mmol/l), or oral sodium supplementation may be required in case of increased body sodium losses with relative high ultrafiltration rates and high renal losses often associated with congenital uropathies. On the other hand, older children and adolescents (especially if anuric) are frequently fluid and salt overloaded, and should benefit from lower sodium chloride concentrations. Beneficial effects of PD solutions with a low sodium concentration (116–125 mmol/l) in adults [29] have not yet been studied in children. As long as respective pediatric data are not available and low sodium PD solutions are not yet admitted on the market careful monitoring of plasma, urine and effluent sodium concentrations and of dietary sodium intake is advised in order to prevent chronic dehydration in infants and persistent salt and fluid overload in older children [8].

Calcium

Longitudinal growth in children requires a positive calcium balance, especially during infancy and the pubertal growth spurt. Therefore, PD fluids with a high calcium concentration (1.75 mmol/l) are usually applied. This need, however, must be counterbalanced against the potential risk of vascular and soft tissue calcifications associated with a high calcium load, and/or a high calcium × phosphate product and should be reduced by the use of calcium-free phosphate binders and PD fluids containing 1.25 mmol/l of calcium. Of note, purely bicarbonate-buffered PD solutions are available with a 1.75-mmol/l calcium concentration only. Close monitoring of serum parathyroid hormone, calcium and phosphate levels is mandatory, especially in infants with a highly dynamic bone metabolism and who even tend to develop hypophosphatemia when fed a low-phosphate formula milk.

Conclusions and Future Prospects

The introduction of various new PD solutions substantially enlarged the therapeutic armamentarium of pediatric nephrologists to tailor the APD prescription to the particular clinical, metabolic and nutritional needs of pediatric patients. These vary greatly with age, body composition and growth. Based on numerous conclusive in vitro and animal studies, and steadily increasing evidence from clinical trials in adult but also in pediatric patients, the use of the modern, more biocompatible PD solutions has generally been recommended in children whenever possible [8]. Differences regarding pH, buffer composition and in GDP profile may at least in part explain discrepancies in study outcomes with the various PD solutions [9]. Increased costs should be offset by the long-term beneficial clinical effects. The latter, however, still remain to be demonstrated. Likewise, randomized comparative trials are needed to define PD schedules combining these solutions and to achieve the best clinical efficacy and the highest level of biocompatibility. An international pediatric PD biopsy study is meanwhile open to all pediatric dialysis centers, timely providing information on individual PD associated alterations of the peritoneal membrane and which should result in more definite answers regarding the specific morphological and functional long-term consequences of the use of PD solutions. Other efforts should include the development of glucose free, nontoxic, nonabsorbable osmotic agents and of PD devices allowing for a more refined adaptation of electrolyte and buffer supply according to individual needs, in order to optimize fluid, mineral and acid base balance and thus to better control long-term sequelae of chronic kidney disease such as bone and cardiovascular disease.

References

1 Fischbach M, Stefanidis CJ, Watson AR, European Paediatric Peritoneal Dialysis Working Group: Guidelines by an ad hoc European committee on adequacy of the paediatric peritoneal dialysis prescription. Nephrol Dial Transplant 2002;17:380–385.

2 Williams JD, Craig KJ, Topley N, Von Ruhland C, Fallon M, Newman GR, Mackenzie RK, Williams GT: Morphologic changes in the peritoneal membrane of patients with renal disease. J Am Soc Nephrol 2002;13:470–479.

3 Yoshino A, Honda M, Fukuda M, et al: Changes in peritoneal equilibration test values during long-term peritoneal dialysis in peritonitis-free children. Perit Dial Int 2001;21:180–185.

4 Schmitt CP, Haraldsson B, Doetschmann R, Zimmering M, Greiner C, Boswald M, Klaus G, Passick-Deetjen J, Schaefer F: Effects of pH-neutral, bicarbonate-buffered dialysis fluid on peritoneal transport kinetics in children. Kidney Int 2002;61:1527–1536.

5 Schmitt CP, von Heyl D, Rieger S, et al: Reduced systemic advanced glycation endproducts in children receiving peritoneal dialysis with low glucose degradation product content. Nephrol Dial Transplant 2007;22:2038–2044.

6 Haag-Weber M, Kramer R, Islam M, et al: Low GDP fluid (Gambrosol trio R) attenuates decline of residual renal function in PD patients. Nephrol Dial Transplant 2010;25:2288–2296.

7 Müller-Krebs S, Kihm LP, Zeier B, Gross ML, Deppisch R, Wieslander A, Henle T, Penndorf I, Oh J, Reiser J, Nawroth PP, Zeier M, Schwenger V: Renal toxicity mediated by glucose degradation products in a rat model of advanced renal failure. Eur J Clin Invest 2008;38:296–305.

8 Schmitt CP, Bakkaloglu SA, Klaus G, Schroeder C, Fischbach M: Solutions for peritoneal dialysis in children: recommendations by the European Pediatric Dialysis Working Group. Pediatr Nephrol 2011;26:1137–1147.

9 Bargman JM: Slouching towards Bethlehem: the beast of biocompatibility. Nephrol Dial Transplant 2010;25:2050–2051.

10 Erixon M, Wieslander A, Lindén T, Carlsson O, Forsbäck G, Svensson E, Jönsson JA, Kjellstrand P: How to avoid glucose degradation products in peritoneal dialysis fluids. Perit Dial Int 2006;26:490–497.

11 De Boer AW, Schröder CH, Van Vliet R, et al: Clinical experience with icodextrin in children: ultrafiltration profiles and metabolism. Pediatr Nephrol 2000;15:21–24.

12 van Hoeck KJ, Rusthoven E, Vermeylen L, et al: Nutritional effects of increasing dialysis dose by adding an icodextrin daytime dwell to Nocturnal Intermittent Peritoneal Dialysis (NIPD) in children. Nephrol Dial Transplant 2003;18:1383–1387.

13 Canepa A, Verrina E, Perfumo F: Use of new peritoneal dialysis solutions in children. Kidney Int 2008;108:S137–S144.

14 Rusthoven E, van der Vlugt ME, van Lingen-van Bueren LJ, et al: Evaluation of intraperitoneal pressure and the effect of different osmotic agents on intraperitoneal pressure in children. Perit Dial Int 2005;25:352–356.

15 Dart A, Feber J, Wong H, et al: Icodextrin re-absorption varies with age in children on automated peritoneal dialysis. Pediatr Nephrol 2005;20:683–685.

16 Gotloib L, Wajsbrot V, Shostak A: Osmotic agents hamper mesothelial repopulation as seen in the doughnut in vivo model. Perit Dial Int 2005;25(suppl 3):S26–S30.

17 Bender TO, Witowski J, Aufricht C, Endemann M, Frei U, Passlick-Deetjen J, Jorres A: Biocompatibility of a bicarbonate-buffered amino-acid-based solution for peritoneal dialysis. Pediatr Nephrol 2008;23:1537–1543.

18 Canepa A, Perfumo F, Carrea A, et al: Long-term effect of amino-acid dialysis solution in children on continuous ambulatory peritoneal dialysis. Pediatr Nephrol 1991;5:215–219.
19 Canepa A, Verrina E, Perfumo F, et al: Value of intraperitoneal amino acids in children treated with chronic peritoneal dialysis. Perit Dial Int 1999;19(suppl 2):S435–S440.
20 Le Poole CY, Welten AG, Weijmer MC, Valentijn RM, van Ittersum FJ, ter Wee PM: Initiating CAPD with a regimen low in glucose and glucose degradation products, with icodextrin and amino acids (NEPP) is safe and efficacious. Perit Dial Int 2005;25(suppl 3):S64–S68.
21 Freida P, Galach M, Divino Filho JC, Werynski A, Lidholm B: Combination of crystalloid (glucose) and colloid (icodextrin) osmotic agents markedly enhances peritoneal fluid and solute transport during the long PD dwell. Perit Dial Int 2007;27:267–276.
22 Akonur A, Leypoldt JK: Three-pore model predictions of 24-hour automated peritoneal dialysis therapy using bimodal solutions. Perit Dial Int 2011;31:537–544.
23 Ogata S, Mori M, Tatsukawa Y, Kiribayashi K, Yorioka N: Expression of vascular endothelial growth factor, fibroblast growth factor, and lactate deydrogenase by human peritoneal mesothelial cells in solutions with lactate or bicarbonate or both. Adv Perit Dial 2006;22:37–40.
24 Yihui Zhai Y, Bloch J, Hömme M, Schaefer J, Hackert T, Philippin B, Schwenger V, Schaefer F, Schmitt CP: Buffer-dependent regulation of aquaporin-1 expression and function in human peritoneal mesothelial cells. Pediatr Nephrol 2012;Mar 1. [Epub ahead of print]
25 Simonsen O, Sterner G, Carlsson O, Wieslander A, Rippe B: Improvement of peritoneal ultrafiltration with peritoneal dialysis solution buffered with bicarbonate/lactate mixture. Perit Dial Int 2006;26:353–359.
26 Fischbach M, Terzic J, Chauvé S, Laugel V, Muller A, Haraldsson B: Effect of peritoneal dialysis fluid composition on peritoneal area available for exchange in children. Nephrol Dial Transplant 2004;19:925–932.
27 Haas S, Schmitt CP, Arbeiter K, Bonzel KE, Fischbach M, John U, Pieper AK, Schaub TP, Passlick-Deetjen J, Mehls O, Schaefer F: Improved acidosis correction and recovery of mesothelial cell mass with neutral-pH bicarbonate dialysis solution among children undergoing automated peritoneal dialysis. J Am Soc Nephrol 2003;14:2632–2638.
28 Rajimakers R, Coester A, Smit W, Krediet RT, Schroeder CH: Free water transport in children on peritoneal dialysis is higher with more biocompatible dialysis solutions, higher with older age and declines with time. Nephrol Dial Transplant 2012;27:1183–1190.
29 Davies S, Carlsson O, Simonsen O, Johansson AC, Venturoli D, Ledebo J, Wieslander A, Chan C, Rippe B: The effects of low-sodium peritoneal dialysis fluids on blood pressure, thirst and volume status. Nephrol Dial Transplant 2009;24:1609–1617.

Enrico Eugenio Verrina, MD
Head, Dialysis Unit, Paediatric Nephrology and Dialysis Department
Giannina Gaslini Institute
Largo G. Gaslini, 5, IT–16148 Genoa (Italy)
Tel. +39 010 563 6276, E-Mail enricoverrina@ospedale-gaslini.ge.it

Ronco C, Rosner MH, Crepaldi C (eds): Peritoneal Dialysis – State-of-the-Art 2012.
Contrib Nephrol. Basel, Karger, 2012, vol 178, pp 23–29

Brazilian Peritoneal Dialysis Multicenter Study (BRAZPD): From Conception to Execution of a National Peritoneal Dialysis Reality Check

José Carolino Divino-Filho[a,b] · Kleyton de Andrade Bastos[c] · Abdul Rashid Qureshi[a] · Miguel Carlos Riella[d] · Roberto Pecoits-Filho[e] · Natália Fernandes[f] on behalf of the Brazilian Peritoneal Dialysis Multicenter Study (BRAZPD) Group

[a]Division of Renal Medicine, CLINTEC, Karolinska Institutet, Stockholm, and [b]Medical- Scientific Office, Diaverum Renal Services Group, Lund, Sweden; [c]Department of Medicine, Federal University of Sergipe, Aracaju, [d]Catholic University of Parana and Pro-Renal Brazil Foundation and [e]Center of Health and Biological Sciences, Catholic University of Paraná, Curitiba, and [f]IMEPEN Foundation and Federal University of Juiz de Fora, Juiz de Fora, Brazil

Abstract

Systematic data collection of patients undergoing renal replacement therapy is critical to the epidemiological and clinical understanding of the treatment. These data may allow more rational use of economic resources and identify interventions to improve treatment and decrease the morbidity and mortality of these patients. The Brazilian Peritoneal Dialysis Multicenter Study (BRAZPD), an observational cohort study of peritoneal dialysis (PD) patients in Brazil, aimed to collect monthly demographics, clinical, laboratory and outcome data of PD patients treated in 114 dialysis clinics around the country, was started in December 2004 and ended in September 2011. BRAZPD has been generating solid and important information, which is very useful as a reality check of the PD therapy for all Brazilian PD centers.

Brazil, with a surface area of 8,500,000 km^2, has more than 190 million inhabitants, divided into five large regions with economic, cultural and geographic differences and is placed among the 10 largest economies of the world.

Unfortunately, there is a scarcity of epidemiological data on the situation of renal disease in the country as well as of the economic, administrative and management aspects of the line services associated with renal therapy as a whole. According to data from the Brazilian Society of Nephrology [1] there was a 28.8% increase in the last 5 years in the need for dialysis therapy with a prevalence of 475 CKD patients/million inhabitants in 2011. However, there is no national registry and therefore the real incidence and prevalence of CKD is unknown.

PD in Brazil, as in most countries, was initially prescribed as a therapy for acute kidney injury and CAPD was introduced to the country in 1980 [2], whereas APD was available in 1989. There are 91,314 dialysis patients (90.6% treated with HD), 54.8% of them living in the

Southeastern region. The most important payer (84.9%) for renal replacement therapy (RRT) is the national government through its Unified Health System (SUS). The low prevalence of PD in Brazil may be related to late referral, patients with lack of information on the different RRT options, nephrologists with no PD experience/training, indication bias, socioeconomic reasons and also economic preference by the treating doctor. PD mortality is 15.5% and is similar to that reported for HD patients (14.7%), according to the 2007 report with data collected in 2004 [1].

Information on PD clinical practice and outcomes has not been abundant in either Brazil or Latin America [3]. The most important PD study is the ADEMEX, a prospective, randomized, controlled clinical trial with 965 Mexican patients [4], whose results led to adjustments in the adequacy guidelines of several guidelines, including the most important one, the ISPD guidelines. Other important studies shedding some light on PD therapy in Latin America have recently been published [5, 6].

Observational studies, which can be exploratory or confirmatory in nature, serve as the important substrate for generating interesting ideas to be tested in appropriate clinical studies to generate medical evidence and, even be used as substrate for guidelines. Paradigm shifts in the field of PD have been influenced by such observational studies [7–11].

Despite being the third country in absolute number of patients on dialysis worldwide, no study of this kind has yet been performed in Brazil. Besides, the absence of a national registry, the lack of PD research during the last 10 years and the biased indication (negative selection) for PD [12] have been considered as motivation to design a prospective observational cohort study. The aim of this study was to develop a national database providing epidemiological and clinical information to be applied to broaden PD knowledge and, consequently, improve the quality of care, serving as a basis for preventive and corrective actions related to the PD programs in Brazil.

Study Design, Data Collection and Analysis

This is a multicenter prospective cohort study, sponsored by Baxter, that started in December 2004 and ended in September 2011. The study included 114 centers each treating more than 10 patients with the Baxter PD system. Each enrolled clinic submitted the project to the local ethics committee for approval. Patients (prevalent and incident) who had signed an informed consent to participate in the study were followed up during the study period. At the moment of the recruitment, data on both prevalent and incident patients were retrieved, including a retrospective analysis of patient history and selected data. They were then followed prospectively collecting data electronically on a monthly basis until an endpoint was achieved.

A software system (PDnet) was especially developed for data collection, designed as two different modules that complement each other. The first module, PDnet offline, was developed in the platform and concept of Java, in which patient information is entered by each center. At the end of each month, the software generates a data file that is sent through a second module, PDnet online. This module is developed using JSP technology, a Tomcat application server and a MySQL database. The secure data received monthly in the coordinating center is then added to the mother database that generated the data for the analysis. The BRAZPD electronic form was designed following the model of the Brazilian Institute of Geography and Statistics, which is the entity responsible for the Brazilian census.

So far, two data extractions have been performed and a third and final one is underway. The first extraction with 3,226 patients, covering the period between December 2004 and February 2007, was used to characterize the cohort with a descriptive analysis [13]. This same data were used to compare the demographic, clinical and laboratory characteristics of the cohort with the PD recommendations proposed by the Spanish PD guidelines [14]. The second extraction with 6,198 patients, covering the period between

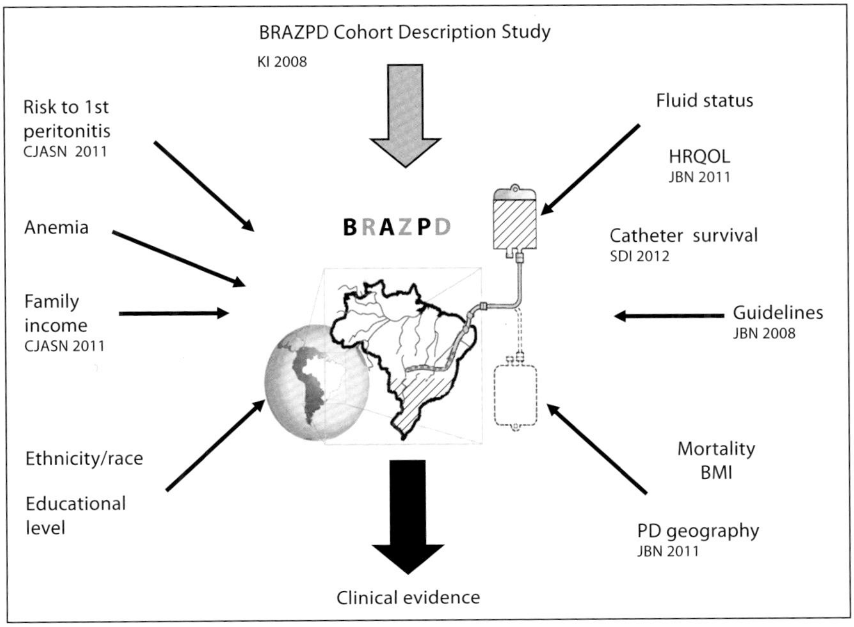

Fig. 1. Published (journal and year) and submitted BRAZPD articles.

December 2004 and October 2007, has been used for all other papers published so far [15–19].

This study was conducted in accordance with the Declaration of Helsinki, and all participants provided written informed consent before enrollment. More details of the study design and the characteristics of the cohort are described elsewhere [13, 20].

Published Papers (fig. 1)

Characterization of the BRAZPD Cohort

In this paper published in *Kidney International* in 2008 [13], the initial results of the BRAZPD, comprising 3,226 PD patients (being 2,094 incident) enrolled in the study between December 2004 and February 2007 were reported. The mean age was 54 ±19 years (37% over 65 years of age), 55% females, 64% Caucasians. APD was the modality utilized in 53% and the peritonitis rate was 1 episode per 30 patient-months. The total dropout rate was 33%, mainly due to deaths. The gross mortality was 17.6% and the main cause of mortality was cardiovascular diseases (40%). The initial BRAZPD results provided a unique opportunity to develop future clinical studies addressing specific PD questions in the Brazilian reality and context (fig. 1).

A Comparative Analysis of the BRAZPD Data with the Spanish Dialysis Guidelines

In a paper published in the *Brazilian Journal of Nephrology* in 2008 [14], the degree of adherence to the therapeutic recommendations proposed by the Spanish dialysis guidelines in the BRAZPD cohort was assessed. The PD patient population and the follow-up period were the same as in the KI paper [13]. Compared to the Spanish guidelines, the BRAZPD patients were older, more diabetic, and presented larger number of comorbidities. The prevalence of infectious complications was low and there was a good fulfillment of recommended laboratorial targets, with the exception of hemoglobin levels. The standards of PD care delivered to the BRAZPD patients are in agreement with those recommended internationally.

Geography of Peritoneal Dialysis (BRAZPD) in Brazil

In a paper published in the *Brazilian Journal of Nephrology* [15] in 2011, the clinical characteristics and outcomes presented by PD patients in different regions of Brazil were analyzed, comprising 5,819 patients (both incident as prevalent) followed up from December 2004 to October 2007. Most patients lived in the Southeast region where the average follow-up time was longer (12.3 months) and with a higher percentage of elderly (36.4%). The prevalence of diabetes was higher in the Southeast and South regions (38.1 and 37%, respectively). Most patients in the North region had previously had HD (66.2%). The mortality was higher in the Northern region (30.1%) as was technique failure (22.3%). The data show different demographic, clinical, mortality and technique failures of PD reflecting the demographic and social peculiarities of Brazil. The geography of PD in Brazil proves to be a mirror of the geography of Brazil.

Factors Associated with the Quality of Life (QoL) of Incident PD Patients in BRAZPD

In a paper published in the *Brazilian Journal of Nephrology* [16] in 2011, the QoL of 1,624 incident patients was assessed with the Karnofsky Index (KI) (assessment by health professionals) and the SF-36 (patient's self-assessment). Patients had low QoL scores in all the SF-36 domains, the 'physical role' domain being the most affected and the 'social functioning' domain having the best score. The KI showed a better QoL as compared with the SF-36 assessment, but similar results were found in the subgroups evaluated: the elderly and the diabetic patients had the worst QoL in both assessments. The results of the present study emphasize the influence of factors such as advanced age and diabetes in the reduction of the QoL parameters of patients undergoing PD. It is worth emphasizing the importance of valuing the patient's perception about his/her own state of health.

Family Income and Survival in BRAZPD: Time to Revisit a Myth?

In a paper published in the *CJASN* in 2011 [17], 1,952 incident PD patients enrolled between December 2004 and October 2007 were divided according to monthly family income. Most of the patients were in CAPD, had not received predialysis care, had <4 school years, and had a monthly family income of <5 minimum wages (80%). There were no differences in technique (log-rank test $\chi^2 = 4.36$) and patient (log-rank test $\chi^2 = 2.92$) survival between the groups. In the multivariate analysis, low family income remained not associated either to worse technique survival (HR = 1.29, 95% CI = 0.91 to 1.84) or to patient survival (HR = 1.40, 95% CI = 0.99–1.99). According to these results, the concept of poverty as a barrier to the choice of PD as RRT should be revisited wherever it is still applied, and for patients wishing to do PD, poverty should not be a reason to deny such therapy.

Geographic and Educational Factors and Risk of First Peritonitis Episode in Incident BRAZPD

In a paper published in the *CJASN* [18] in 2011, incident PD patients (n = 2,032) enrolled between December 2004 and October 2007 were followed up until their first peritonitis. Cox proportional model was used to determine independent factors associated with peritonitis. In a cumulative follow-up of 22,026 patient months, 474 (23.3%) presented a first peritonitis episode. This study has identified educational level as a strong risk predictor for the first peritonitis episode, independent of socioeconomic status, PD modality, and co-morbidities. These results reinforce the need for further studies looking at factors that influence peritonitis incidence, including those which are considered non-modifiable today, to identify intervention alternatives and thereby improve PD outcomes.

Similar Outcomes of Catheters Implanted by Nephrologists and Surgeons: Analysis of the BRAZPD Cohort

In a paper published in *Seminars in Dialysis* [19] in 2012, the impact of the PD catheter insertion operator (nephrologist vs. surgeon) on early catheter complications and on technique survival was explored. Valid data obtained from 736 catheter implantations performed in 93 centers were analyzed. Mechanical (HR = 0.99; 95% CI 0.56–1.76; p = 0.98) and infectious (HR = 0.63, 95% CI 0.32–1.23; p = 0.17) early complication rates as well as long-term survival were similar between groups, defined by operator profile, supporting the role of interventional nephrology in the placement of PD catheters.

Unpublished Data

A number of papers analyzing different aspects of the BRAZPD cohort have been submitted for publication and await reply from the Journals (fig. 1).

Gonçalves' group look into predictors of anemia and the impact of hemoglobin and its variability on patients' outcome.

Fernandes and coworkers evaluate the role played by body size and longitudinal body weight (BW) changes in the survival of incident PD patients (n = 1,911). Survival analyses were performed using Kaplan-Meier survival curves and the Cox proportional hazards. Competing risk analysis was used to study the influence of BMI on survival. Two sensitivity analyses were also carried out. Restricted cubic splines were used to evaluate nonlinear relationships between BMI levels and mortality.

The presence of a simple and easily detectable sign of peripheral edema is a very relevant tool not only to assess the patient's clinical hypertensive status but also the PD prescription and patient compliance. In a third submitted paper, Ferreira's group evaluate the association of pitting edema with blood pressure behavior in 1,089 incident hypertensive BRAZPD patients during 12 months.

Health-related quality of life (HRQOL) is an important outcome parameter for monitoring quality of care delivered to maintenance dialysis patients. Grincenkov and coworkers assess if educational level and family income are associated with baseline and longitudinal changes in HRQOL scores during the first year. A total of 1,624 incident BRAZPD patients were evaluated at baseline whereas 486 of these patients were also assessed after 12 months.

The Brazilian population is one of the most heterogeneous populations in the world as a result of five centuries of admixture between its ancestral roots. There are no available epidemiological studies about the influence of ethnicity/race on outcomes of PD patients in South America. Fernandes and colleagues assess the influence of ethnicity on mortality of incident BRAZPD patients.

There is evidence that limited educational level (EL) contributes to differences in health outcomes. Bastos and coworkers assess the effect of EL on survival in the BRAZPD incident patients (n = 1,952) enrolled from December 2004 to October 2007 and divided according to EL (in school years).

In a cross-sectional, national, ecologic study, Fernandes and coworkers investigate the relationship between all-cause and cardiovascular mortality rates in BRAZPD patients and their respective general population.

Future Studies, Postgraduate Studies and International Cooperation

The BRAZPD has stimulated young nephrologists and nurses to work with the data and this has, so far, led to the accomplishment of three PhD theses by nephrologists and two master degrees (one renal nurses and one psychologist) in four different universities and states of the country.

Meanwhile, BRAZPD is certainly contributing to the understanding of PD at the national level, and not less, generating specific PD questions, which may lead to the development of cooperative studies among the different national and regional PD registries across the world.

Conclusions

Nine years have passed since the conception of the BRAZPD and, looking back, we can say that

BRAZPD has been accomplishing what it was created for: to generate solid and important information, which is very useful as a reality check of the PD therapy for all Brazilian PD centers. All these efforts have contributed to a better understanding of PD therapy, a stimulus for clinical research and to a better care of the PD patient in Brazil, especially in the centers participating in the study. Without the support, determination and enthusiasm of all patients, nurses and doctors, none of this could have been achieved. We should here also register our gratitude to Baxter Health Care Brazil for their support of this project; without it BRAZPD would not have existed.

It is with sorrow that we received the news that the support to BRAZPD has been terminated; however, the investigators deeply involved from the conception and start of this cohort study will continue pursuing the execution of the data gathered throughout these years with a pure and uncompromised sense of bringing forth as much information as possible in order to continuously improve the PD therapy and care in Brazil.

Acknowledgements

We thank the renal multi-professional team and patients from all centers participating in the BRAZPD, Ed Vonesh, Bengt Lindholm and Baxter Novum, the Brazilian Baxter Renal team, and especially Debora Ramos, Regina Fortes, Angela Tosi and Daniel Rimoli for their important contribution to this project.

Disclosure Statement

Baxter Healthcare Corporation Brazil has sponsored this study. During the data collection and analysis, José Carolino Divino-Filho was employed by Baxter; his employment by Baxter ended on March 31, 2011. Roberto Pecoits-Filho and Miguel Carlos Riella have received consulting fees and speaker honorarium from Baxter Healthcare.

References

1 Sociedade Brasileira de Nefrologia: www.sbn.org.br accessed 27 February 2012.
2 Riella MC, et al: Diálise Peritoneal ambulatorial contínua (CAPD): experiência preliminar. J Bras Nefrol 1982;4:45–52.
3 Pecoits-Filho R, Abensur H, Cueto-Manzano AM, et al: Overview of peritoneal dialysis in Latin America. Perit Dial Int 2007;27:316–321.
4 Paniagua R, Amato D, Vonesh E, et al: Effects of increased peritoneal clearences on mortality rates in peritoneal dialysis: ADEMEX, a prospective, randomized, controlled trial. J Am Soc Nephrol 2002;13:1307–1320.
5 Sanabria M, Munoz J, Trillos C, et al: Dialysis outcomes in Colombia (DOC) study: a comparison of patient survival on peritoneal dialysis vs hemodialysis in Colombia. Kidney Int Suppl 2008;108:S165–S172.
6 Moretta G, Locatelli AJ, Gadola L, De AJ, Sola L, Caporale N, Schargorodsky J, Ducasse E, Pastorino G, Marchetta N, Espeche W, Ortiz Z: Rio de La Plata study: a multicenter, cross-sectional study on cardiovascular risk factors and heart failure prevalence in peritoneal dialysis patients in Argentina and Uruguay. Kidney Int Suppl 2008;108:S159–S164.
7 Churchill DN, Thorpe KE, Vonesh EF, Keshaviah PR: Lower probability of patient survival with continuous peritoneal dialysis in the United States compared with Canada. Canada-USA (CANUSA) Peritoneal Dialysis Study Group. J Am Soc Nephrol 1997;8:965–971.
8 Jager KJ, Merkus MP, Boeschoten EW, et al: Dialysis in the Netherlands: the clinical condition of new patients put into a European perspective. NECOSAD study group. Netherlands cooperative study on the adequacy of dialysis phase 1. Nephrol Dial Transplant 1999;14:2438–2444.
9 Garcia-Garcia G, Monteon-Ramos JF, Garcia-Bejarano H, Gomez-Navarro B, Reyes IH, Lomeli AM, Palomeque M, Cortes-Sanabria L, Breien-Alcaraz H, Ruiz-Morales NM: Renal replacement therapy among disadvantaged populations in Mexico: a report from the Jalisco Dialysis and Transplant Registry (REDTJAL). Kidney Int Suppl 2005;97:S58–S61.
10 Brown EA, Davies SJ, Rutherford P, Meeus F, Borras M, Riegel W, Divino Filho JC, Vonesh E, van BM: Survival of functionally anuric patients on automated peritoneal dialysis: the European APD Outcome Study. J Am Soc Nephrol 2003;14:2948–2957.
11 Lam MF, Tang C, Wong AK, Tong KL, Yu AW, Li CS, Cheung KO, Lai KN: ASPD: a prospective study of adequacy in Asian patients on long term, small volume, continuous ambulatory peritoneal dialysis. Perit Dial Int 2006;26:466–474.

12 Rocha PN, Sallenave M, Casqueiro V, Campelo Neto B, Presídio S: Motivo de 'escolha' de diálise peritoneal: exaustão de acesso vascular para hemodiálise. J Bras Nefrol 2010;32:23–28.
13 Fernandes N, Bastos MG, Cassi HV, Machado NL, Ribeiro JA, Martins G, et al: The Brazilian Peritoneal Dialysis Multicenter Study (BRAZPD): characterization of the cohort. Kidney Int Suppl 2008;108:S145–S151.
14 Fernandes N, Bastos MG, Pecoits-Filho R, et al: Sucessos e Fracassos – Uma Análise dos Dados do BRAZPD Comparados às Diretrizes Espanholas. J Bras Nefrol 2008;30:22–31.
15 Fernandes NM, Chaoubah A, Bastos KA, et al: Geography of peritoneal dialysis in Brazil: analysis of a cohort of 5,819 patients (BRAZPD). J Bras Nefrol 2011;32:268–274.
16 Grincenkov FR, Fernandes N, Chaoubah A, et al: Factors associated with the quality of life of incident patients on PD in Brazil (BRAZPD). J Bras Nefrol 2011;33:38–44.
17 Bastos KA, Qureshi AR, Lopes AA, et al: Family income and survival in Brazilian Peritoneal Dialysis Multicenter Study Patients (BRAZPD): time to revisit a myth? Clin J Am Soc Nephrol 2011;6:1676–1683.
18 Martin LC, Caramori JC, Fernandes N, Divino-Filho JC, Pecoits-Filho R, Barretti P: Geographic and educational factors and risk of the first peritonitis episode in brazilian peritoneal dialysis study (BRAZPD) patients. Clin J Am Soc Nephrol 2011;6:1944–1951.
19 Moraes TP, Campos R, Tokunaga de Alcantara M, Chula D, Vieira MA, Riella MC, Olandowski M, Divino-Filho JC, Pecoits-Filho R: Similar outcomes of catheters implanted by nephrologists and surgeons: analysis of the Brazilian Peritoneal Dialysis Multicentric study. Semin Dialysis 2012 Feb 24. doi: 10.1111/j.1525-139X.2012.01050.x. [Epub ahead of print].
20 Fernandes N: Peritoneal dialysis in Brasil: description of a cohort and risk factors associated to patient and technique survival; PhD thesis, Universidade Federal de Juiz de Fora, Brasil, 2009.

José Carolino Divino-Filho, MD, PhD
Diaverum Renal Services Group
Barerstrasse 7
D–80333 Munich (Germany)
Tel. +49 1728479237, E-Mail jose.divino@diaverum.com

Ronco C, Rosner MH, Crepaldi C (eds): Peritoneal Dialysis – State-of-the-Art 2012.
Contrib Nephrol. Basel, Karger, 2012, vol 178, pp 30–34

Comparing Outcomes of Hemodialysis and Peritoneal Dialysis Patients: Consider the Pitfalls

Rajnish Mehrotra

Los Angeles Biomedical Research Institute at Harbor-UCLA, Torrance, Calif., and David Geffen School of Medicine at UCLA, Los Angeles, Calif., USA

Abstract

Patients with end-stage renal disease have a limited life expectancy. It is primarily for this reason that there is interest in determining whether one form of dialysis therapy provides any survival advantage over another in different subgroups of individuals. Randomized controlled clinical trials are the gold standard in answering such a question. However, in-center hemodialysis and home peritoneal dialysis require profoundly significant but different effects on patients' lifestyle and it is not surprising that most patients don't want to leave that choice to chance and refuse to participate in such clinical trials. Thus, we have to depend upon observational data to compare outcomes with the two different dialysis therapies. Yet such studies are not without pitfalls, particularly those arising from selection bias, confounding by indication, and residual confounding. These pitfalls and potential methods to overcome them are discussed in this paper. Despite such adjustments, it is impossible to determine if the differences in survival, if any, are a direct result of the dialysis modality or from differences in the characteristics of the patients who are treated with these therapies. Juxtaposing this limitation with the profound impact of dialysis therapies on patients' lives, it is prudent to leave the decision of selection of dialysis modality to the patients themselves and healthcare providers should offer decision support for individuals attempting to make such a selection.

For almost 50 years now, maintenance dialysis therapies have allowed us to prolong the lives of patients with end-stage renal disease. Furthermore, despite substantially expanding the pool of patients eligible to receive maintenance dialysis (namely elderly and diabetics), the annual mortality rates of dialysis patients in 2009 in the United States were almost 25% lower than they were in the mid-1980s [1]. Yet, substantial challenges remain. The median life expectancy of patients starting maintenance dialysis ranges from only 3–5 years in different parts of the world [1, 2]. Thus, there is considerable interest in identifying modifiable determinants of patient survival. Dialysis modality has been considered to be one such modifiable determinant and a large number of studies have been undertaken to compare the survival of patients treated with in-center hemodialysis (HD) and home peritoneal dialysis (PD).

The greatest threat to the internal validity of any study is confounding – systematic differences in the distribution of one or more factors prognostically related to the outcome of interest (namely death) between individuals treated with two therapies. Randomized, controlled trials are the best way to control for confounding as randomization assures equal distribution of not only known but also unknown confounders. However, in-center HD and PD have substantial and disparate effects on patients' life style and when explained about the two therapies, patients in the developed world have been unwilling to leave the choice between two therapies simply to chance (or random allocation). It is for this reason that enrollment for the most recent attempt to compare in-center HD with PD in the Netherlands failed spectacularly and was able to randomize only 38 subjects despite identifying 773 individuals who met all inclusion and exclusion criteria [3]. Investigators in China have taken up this challenge and have recently launched a randomized, controlled clinical trial to compare the two therapies with the goal of enrolling 1,370 subjects (clinicaltrials.gov identifier: NCT01413074). However, the results of this clinical trial are unlikely to be available before 2017 and up until then, one would need to depend only on observational studies to compare the outcomes of in-center HD and PD. While these studies provide useful information, it is important to consider the pitfalls to better understand how to apply the results of these studies in clinical practice.

Adjusting Inter-Modality Comparisons for Confounding from Baseline and Time-Varying Differences in Patients Who Dialyze In-Center or at Home

Over the last three decades, inter-modality comparisons have evolved from using information about patients treated in single centers to those that use data from national registries. Undoubtedly, this has enhanced the external validity of the comparisons. It is evident from these registry studies that there are systematic differences in patients who are treated with in-center HD or PD but these differences vary from one part of the world to the other. Thus, while in the United States PD patients are younger and healthier than those treated with in-center HD, it is the opposite in Australia, New Zealand, and France [2, 4, 5]. It is important to keep these differences in mind when evaluating studies from different parts of the world.

The conventional way to control for confounding is by including a variety of variables as covariates in time-to-event survival analyses. The variables included as covariates generally are believed to be important risk factors for the event of interest (namely death) that may or may not be differentially distributed in patients treated with the two dialysis therapies. This allows one to estimate adjusted hazards ratio for death for patients treated with one dialysis therapy with the other group as a reference. However, conventional survival models are insufficient to account for the complexities when comparing dialysis therapies. Studies over the last 15 years have highlighted the importance of considering 'interactions', where the relationship of death risk to dialysis modality varies by subgroup. At least five such 'interactions' have been identified: (1) with time, whereby the death risk for PD patients is reportedly lower (relative to in-center HD) in the first 1–3 years of start of dialysis followed by a higher long-term risk; (2) with age, whereby the death risk for PD patients is lower for the young but higher for the elderly; (3) with diabetic status, whereby the death risk for PD patients is lower for the non-diabetics but higher for diabetics; (4) with cardiovascular co-morbidity whereby the death risk for PD patients is lower for those with no such co-existing illness but higher for those with coexisting illness, and (5) with era, whereby the improvements in PD outcomes in many different parts of the world have outpaced those with seen for HD patients [6, 7]. Studies that have failed to account for these interactions in survival analyses have produced results that appear to be contradictory but are essentially misleading [8, 9].

Despite the inclusion of covariates and consideration of interactions, the risk for 'residual confounding' – our inability to completely adjust for important differences in two groups of patients – remains. It is because we can only adjust for the potential confounders for which data are available. Many registry studies do not have data for important baseline confounders, most analyses don't include confounders that may differentially appear after start of dialysis, and it is likely that there are many potential confounders that science today is simply unaware of. The importance of residual confounding is evident from some recent inter-modality comparisons. Most contemporary studies from different parts of the world show remarkably similar survival of patients treated with in-center HD or PD patients; studies from Australia, New Zealand and France, where PD patients are generally older and sicker than those treated with in-center HD, are the only ones that show higher death risk with the therapy [4, 5, 10]. Similarly, the long-term death risk is higher when one compares all PD patients with potentially the healthiest patients that start treatment with in-center HD, the ones with an arteriovenous fistula [11]. Conversely, patients who have had no pre-dialysis nephrology care have a significantly higher death risk and this population is disproportionately reflected in the HD cohort. This higher death risk may be the reason for the apparent 'early survival advantage' seen in patients who start treatment with PD [12]. Indeed, this survival advantage with PD is not apparent in analyses that exclude 'late-referred' patients [13].

There is increasing interest in using propensity scores when comparing dialysis modalities [14, 15]. The first step is to build a best-fit logistic regression model to predict an individual patients' probability of starting treatment with PD based upon the baseline demographic, clinical, and laboratory characteristics; this probability is expressed numerically for each patient and is called the propensity score. Inter-modality comparisons can then be done in each tertile, quartile, or quintile of propensity scores, or patients can be matched using these scores, or they can be included as covariates in survival analyses. Undoubtedly, this approach is superior to conventional survival analyses but it is important to be cognizant of the limitations of this approach as well – propensity scores can be calculated using only the known baseline confounders. In a systematic analysis of predictors of treatment with PD in the United States, known confounders could explain only 25% of the variability in use of the therapy [16]. Thus, while the use of propensity scores attenuates the problem of residual confounding, it does not eliminate the problem.

Marginal structural modeling is a causal inference approach that further refines the comparison of two therapies and recently has been applied to inter-modality comparisons. This approach can account for baseline confounding but also time-varying confounding. An important time-varying confounding that is often not accounted for is differential transplant rates. In the United States, the adjusted transplant rate of PD patients is about 50% higher than for in-center HD patients [2]. Thus, the healthiest patients leave the PD cohort at a faster rate than the in-center HD cohort and this is a potential explanation for the apparently higher long-term risk seen with PD in earlier cohorts. Marginal structural models allows one to calculate 'weights' or adjusters to be included in statistical models for individual patients using the propensity of being treated with a given therapy based upon baseline characteristics and the probability of being censored for transplantation or for other reasons [2]. This refinement is clearly superior to the use of propensity scores but still does not eliminate the problem of residual confounding.

It is thus evident that even the most sophisticated statistical models cannot determine if differences in survival with two therapies, if any, are attributable to the dialysis modality or to the patients who choose the particular renal replacement therapy. This uncertainty is important to acknowledge when evaluating inter-modality comparisons.

Contemporary Comparisons of HD and PD Survival

In the United States, the improvements in survival of patients starting treatment with PD has outpaced those seen for individuals treated with in-center HD [7]. Two studies – one using propensity score matching, and the other with marginal structural models – have shown similar 4- and 5-year survival, respectively, of patients starting treatment with either of the two therapies [2, 15]. Furthermore, data from the USRDS shows similar 10-year survival for patients treated with the two therapies [1]. Lack of statistical significance of difference in survival in studies that have included hundreds of thousands of patients is reassuring and implies truly an equivalent survival with the two therapies.

Greater improvements in survival of PD patients have also been reported from other parts of the world. Thus, greater improvements in survival of PD patients are evident from Canada, France, Australia and New Zealand [4, 17, 18]. Similar trends have been reported from presently unpublished observations from Denmark and Taiwan. The reasons for this differential improvement in outcomes with the two dialysis modalities are not readily evident. This could be a result of greater attention to prescription management, substantial reduction in infection risk, or implementation of quality improvement programs; given lack of data, these remain speculative.

It has been argued that since improvement in PD outcomes has occurred at a time when utilization of the therapy has declined, the reduction in death risk may be a result of more selective assignment of patients to the therapy. While this possibility cannot be entirely excluded, it is reassuring to note that equivalency of outcomes with the two therapies has been reported from countries with much greater use of PD than the United States: Canada 18%, Australia and New Zealand 25%, and Colombia 53% [4, 17, 19]. Furthermore, excellent long-term outcomes have been reported from Hong Kong, a country where over 80% of the patients are treated with PD [20]. These considerations suggest that as long as attention is paid to practice patterns, we should be able to expect similar outcomes with the two dialysis therapies.

How Should the Data from Survival Studies Be Used to Make Treatment Recommendations for Patients?

The treatment of end-stage renal disease requires patients to make more adjustments in their lifestyle – the need to come to a dialysis facility thrice weekly or perform the therapy at home – than are asked of patients with virtually any other chronic disease [21]. The patients are also asked to adapt to these changes in lifestyle at a time of great stress for them and their families. Patients with a recent diagnosis of end-stage renal disease report confronting death, are weighing the impact of their disease on their loved ones, and want choices [22]. Up to 10% of patients develop such extreme anxiety that it meets the diagnostic criteria for post-traumatic stress disorder [23]. If one juxtaposes the anxiety and stress in a patient who has just been told that they need dialysis to the uncertainties in the interpretation of survival studies and the difficulties in attributing differences in survival, if any, to the dialysis modality, it would be prudent to leave this choice to the patients [21]. Put differently, the differences in survival of patients treated with in-center HD or PD are small, if any, and they are as likely to be a result of the differences in the characteristics of the patients who are treated with the two therapies as a direct effect of the dialysis modality. Given this uncertainty, it is best for patients to undergo comprehensive CKD education to provide decision support for patients to select the dialysis modality which they believe will work best for them given their expectations and desires for their personal lives.

Disclosure Statement

Rajnish Mehrotra has received grant support, honoraria, and/or has served as an ad hoc consultant for Baxter Healthcare and DaVita, Inc.

References

1 United States Renal Data System: Annual Data Report. Bethesda, US Department of Public Health and Human Services, Public Health Service, National Institutes of Health, 2011.

2 Mehrotra R, Chiu YW, Kalantar-Zadeh K, Bargman J, Vonesh E: Similar outcomes with hemodialysis and peritoneal dialysis in patients with end-stage renal disease. Arch Intern Med 2011;171:110–118.

3 Korevaar JC, Feith GW, Dekker FW, van Manen JG, Boeschoten E, Bossuyt PMM, Krediet RT, Group, ftNS: Effect of starting hemodialysis compared with peritoneal dialysis in patients new on dialysis treatment: a randomized controlled trial. Kidney Int 2003;64:2222–2228.

4 McDonald SP, Marshall MR, Johnson DW, Polkinghorne KR: Relationship between dialysis modality and mortality. J Am Soc Nephrol 2009;20:155–163.

5 Sens F, Schott-Pethelaz AM, Labeeuw M, Colin C, Villar E: Survival advantage of hemodialysis relative to peritoneal dialysis in end-stage renal disease patients with congestive heart failure. Kidney Int 2011;80:970–977. doi: 10.1038/ki.2011.233. Epub 2011 Jul 20.

6 Vonesh EF, Snyder JJ, Foley RN, Collins AJ: The differential impact of risk factors on mortality in hemodialysis and peritoneal dialysis. Kidney Int 2004;66:2389–2401.

7 Mehrotra R, Kermah D, Fried L, Kalantar-Zadeh K, Khawar O, Norris K, Nissenson A: Chronic peritoneal dialysis in the United States: declining utilization despite improving outcomes. J Am Soc Nephrol 2007;18:2781–2788.

8 Ganesh SK, Hulbert-Shearon T, Port FK, Eagle K, Stack AG: Mortality differences by dialysis modality among incident ESRD patients with and without coronary artery disease. J Am Soc Nephrol 2003;14:415–424.

9 Stack AG, Molony DA, Rahman NS, Dosekun A, Murthy B: Impact of dialysis modality on survival of new ESRD patients with congestive heart failure in the United States. Kidney Int 2003;64:1071–1079.

10 Chiu YW, Jiwakanon S, Lukowsky L, Duong U, Kalantar-Zadeh K, Mehrotra R: An update on the comparisons of mortality outcomes of hemodialysis and peritoneal dialysis patients. Semin Nephrol 2011;31:152–158.

11 Perl J, Wald R, McFarlane P, Bargman JM, Vonesh E, Na Y, Jassal SV, Moist L: Hemodialysis vascular access modifies the association between dialysis modality and survival. J Am Soc Nephrol 2011;22:1113–1121.

12 Fenton SS, Schaubel DE, Desmeules M, Morrison HI, Mao Y, Copleston P, Jeffery JR, Kjellstrand CM: Hemodialysis versus peritoneal dialysis: a comparison of adjusted mortality rates. Am J Kidney Dis 1997;30:334–342.

13 Quinn RR, Hux JE, Oliver MJ, Austin PC, Tonelli M, Laupacis A: Selection bias explains apparent differential mortality between dialysis modalities. J Am Soc Nephrol 2011;22:1534–1542.

14 Jaar BG, Coresh J, Plantinga LC, Fink NE, Klag MJ, Levey AS, Levin NW, Sadler JH, Kliger A, Powe NR: Comparing the risk for death with peritoneal dialysis and hemodialysis in a national cohort of patients with chronic kidney disease. Ann Intern Med 2005;143:174–183.

15 Weinhandl ED, Foley RN, Gilbertson DT, Arneson TJ, Snyder JJ, Collins AJ: Propensity-matched mortality comparison of incident hemodialysis and peritoneal dialysis patients. J Am Soc Nephrol 2010;21:499–506.

16 Stack AG: Determinants of modality selection among incident US dialysis patients: results from a national study. J Am Soc Nephrol 2002;13:1279–1287.

17 Yeates K: Personal communication.

18 Greneche S, D'Andon A, Jacquelinet C, Faller B, Fouque D, Laville M: [Choosing between peritoneal dialysis and haemodialysis: a critical appraisal of the literature]. Nephrol Ther 2005;1:213–220.

19 Sanabria M, Munoz J, Trillos C, Hernandez G, Latorre C, Diaz CS, Murad S, Rodriguez K, Rivera A, Amador A, Ardila F, Caicedo A, Camargo D, Diaz A, Gonzalez J, Leguizamon H, Lopera P, Marin L, Nieto I, Vargas E: Dialysis outcomes in Colombia (DOC) study: a comparison of patient survival on peritoneal dialysis vs hemodialysis in Colombia. Kidney Int Suppl 2008;108:S165–S172.

20 Li PK, Szeto CC: Success of the peritoneal dialysis programme in Hong Kong. Nephrol Dial Transplant 2008;23:1475–1478.

21 Mehrotra R: Choice of dialysis modality. Kidney Int 2011;80:909–911.

22 Morton RL, Tong A, Howard K, Snelling P, Webster AC: The views of patients and carers in treatment decision making for chronic kidney disease: systematic review and thematic synthesis of qualitative studies. BMJ 2010;340:c112.

23 Tagay S, Kribben A, Hohenstein A, Mewes R, Senf W: Posttraumatic stress disorder in hemodialysis patients. Am J Kidney Dis 2007;50:594–601.

Prof. Rajnish Mehrotra
Los Angeles Biomedical Research Institute at Harbor-UCLA
1124 W Carson Street
Torrance, CA 90502 (USA)
Tel. +1 310 222 3891, E-Mail rmehrotra@labiomed.org

Ronco C, Rosner MH, Crepaldi C (eds): Peritoneal Dialysis – State-of-the-Art 2012.
Contrib Nephrol. Basel, Karger, 2012, vol 178, pp 35–39

Hypogonadism in Males with Chronic Kidney Disease: Another Cause of Resistance to Erythropoiesis-Stimulating Agents?

Peter Stenvinkel · Peter Bárány

Division of Renal Medicine, Department of Clinical Science, Intervention and Technology, Karolinska Institutet, Stockholm, Sweden

Abstract

Anemia, inflammation, resistance to erythropoiesis-stimulating agents (ESA) and hypogonadism (testosterone deficiency) are highly prevalent conditions, which heralds poor prognosis, in chronic kidney disease (CKD). It has been speculated that testosterone stimulates erythropoiesis via production of hematopoietic growth factors and possibly improvement of iron bioavailability. Whereas inflammation stimulates synthesis of the liver-derived iron regulatory protein hepcidin, a recent study suggests that testosterone inhibits hepcidin synthesis, thus offering a possible novel mechanism for testosterone-induced erythropoiesis. As any agent that lowers hepcidin may be an effective strategy to normalize iron homeostasis and overcome renal anemia, testosterone deficiency should be considered in this patient group. Indeed, a recent study in males with CKD showed that hypogonadism may be an additional cause of anemia and reduced ESA responsiveness. Thus, a randomized controlled trial is needed to test the possibility that restoration of testosterone levels in hypogonadal CKD males may translate into lower prevalence of anemia, better ESA responsiveness and better quality of life.

Although testosterone deficiency, usually accompanied by elevation of serum gonadotropin concentrations, is present in up to 60% of men with chronic kidney disease (CKD) [1, 2], hypogonadism has so far received relatively little attention among nephrologists. It has recently been shown that levels of testosterone decrease as renal function declines and in CKD males, low testosterone levels is associated with inflammation [2], endothelial dysfunction [3], cardiovascular comorbidity and poor outcome [1, 2]. Although the exact reason(s) for a reduction in free testosterone levels in CKD are not fully evident it could be speculated that prolactin retention and subsequent inhibition of gonadotropins contribute [4].

High Prevalence of ESA Resistance in Dialysis Patients

Anemia and hyporesponsiveness to erythropoiesis-stimulating agents (ESA) are commonly observed in CKD patients and are associated with increased morbidity, mortality and a significant health-care economic burden [5]. Many reasons for ESA resistance have been proposed, the most important being blood loss, poor adherence, iron-restricted erythropoiesis and inflammation [6, 7]. In addition to these well-recognized factors, reports in the literature also suggest that some additional factors (or conditions) modify ESA responsiveness, such as hematological diseases and variants of hemoglobin phenotypes, malignancies, secondary hyperparathyroidism with bone marrow fibrosis, high altitude, insulin resistance, statins, renin-angiotensin inhibitors (ACEi) and vitamin D deficiency [8].

Androgens Stimulate Erythropoiesis

The fact that androgens increase erythropoiesis was reported already in the early 1960s [9]. In a representative sample of 905 persons above 65 years without cancer, CKD or anti-androgenic treatment both males and females with low testosterone levels had a higher risk of anemia [10]. In accordance, a recent study of older individuals with anemia of unknown etiology showed that impaired ESA response and lower testosterone levels were significantly more common in the anemic group [11]. As a meta-analysis of 51 studies in the nonrenal population demonstrated that testosterone treatment was associated with a significant mean weight difference in hemoglobin of 8 g/l, the anti-anemic effect of testosterone seems to be of clinical significance [12]. Indeed, a well-known side effect of testosterone therapy in the nonrenal population is polycythemia, and orchiectomy has been reported to cause a decrease in hemoglobin levels of about 12 g/l [13]. Although testosterone treatment and orchiectomy has such a significant effect on hemoglobin levels, the exact mechanisms by which testosterone stimulate erythropoiesis are not evident. It has been suggested that testosterone stimulates erythropoietin production and erythroid progenitor cells [14]. However, one study showed that although testosterone was associated with an increase in hemoglobin, erythropoietin levels did not change [15]. Moreover, a study by Kim et al. [16] reported that the growth-stimulatory effects of androgens on hematopoietic progenitor cells are minimal and mostly restricted to mature erythroid progenitors. The myelostimulating effects of androgens in this study could be attributed, at least in part, to the stimulation of production of hematopoietic growth factors in bone marrow stromal cells. Given the reported minimal effect of testosterone on erythroid precursors recent evidence suggesting that this hormone acts on iron metabolism is intriguing. We observed an association between low testosterone levels and high levels of hypochromic red blood cells [8], an indicator of functional iron deficiency. Moreover, a recent study showed that testosterone influences iron bioavailability by suppression of hepcidin by more than 50% in males and that early changes in hepcidin levels predicted changes in hemoglobin [17]. Elevated levels of hepcidin contribute to the dysregulation of iron homeostasis in CKD and whereas anemia and hypoxia suppress hepcidin production, inflammatory cytokines, such as interleukin-6 stimulate this liver-derived protein [18]. It has been speculated that an agent that lower hepcidin (or inhibit its actions) may be an effective strategy to restore normal iron homeostasis and overcome uremic anemia [19]. Thus, if testosterone proves to suppress hepcidin production also in the inflamed uremic milieu, it may be an effective adjuvant to ESA in the treatment of renal anemia.

Before the introduction of ESA into clinical practice in the late 1980s, some nephrologists used androgens for treatment of renal anemia [20]. Moreover, small studies with androgens have suggested that testosterone can be used as an adjuvant to ESA in the treatment of renal anemia. Gaughan et al. [21] showed in a 6-month, prospective, randomized trial of 19 HD patients that low-dose ESA in combination with androgens increased hematocrit more compared to the group that only received ESA. Moreover, Ballal et al. [22] showed in 15 male HD patients that androgen therapy significantly augments the action of exogenous ESA. In a study of 17 anemic HD patients, Lee et al. [23] showed that adjuvant androgen therapy was effective for the treatment of anemia even in patients continuously treated with low-dose ESA. Finally, the hypothesis that low testosterone is a significant contributor to renal anemia and ESA resistance is indirectly supported by a study that showed that ACEi treatment causes ESA resistance via a reduction of free testosterone levels [24].

Hypogonadism: A Neglected Cause of ESA Resistance?

Based on the well-documented effects of testosterone on erythropoiesis in the general population

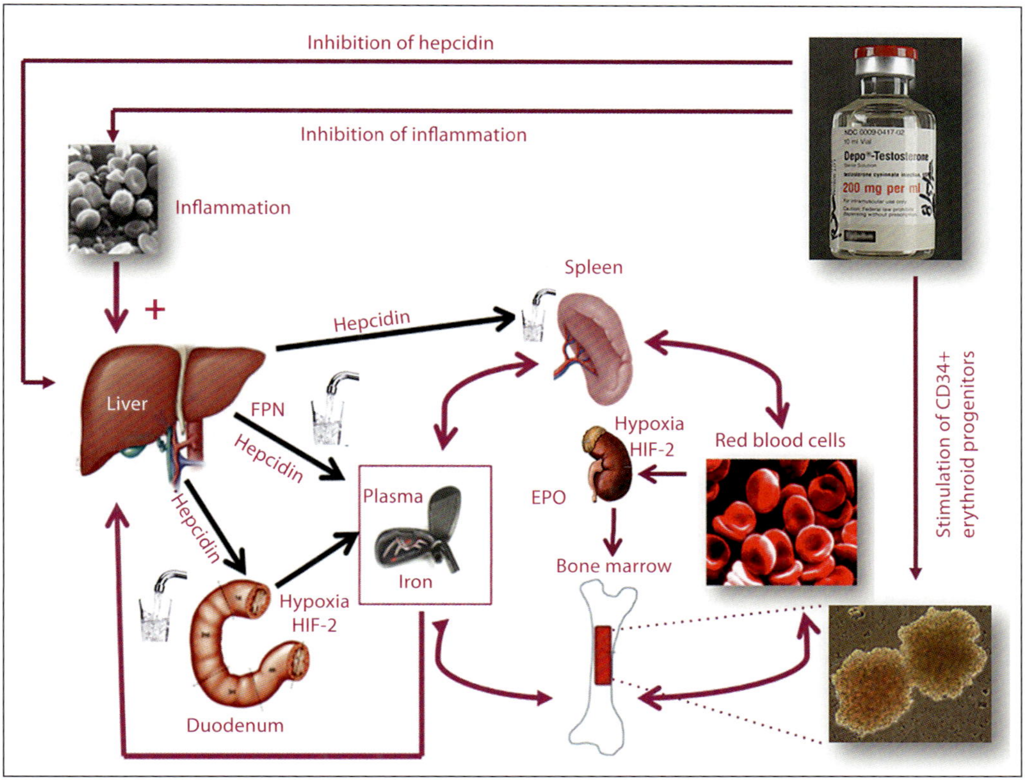

Fig. 1. Overview of suggested testosterone actions on iron metabolism and erythropoiesis. Testosterone stimulates erythroid progenitors in the bone marrow, inhibits hepcidin synthesis in the liver and acts on the immune system reducing the inflammatory response.

and previous small studies indicating that androgens may be used as an adjuvant for treatment of renal anemia, we hypothesized that low testosterone levels are associated with ESA resistance. Testosterone levels were measured in one group of 239 ESA-naïve CKD stage 1–5 male patients from Turkey and a prevalent group of 126 ESA-treated men undergoing HD in Sweden [8]. The study demonstrated that ESA-naïve CKD stage 1–5 patients with testosterone deficiency were five times more likely to be anemic than CKD patients with normal testosterone levels. In addition, as low testosterone levels predicted high ESA doses in male HD patients our data support the hypothesis that hypogonadism promote ESA resistance. The data accord with studies in type 2 diabetes, demonstrating an association between testosterone levels and hemoglobin [25]. Our results raise the question of whether restoration of testosterone levels to the normal range may translate into better ESA responsiveness. The observation that the significant association between testosterone levels and ESA dose in our study was lost when indices of iron status (i.e. iron medication and hypochromic red blood cells) were introduced into the model suggests that reduced iron availability for erythropoiesis contributes. Indeed, it has previously been demonstrated in CKD patients that testosterone supplementation improved iron reutilization [26] and replenished bone marrow iron stores [27]. Based on these reports and the recent finding by Bachman et al. [17] that testosterone supplementation via suppression of hepcidin promotes erythropoiesis, it could be speculated that testosterone supplementation could be a valuable adjuvant to ESA for the treatment of renal anemia (fig. 1). Moreover, as testosterone replacement shifts the cytokine balance to a state of reduced inflammation it could be speculated that this indirectly may lead to less ESA resistance (fig. 1). It should be mentioned that testosterone supplementation in hypogonadal males on dialysis may have several beneficial effects beyond anemia, such as reducing inflammation [28], enhancing mood [29] and cognition [30] as well as promoting better bone strength [31], insulin sensitivity [32], endothelial function [33] and muscle strength [34]; changes that together may translate into better life quality.

Hypogonadism and Vitamin D: Is There a Link?

An intriguing novel mechanism by which testosterone indirectly may affect ESA resistance are recent reports on an association between 25(OH)-D-vitamin and testosterone levels and a concordant pattern of seasonal variations between these two hormones [35]. Although Nimptsch et al. [36] did not observe parallel seasonal variation patterns their study supports the positive association between 25(OH)-D-vitamin and testosterone levels. In a study of 3,369 community-dwelling males, Lee et al. [37] confirmed that hypogonadism was associated with vitamin D deficiency. Finally, Pilz et al. [38] demonstrated that daily vitamin D supplementation (3,332 IU) increased testosterone levels from 10.7 ± 3.9 to 13.4 ± 4.7 nmol/l ($p < 0.001$) in 165 males without renal disease. Thus, further studies are needed to confirm if these associations exist also in males with CKD and to test if vitamin D supplementation can normalize testosterone levels in this patient group.

Conclusion

Hypogonadism may be an additional and among nephrologists neglected (or forgotten) cause of renal anemia and reduced ESA responsiveness. It can be speculated that the beneficial effects of testosterone on erythropoiesis occur through mechanisms that may involve suppression of hepcidin and better iron availability. The hypothesis that correction of hypogonadism improves ESA responsiveness and increase quality of life in male dialysis patients needs to be tested in an interventional trial.

Disclosure Statement

Bayer supports a randomized controlled trial on testosterone undecanoate to be conducted by the authors.

References

1 Carrero JJ, Qureshi AR, Nakashima A, et al: Prevalence and clinical implications of testosterone deficiency in men with end-stage renal disease. Nephrol Dial Transplant 2011;26:184–190.

2 Carrero JJ, Qureshi AR, Parini P, et al: Low serum testosterone increases mortality risk among male dialysis patients. J Am Soc Nephrol 2009;20:613–620.

3 Yilmaz MI, Sonmez A, Qureshi AR, et al: Endogenous testosterone, endothelial dysfunction, and cardiovascular events in men with nondialysis chronic kidney disease. Clin J Am Soc Nephrol 2011;6:1617–1625.

4 Carrero JJ, Kyriazis J, Sonmez A, et al: Prolactin levels, endothelial dysfunction, and the risk of cardiovascular events and mortality in patients with CKD. Clin J Am Soc Nephrol 2012;7:207–215.

5 Solomon SD, Uno H, Lewis EF, et al: Erythropoietic response and outcomes in kidney disease and type 2 diabetes. N Engl J Med 2010;363:1146–1155.

6 Barany P, Divino-Filho JC, Bergström J: High C-reactive protein is a strong predictor of resistance to erythropoietin in hemodialysis patients. Am J Kidney Dis 1997;29:565–568.

7 Elliott J, Mishler D, Agarwal R: Hyporesponsiveness to erythropoietin: causes and management. Adv Chronic Kidney Dis 2010;16:94–100.

8 Carrero JJ, Bárány P, Yilmaz MI, Qureshi AR, Sonmez A, Heimbürger H, et al: Testosterone deficiency is a cause of anemia and reduced responsiveness to erythropoiesis stimulating agents in men with chronic kidney disease. Nephrol Dial Transpl 2012;27:709–715.

9 Thomas K: On a new observation on the hematotrophic effect of testosterone derivatives. Klin Wochenschr 1961;39:55–56.

10 Ferrucci L, Maggio M, Bandinelli S, Basaria S, Lauretani F, Ble A, et al: Low testosterone levels and the risk of anemia in older men and women. Arch Intern Med 2006;166:1380–1388.
11 Waalen J, von Lohneysen K, Lee P, Xu X, Friedman JS: Erythropoietin, GDF15, IL6, hepcidin and testosterone levels in a large cohort of elderly individuals with anaemia of known and unknown cause. Eur J Haematol 2011;87:107–116.
12 Fernandez-Balsells MM, Murad MH, Lane M, et al: Clinical review. 1. Adverse effects of testosterone therapy in adult men: a systematic review and meta-analysis. J Clin Endocrinol Metab 2010;95:2560–2575.
13 Fonseca R, Rajkumar SV, White WL, Tefferi A, Hoagland HC: Anemia after orchiectomy. Am J Hematol 1998;59:230–233.
14 Mirand EA, Gordon AS, Wenig J: Mechanism of testosterone action in erythropoiesis. Nat Genet 1965;206:270–272.
15 Coviello AD, Kaplan B, Lakshman KM, Chen T, Singh AB, Bhasin S: Effects of graded doses of testosterone on erythropoiesis in healthy young and older men. J Clin Endocrinol Metab 2008;93:914–919.
16 Kim SW, Hwang JH, Cheon JM, et al: Direct and indirect effects of androgens on survival of hematopoietic progenitor cells in vitro. J Korean Med Sci 2005;20:409–416.
17 Bachman E, Feng R, Travison T, et al: Testosterone suppresses hepcidin in men: a potential mechanism for testosterone-induced erythrocytosis. J Clin Endocrinol Metab 2010;95:4743–4747.
18 Nemeth E, Rivera S, Gabayan V, et al: IL-6 mediates hypoferremia of inflammation by inducing the synthesis of the iron regulatory hormone hepcidin. J Clin Invest 2004;113:1271–1276.
19 Coyne DW: Hepcidin: clinical utility as a diagnostic tool and therapeutic target. Kidney Int 2011;80:240–244.
20 Richardson JR Jr, Weinstein MB: Erythropoietic response of dialyzed patients to testosterone administration. Ann Intern Med 1970;73:403–407.
21 Gaughan WJ, Liss KA, Dunn SR, et al: A 6-month study of low-dose recombinant human erythropoietin alone and in combination with androgens for the treatment of anemia in chronic hemodialysis patients. Am J Kidney Dis 1997;30:495–500.
22 Ballal SH, Domoto DT, Polack DC, Marciulonis P, Martin KJ: Androgens potentiate the effects of erythropoietin in the treatment of anemia of end-stage renal disease. Am J Kidney Dis 1991;17:29–33.
23 Lee MS, Ahn SH, Song JH: Effects of adjuvant androgen on anemia and nutritional parameters in chronic hemodialysis patients using low-dose recombinant human erythropoietin. Korean J Intern Med 2002;17:167–173.
24 DeLong M, Logan JL, Yong KC, Lien YH: Renin-angiotensin blockade reduces serum free testosterone in middle-aged men on haemodialysis and correlates with erythropoietin resistance. Nephrol Dial Transplant 2005;20:585–590.
25 Grossmann M, Panagiotopolous S, Sharpe K, et al: Low testosterone and anaemia in men with type 2 diabetes. Clin Endocrinol (Oxf) 2009;70:547–553.
26 Haurani FI, Green D: Primary defective iron reutilization. Response to testosterone therapy. Am J Med 1967;42:151–158.
27 Schustack A, Meshiaj D, Waiss Z, Gotloib L: Intramuscular iron replenishment and replacement combined with testosterone enanthate in maintenance hemodialysis anemia: a follow-up of up to 8 years on 16 patients. Clin Nephrol 1985;23:303–306.
28 Kalinchenko SY, Tishova YA, Mskhalaya GJ, Gooren LJ, Giltay EJ, Saad F: Effects of testosterone supplementation on markers of the metabolic syndrome and inflammation in hypogonadal men with the metabolic syndrome: the double-blinded placebo-controlled Moscow study. Clin Endocrinol (Oxf) 2010;73:602–612.
29 Almeida OP, Yeap BB, Hankey GJ, Jamrozik K, Flicker L: Low free testosterone concentration as a potentially treatable cause of depressive symptoms in older men. Arch Gen Psychiatry 2008;65:283–289.
30 Yeap BB, Almeida OP, Hyde Z, Chubb SA, Hankey GJ, Jamrozik K, et al: Higher serum free testosterone is associated with better cognitive function in older men, while total testosterone is not. The Health In Men Study. Clin Endocrinol (Oxf) 2008;68:404–412.
31 Fink HA, Ewing SK, Ensrud KE, Barrett-Connor E, Taylor BC, Cauley JA, et al: Association of testosterone and estradiol deficiency with osteoporosis and rapid bone loss in older men. J Clin Endocrinol Metab 2006;91:3908–3915.
32 Malkin CJ, Jones TH, Channer KS: The effect of testosterone on insulin sensitivity in men with heart failure. Eur J Heart Fail 2007;9:44–50.
33 Malkin CJ, Jones RD, Jones TH, Channer KS: Effect of testosterone on ex vivo vascular reactivity in man. Clin Sci (Lond) 2006;111:265–274.
34 Kenny AM, Kleppinger A, Annis K, Rathier M, Browner B, Judge JO, et al: Effects of transdermal testosterone on bone and muscle in older men with low bioavailable testosterone levels, low bone mass, and physical frailty. J Am Geriatr Soc 2010;58:1134–1143.
35 Wehr E, Pilz S, Boehm BO, Marz W, Obermayer-Pietsch B: Association of vitamin D status with serum androgen levels in men. Clin Endocrinol (Oxf) 2010;73:243–248.
36 Nimptsch K, Platz EA, Willett WC, Giovannucci E: Association between plasma 25-OH vitamin D and testosterone levels in men. Clin Endocrinol (Oxf) 2012 Jan 2. doi: 10.1111/j.1365-2265.2012.04332.x. [Epub ahead of print].
37 Lee DM, Tajar A, Pye SR, et al: Association of hypogonadism with vitamin D status: the European Male Ageing Study. Eur J Endocrinol 2012;166:77–85.
38 Pilz S, Frisch S, Koertke H, et al: Effect of vitamin D supplementation on testosterone levels in men. Horm Metab Res 2011;43:223–225.

Peter Stenvinkel, MD, PhD
Division of Renal Medicine, K56, Karolinska University Hospital at Huddinge
SE–141 86 Stockholm (Sweden)
Tel. +46 8 58582532, E-Mail peter.stenvinkel@ki.se

Ronco C, Rosner MH, Crepaldi C (eds): Peritoneal Dialysis – State-of-the-Art 2012.
Contrib Nephrol. Basel, Karger, 2012, vol 178, pp 40–46

Getting the Right Patient on the Right Renal Replacement Therapy

Miguel Pérez Fontán · Ana Rodríguez-Carmona · Andrés López-Muñiz · Teresa García-Falcón

Division of Nephrology, University Hospital of A Coruña, A Coruña, Spain

Abstract

Adequate selection of the modality of renal replacement therapy (RRT), ideally based on well-planned predialysis care, informed decision by the patient and timely initiation of dialysis, is essential to optimize the outcome of patients with chronic kidney disease. However, there are important practical limitations to the success of this process. A major consequence is the underutilization of home-based dialysis therapies, including peritoneal dialysis (PD). A wide array of medical and social factors have been invoked as contraindications to PD, but well-designed studies have shown that most patients (probably >70%) starting dialysis are suitable for this technique. PD is feasible and may be preferred by a significant proportion of patients in many claimed unfavorable settings. The practicing nephrologist should be able to: disclose which are insurmountable barriers to PD, clarify the significance of relative contraindications in individual cases, and identify favorable and unfavorable settings for home dialysis. These abilities will permit quality education, justified advice, well-targeted informed decision and, predictably, successful selection of the modality of RRT. This article provides some clues to approach these issues in three different settings: planned start of RRT after predialysis care, unplanned start of dialysis and programmed changes of modality during follow-up.

Management of end-stage kidney disease (ESKD) demands systematic approaches to optimize care and limit the economic burden of renal replacement therapies (RRT). An integrative view of the different modalities is essential to ensure that patients may benefit from the best possible therapy during their progress. This itinerary must start before the initiation of dialysis. All individuals with advanced chronic kidney disease (CKD) should undergo structured predialysis care, oriented to delay the progression of CKD, prevent its complications and, importantly, permit education on the characteristics of different techniques of RRT, oriented to select the most appropriate and prepare the patient for its initiation. On the other hand, the right to informed decision should not stop with the start of RRT, because changes in the circumstances of the patient can make convenient a mode of RRT different to the initially chosen.

In the present article, we shall give some clues to help patients target their most convenient modality of RRT in three different scenarios.

Targeting RRT in the Patient Receiving Predialysis Care

This favorable setting permits a fruitful cooperation between the patient, his/her relatives and the attending team to select the most convenient modality of RRT. In some cases, usually associated with a short life expectancy or irreversible loss of the quality of life, the choice will be conservative management. A small proportion of individuals will have access to preemptive kidney transplantation (KT). Finally, in the majority of cases dialysis will be the only possible path. A proportion of patients in this latter group will still be eligible for KT but, even in these, dialysis will be necessary for variable, often prolonged periods of time.

An important issue at the time of planning modality selection is that information and advice should be objective and, whenever possible, based on scientific evidence, but not necessarily neutral. Of course, the educator has the right to manifest his preferable option, but must present orderly clinical and social arguments to support the recommendation. Unfortunately, and despite the abundance of information oriented to facilitate these decisions, many issues remain controversial, due to a paucity of quality evidence.

Many nephrologists still have a perception that a majority of ESKD patients present clinical or social contraindications to home dialysis, including peritoneal dialysis (PD), and that the latter technique is globally inferior to hemodialysis (HD) [1, 2]. However, well-designed studies have shown that more than 70% of patients starting RRT are suitable for PD, as compared with 95% in the case of HD [3–5]. Moreover, PD and HD appear globally equivalent in terms of patient survival. Remarkably, the last years have contemplated a significant improvement in the results reported for PD, driven by technical advances and the maturity gained during the 1990s. Current registry data suggest that the comparability between PD and HD persists now at least until the fifth year of follow-up [6, 7]. Technique survival is still lower in PD although, in this case too, results have improved markedly, and median survival rates of five years or more are now a realistic target. On the other hand, for decades PD has suffered the label of infection-prone technique. The progressive decrease in the incidence of peritoneal infections and the excess use of central venous catheters (CVC) for HD has reversed this situation, and CVC-related bacteremia is currently the main infectious threat to dialysis patients [8]. There is no evidence of a generic superiority of either PD or HD in terms of quality of life [9]. The latter depends more likely on a right modality selection than on the modality itself.

Absolute Contraindications and Indications for PD

There are few unquestionable medical contraindications for PD. These include lack of a suitable peritoneal membrane (extensive surgical resection, peritoneal sclerosis), inability of the abdominal cavity to sustain the mechanics of the process (peritoneal compartmentalization, uncorrectable hernias or pleuroperitoneal leaks) or conditions bringing an unacceptable risk of infection (active inflammatory bowel disease, recurrent diverticulitis). Social contraindications are more frequent in clinical practice. Refusal by the patient to take on self-care is the most common one. This argument is currently challenged in some countries due to financial constraints [10] but, in general, few nephrologists would pressure a patient who overtly rejects self-care dialysis. The combination of an inability for self-care and lack of support by either relatives or the health care system is another insuperable barrier to home dialysis selection. On the other hand, aside from the unusual case of an impossibility to sustain any type of vascular access, there are few unequivocal medical or social indications for PD.

Controversial Contraindications and Indications for PD

Some patients suffer medical conditions which may interfere with the success of PD, but should not be considered generic contraindications to this technique. Adult polycystic kidney disease may compromise PD through complicated catheter insertion, increased prevalence of hernias and diverticulosis or inability to meet adequacy targets, due to the conflict of space created by the enlarged kidneys. However, PD has been used extensively in this condition [11], and should probably be discouraged only in patients who associate giant kidneys with other risk factors for inadequacy (e.g. large patients with absent residual renal function RRF) or mechanical complications (e.g. recurrent hernias).

Morbid obesity is often quoted as a contraindication to PD, due to complicated catheter insertion, increased risks of hernias and infections, and worsening metabolic derangements. Despite these drawbacks, there is no consistent evidence that PD is inferior to HD in these patients [12].

Former claims about the inconvenience of PD to treat ESKD individuals with advanced cirrhosis and ascites were based on the potential risks of peritoneal infection and worsening malnutrition (protein leak). However, this technique also permits a gentle control of volemia and alleviates tense ascites in these patients. Clinical experience supports the use of PD in this setting [13].

Diverticulosis has been claimed to confer an increased risk of enteric peritonitis, but this fear has not been clearly substantiated by clinical experience. Chronic obstructive pulmonary disease, lumbar spine disorders or malnutrition may deserve specific prescription strategies, but do not represent contraindications to PD. Other less-frequent medical conditions which may hamper the use of PD include ostomies, recurrent correctable hernias or dormant inflammatory bowel disease.

There are some relative social contraindications to PD. Patients with a background of noncompliance, limited ability for self-care and poor family support, or unstable home conditions should be carefully evaluated with the help of social workers and psychologists before home dialysis is considered.

Some medical reasons to recommend PD over HD in the predialysis stage include recurrent thrombosis of planned vascular accesses, hypercoagulability syndromes, antecedents of cholesterol embolism or bleeding diatheses. Long distance to the nearest HD center, poor mobility or convenience of a stable home environment (e.g. children) are frequently quoted, relative social indications for PD.

Favorable and Unfavorable Settings for PD

Well-planned predialysis care followed by informed decision is, undoubtedly, the most important factor for selection of PD by patients incident on RRT, as shown by different registry [3, 14–16] and cohort studies [5, 17], and even randomized trials [18]. In general, attempts to predict from demographic data which patients will be inclined to home dialysis have found a limited success. Male sex, pediatric age, low comorbidity, motivated individuals with an interest in an independent lifestyle, active workers, persons with a high educational level, and availability of family support have all been quoted as conditions favoring home PD, while older age, comorbidity and lack of family support are common arguments to prefer in-center HD [3, 5, 14, 19, 20]. PD and home HD patients also present differentiated patterns [20]. Overall, the predictive capacity of these profiles is poor and they cannot substitute individual informed decision.

In patients with ESKD and no apparent contraindication for any modality of RRT, predialysis education should include the proposal of an orderly planned RRT. This integrative approach to RRT [21] has a natural extension in the 'PD-first' strategy [22]. The seminal argument is the time-dependent risk relationship between PD and HD, the former yielding better results during the first years of RRT. In addition, PD is particularly fit for initiation with low-dose schedules (incremental prescription), which optimize quality of life and decrease the economic cost of therapy. Later on, many patients will still do well on PD while, for those announcing complications such as inadequacy or membrane dysfunction, a timely change to HD will permit continuation of quality RRT. There is some evidence that this strategy provides better outcomes than HD-only approaches [21]. On the contrary, late transfer to PD of patients previously treated with HD is feasible, but yields poorer results. The reasons are not totally clear, but better preservation of RRF and greater dependence on it for success in the case of PD are important factors.

Incident patients who are eligible for KT represent a paradigm of the benefits of a well-planned strategy of RRT. Their life expectancy is long and the waiting time for transplantation is variable, and usually unpredictable. After KT, long term graft failure will occur in a significant proportion of cases, meaning reinitiation of dialysis, often indefinitely. The benefits of the PD-first approach will be maximal in this long-term scenery. Importantly, PD will prevent or delay the need for a vascular access, avoiding drawbacks which could persist after KT. Thus, CVC associate an important risk of infection while in place and may injure central veins irreversibly, internal vascular grafts are both a potential source of infection and inflammation, and functioning internal fistulas may carry cardiovascular consequences, including left ventricular hypertrophy. On the other hand, the risk of peritonitis is specific of PD, but there is no evidence that the overall incidence of severe infection after KT is higher in PD than in HD patients. Finally, registry data suggest that PD patients do at least as well, and probably better after KT than HD patients, presenting lower delayed graft function [23] and better patient and graft survival rates [24, 25]. Only primary graft thrombosis appears more frequent in PD than in HD patients. As refers to the latter findings, some of them may be the consequence of selection biases, rather than of specific effects of the modality of dialysis.

Older age associates frequently unfavorable conditions for home PD, including inability for self-care, lack of family support and associated comorbidities which may hamper the success of this technique [3–5, 16, 19]. The combination of older age with diabetes or cardiovascular comorbidity has been claimed to boost an increased risk of mortality on PD, when compared with HD [26]. Even if these limitations are considered, PD may still be underutilized in the elderly. Many of these patients could benefit from this technique, which provides home-based, gentle dialysis to individuals who often display a poor tolerance to HD and in whom maintaining a well-functioning internal vascular access may be a challenge. PD is a good alternative to permanent CVC for HD, particularly in older patients with longer life expectancy [27]. Home or center-based assisted PD facilities have proved efficient to provide PD to older patients who prefer home dialysis but are unable to do self-care [28].

Some registry data have put under question the convenience of PD in subjects with diabetes or cardiovascular disease [6, 26]. The unpredictability of the capacity of ultrafiltration and of the pace of decline of RRF cast doubt on the consistency of PD to guarantee an adequate volume control, which may be critical in these patients. Moreover, the use of glucose as an osmotic agent and the peritoneal protein leak may contribute to an aggravation of metabolic disturbances. These drawbacks downplay the old claimed advantage over HD of continuous, gentle volume control in these cases. However, current PD practice offers instruments to approach these inconveniences, including automated techniques, icodextrin and, in general, glucose-sparing strategies. There is still a concern that some subsets of patients, including those with an antecedent of congestive heart failure, may do not as well in PD as in HD [29]. Interestingly, PD is viewed as a resource for management of patients with severe heart failure and nonterminal CKD [30]. Overall, diabetes and cardiovascular disease should not be considered unfavorable settings for PD, but neither the former view of this technique as a preferable option when these conditions are present is sustained by current data.

Planning RRT in the Patient Who Starts Unplanned

Unplanned start of RRT is an undesirable setting, leading to prolonged hospital admissions, high incidence of early infectious and noninfectious complications and increased mortality rates [15]. Many patients initiating dialysis by this route present unfavorable social and medical characteristics, and a majority have not undergone adequate predialysis care. Most will finally be managed with in-center HD, using CVC for variable, usually prolonged, often indefinite periods of time [31].

The feasibility of PD in patients who start unplanned RRT has been advocated by several studies [32, 33]. At first sight, PD is not attractive in this setting, for several reasons. First, urgent catheter insertion and initiation of PD demand specific resources. Moreover, PD is not efficient for emergency dialysis (hyperkalemia, volume overload, pericarditis, etc.). Thirdly, acute-start PD may associate a high incidence of technical complications, including catheter malfunction and dialysate leaks. Finally, the majority of patients in this situation will prefer in-center HD. However, these arguments should not deter from considering PD for an unplanned start. First, this approach will permit patients to view PD as a realistic alternative. In addition, PD will prevent some risks brought by emergency HD, particularly early infections. Unplanned PD does not carry a significant risk of peritonitis [32, 33], while the incidence of septicemia is markedly lower than in unplanned HD [8]. Even if the patient finally prefers HD, PD may perform as a bridge until maturation of a permanent vascular access. Overall, the PD option should be considered during unplanned initiation of RRT. This approach may be particularly convenient in areas where CVC-related infections represent a major problem.

Anticipating Failure with Planned Technique Transfer

Integral management of ESKD implies that the convenience of any modality of RRT may expire should the personal or medical circumstances of the patient change. The traditional approach was to undertake modality changes only after overt failure of the original technique. The current perception is that a proactive change, before clinical complications appear, may be more beneficial [21]. In practice, the pathway from PD to HD is relatively well established, and planned transfer of patients with impending PD failure (borderline adequacy, ongoing membrane dysfunction) is being increasingly advocated. On the contrary, programmed transfers from HD to PD are less frequent. This may be partly a consequence of the superior technique survival of HD, but many patients who, for different reasons, do not do well on HD are not offered the possibility of changing to PD. Potential indications include exhaustion of vascular accesses, recurrent complications associated to CVC, poor hemodynamic tolerance to HD, recurrent bleeding and changes in the personal conditions of the patient which may benefit from home-based therapies (home HD should be particularly considered in the latter case). PD will do worse as a second-line therapy than as a primary option, but may preferable to continuation of HD under adverse conditions.

Patients who start dialysis after failure of a KT represent a high-risk subgroup, due to frequently delayed reinitiation of dialysis, accumulated immunosuppression, sequelae of complications during primary dialysis and KT and rapid decline of RRF. The latter circumstance could argue against the use of PD in this setting, but the limited information available does not indicate that the modality of RRT has an influence on the outcome of these patients [34]. Remarkably, the incidence of severe infections may be higher in patients re-started on HD, particularly if CVC are used as vascular access [35].

Conclusions

Predialysis care, informed decision by the patient and timely initiation of dialysis are keystones to a successful selection of the modality of RRT

More than 70% of the patients with ESKD are suitable for PD, as compared with (approx.) 95% in the case of HD. Many medical and social factors have been invoked to discourage the selection of PD as a modality of RRT, but this technique can be used successfully in the majority of these settings.

The PD-first approach has a solid theoretic background, and the suitable patient must be made aware of its potential advantages. Patients with a prolonged life expectancy, and particularly those eligible for KT, may benefit most from this strategy.

Older age associates frequently adverse social and medical conditions for home dialysis. Home or center-based assisted PD facilities have a potential to improve the utilization of PD, in this setting.

There is no conclusive evidence that the presence of diabetes or cardiovascular disease settle a specific preference either for PD or HD.

The majority of patients undergoing unplanned start of dialysis are treated with in-center HD, due both to their characteristics and to care protocols oriented to this modality. Use of PD for an unplanned start may help reduce the incidence of CVC-associated infections, and permit a higher utilization of this technique.

Timely changes of the technique of dialysis should be submitted to the consideration of patients, whenever a complicated course under the current modality is predicted. Inadequacy, ongoing membrane dysfunction (PD to HD), recurrent infections or dysfunction of the vascular access and poor hemodynamic tolerance to HD (HD to PD) are potential settings for this approach.

References

1 Johansen KL: Choice of dialysis modality in the United States. Arch Intern Med 2011;171:107–109.
2 Lameire N, van Biesen W: Epidemiology of peritoneal dialysis: a story of believers and nonbelievers. Nat Rev Nephrol 2010;6:75–82.
3 Jager K, Korevaar JC, Dekker FW, Krediet RT, Boeschoten EW: The effect of contraindications and patient preference on dialysis modality selection in ESRD patients in the Netherlands. Am J Kidney Dis 2004;43:891–899.
4 Mendelssohn DC, Mujais SK, Soroka SD, Brouillette J, Takano T, Barre PE, Mittal BV, Singh A, Firanek C, Story K, Finkelstein FO: A prospective evaluation of renal replacement therapy modality elegibility. Nephrol Dial Transplant 2009;24:555–561.
5 Oliver MJ, Garg AX, Blake PG, Johnson JF, Verrelli M, Zacharias JM, Pandeya S, Quinn RR: Impact of contraindications, barriers to self-care and support on incident peritoneal dialysis utilization. Nephrol Dial Transplant 2010;25:2737–2744.
6 Weinhandl ED, Foley RN, Gilbertson DT, Arneson TJ, Snyder JJ, Collins AJ: Propensity-matched mortality comparison of incident hemodialysis and peritoneal dialysis patients. J Am Soc Nephrol 2010;21:499–506.
7 Mehrotra R, Chiu WC, Kalantar-Zadeh K, Bargman J, Vonesh E: Similar outcomes with hemodialysis and peritoneal dialysis in patients with end-stage renal disease. Arch Intern Med 2011;171:110–118.
8 Ishani A, Collins AJ, Herzog CA, Foley RN: Septicemia, access and cardiovascular disease in dialysis patients: the USRDS wave 2 study. Kidney Int 2005;68:311–318.
9 Boateng EA, East L: The impact of dialysis modality on quality of life: a systematic review. J Ren Care 2011;37:190–200
10 Yu AW, Chau KF, Ho YW, Li PK: Development of the 'peritoneal dialysis first' model in Hong Kong. Perit Dial Int 2007;27(suppl 2):S53–S55.
11 Lobbedez T, Touam M, Evans D, Ryckelynck JP, Knebelman B, Verger C: Peritoneal dialysis in polycystic kidney disease patients. Report from the French peritoneal dialysis registry. Nephrol Dial Transplant 2011;26:2332–2339.
12 Abbott KC, Oliver DK, Hurst FP, Das NP, Gao SW, Perkins RM: Body mass index and peritoneal dialysis: 'exceptions to the exception' in reverse epidemiology? Semin Dial 2007;20:561–565.
13 Guest S: Peritoneal dialysis in patients with cirrhosis and ascites. Adv Perit Dial 2010;26:82–87.
14 Kutner NG, Zhang R, Huang Y, Wasse H: Patient awareness and initiation of peritoneal dialysis. Arch Intern Med 2011;171:119–124.
15 Lacson E, Wang W, DeVries C, Leste K, Hakim RM, Lazarus M, Pulliam J: Effects of nationwide predialysis educational program on modality choice, vascular access and patient outcomes. Am J Kidney Dis 2011;58:235–242.
16 van de Luijtgaarden MWM, Noordzij M, Stel VS, Ravani p, Jarraya F, Collart F, Schön S, Leivestad T, Puttinger H, Wanner C, Jager KJ: Effects of comorbid and demographic factors on dialysis modality choice and related patient survival in Europe. Nephrol Dial Transplant 2011;26:2940–2947.
17 Marron B, Ortiz A, Sequera P, Martín-Reyes G, de Arriba G, Lamas JM, Martínez Ocaña JC, Arrieta J, Martinez F: Impact of end-stage renal disease care in planned dialysis start and type of renal replacement therapy – a Spanish multicentre experience. Nephrol Dial Transplant 2006;21(suppl. 2):ii51–ii55.
18 Manns BJ, Taub K, Vanderstraeten C, Jones J, Mills C, Visser M, McLaughlin K: The impact of education on chronic kidney disease patients' plans to initiate dialysis with self-care dialysis: a randomized trial. Kidney Int 2005;68:1777–1783.

19 Chanouzas D, Ng KP, Fallouh B, Baharani J: What influences patient choice of treatment modality at the predialysis stage? Nephrol Dial Transplant 2002;22:184–190.
20 Rioux JP, Bargman JM, Chan CT: Systematic differences among patients initiated on home hemodialysis and peritoneal dialysis: the fallacy of potential competition. Nephrol Dial Transplant 2010;25:2364–2367.
21 van Biesen W, Vanholder RC, Veys N, Dhondt A, Lameire NH: An evaluation of an integrative care approach for end-stage renal disease patients. J Am Soc Nephrol 2000;11:116–125.
22 Chaudhary K, Sangha H, Khanna R: Peritoneal dialysis first: rationale. Clin J Am Soc Nephrol 2011;6:447–456.
23 Bleyer AJ, Burkart JM, Russell GB, Adams PL: Dialysis modality and delayed graft function after cadveric kidney transplantation. J Am Soc Nephrol 1999;10:154–159.
24 Goldfarb-Rumyantzev AS, Hurdle JF, Scandling JD, Baird BC, Cheung AK: The role of pretransplantation renal replacement therapy modality in kidney allograft and recipient survival. Am J Kidney Dis 2005;46:537–549.
25 Molnar MZ, Mehrotra R, Duong U, Bunnapradist S, Lukowsky LR, Krishnan M, Kovesdy CP, Kalantar-Zadeh K: Dialysis modality and outcomes in kidney transplant recipients. Clin J Am Soc Nephrol 2012;7:332–341.
26 Vonesh EF, Snyder JJ, Foley RN, Collins AJ: Mortality studies comparing peritoneal dialysis and hemodialysis: what do they tell us? Kidney Int 2006;suppl 103:S3–S11.
27 Tamura MK, Tan JC, O'Hare AM: Optimizing renal replacement therapy in older adults: a framework for making individualized decisions. Kidney Int 2011;doi: 10.1038/ki.2011.384
28 Brown E: How to address barriers to peritoneal dialysis in the elderly. Perit Dial Int 2011;31(suppl 2):S83–S85.
29 Sens F, Schott-Pethelaz AM, Labeeuw M, Colin C, Villar E: Survival advantage of hemodialysis relative to peritoneal dialysis in patients with end-stage renal disease and congestive heart failure. Kidney Int 2011;80:970–977.
30 Mehrotra R, Kathuria P: Place of peritoneal dialysis in the management of treatment-resistant congestive heart failure. Kidney Int 2006;(suppl 103): S67–S71.
31 Perl J, Wald R, McFarlane P, Bargman JM, Vonesh E, Na Y, Jassal SV, Moist L: Hemodialysis vascular access modifies the association between dialysis modality and survival. J Am Soc Nephrol 2011;22:1113–1121.
32 Povlsen JV, Ivarsen P: How to start the late referred ESRD patient urgently on chronic APD. Nephrol Dial Transplant 2006;21(suppl 2):ii56–ii59.
33 Lobbedez T, Lecouf A, Ficheux M, Henri P, Hurault de Ligny B, Ryckelynck JP: Is rapid initiation of peritoneal dialysis feasible in unplanned dialysis patients? A single-centre experience. Nephrol Dial Transplant 2008;23:3290–3294.
34 Perl J, Hasan O, Bargman JM, Jiang D, Na Y, Gill JS, Jassal SV: Impact of dialysis modality on survival after kidney transplant failure. Clin J Am Soc Nephrol 2011;6:582–590.
35 Johnston O, Zalunardo N, Rose C, Gill JS: Prevention of sepsis during the transition to dialysis may improve the survival of transplant failure patients. J Am Soc Nephrol 2007;18:1331–1337.

Miguel Pérez Fontán, MD
Division of Nephrology, University Hospital of A Coruña
Xubias 84
ES–15006 A Coruña (Spain)
Tel. +34 981 178159, E-Mail Miguel.Perez.Fontan@sergas.es

Ronco C, Rosner MH, Crepaldi C (eds): Peritoneal Dialysis – State-of-the-Art 2012.
Contrib Nephrol. Basel, Karger, 2012, vol 178, pp 47–52

Doubts on the Long-Term Survival of Peritoneal Dialysis Patients Are No Longer a Medical Barrier to Home Dialysis

Norbert Lameire · Wim Van Biesen

University Hospital, Ghent, Belgium

Abstract

Remarkable differences in the utilization of peritoneal dialysis (PD) versus other forms of renal replacement therapy (RRT) exist between different continents, countries and even different regions in a given country. Since many years a number of medical and nonmedical barriers against home dialysis, notably PD have been recognized. One of the reasons for the low utilization of home (peritoneal) dialysis is the incomplete presentation of treatment options to the patient with ESRD. This review updates some recent data on the long-term survival of PD patients in comparison with long-term hemodialysis. Doubts on the long-term survival results on PD are still one of the major medical systematic barriers preventing the expansion of PD for the treatment of ESRD. These recent survival results show that even over a long follow-up time, PD, at least in patients who are starting RRT in a planned way, has the same survival as patients starting on chronic hemodialysis.

As outlined in a previous paper [1], and very recently summarized in a review paper [2], according to a survey amongst nephrologists, the optimal utilization rate for peritoneal dialysis (PD) is around 25–30%, which is much higher than the rate that is currently achieved, revealing a discrepancy between what is considered 'optimal' and what is actually observed in practice. In addition, we pointed out that remarkable differences in the utilization of PD versus other forms of renal replacement therapy (RRT) exist between different continents, countries and even different regions in a given country [1]. An example of strong regional differences in PD utilization in a country is France [3]. In a recent study of the 22 French regions, 2 regions with a high rate of PD utilization (prevalence >15%) and 3 regions with a low rate of PD utilization (prevalence <10%) were selected. A survey among the nephrologists in these regions revealed that opinions on the optimal rate of PD for prevalent and incident dialysis patients were significantly different between 'high-prevalence' and 'low-prevalence' groups. Remarkably, and confirming previous observations [1], there was a significant difference concerning the optimal rate of PD in incident dialysis patients between nephrologists working in public centers (29 ± 15%), those working in nonprofit clinics (27 ± 12%) and nephrologists working in the private sector (14 ± 8%).

In the US, some nephrologists think that >20% of prevalent patients with ESRD should receive PD, whereas only 7% currently do [4,

5]. At this time, over 90% of dialysis patients in the United States are treated with in-center hemodialysis; the overwhelming majority of the remainder are treated with home PD [6]. The utilization of PD in the United States is substantially lower than in other countries in North America (Canada and Mexico), western Europe (namely UK, Netherlands, Sweden, Denmark, Finland, Iceland), and Australia-New Zealand.

It is sometimes suggested that many patients even though they could physically and psychologically be able to dialyze at home do not want to do this.

However, surveys collected data from a great number of dialysis units in ESRD Network 18 between April 1, 2002 and May 31, 2002. A substantial proportion of patients were unaware of their kidney disease (36%) or were not even seeing a nephrologist (36%) until <4 months before first dialysis. The presentation of treatment options was delayed and the majority of ESRD patients were not presented with chronic PD, home hemodialysis, or renal transplantation as options (66, 88 and 74%, respectively). There was no relationship between the medical conditions of the patients and the probability of PD being offered among patients who had been seeing a nephrologist for over a year. Variables significantly associated with selection of chronic PD as dialysis modality were the probability of chronic PD being presented as a treatment option and the time spent on patient education [7]. A more recent report confirms that the large majority of US patients with advanced chronic kidney disease are unaware of the possibility of dialyzing at home [8].

It thus seems that an incomplete presentation of treatment options is an important factor in the underutilization of home dialysis therapies, notably PD. In some Belgian units, patients who progress towards ESRD are offered a structured predialysis education program. A high percentage of patients exposed to this education program start with a self-care modality of renal replacement therapy, such as PD [9]. The question as to why all physicians do not provide such education remains unanswered, although several possible answers exist. One possibility is that physicians themselves may not feel comfortable with PD, as is indicated by the large list of 'potential contraindications' for PD' [10].

In this review, we will update some data on the long-term survival of PD patients in comparison with long-term hemodialysis. Doubts on the long-term survival results on PD are still one of the major medical systematic barriers preventing the expansion of PD for the treatment of ESRD. Some, but not all of the barriers against PD are the same as for home hemodialysis but for reasons of space we will limit this discussion to PD.

There is a large body of data allowing the conclusion that many of the barriers to PD are nonmedical [1, 2]. These barriers lie within the healthcare system, and the local availability of the different dialysis modalities in a given country, very frequently dictated by economic factors such as the reimbursement of the different modalities, other more subtle economic factors, lack of education of both nephrologists and patients, the referral pattern of the patient, and the experience of the treating team with PD. Many of these factors have been discussed in more detail by us [1, 11] and recently by Golper et al. [2] elsewhere. These nonmedical barriers are probably the most important to explain why the PD take-up rate does not reflect patient choice. Whereas it is easy to accept that in many of the countries where its penetration is low, PD is often not offered to the patient, also at the other end of the spectrum in countries where PD is very frequently used, like in Hong Kong, patients are also not free to select their dialysis modality [12, 13]. This 'paradox' makes us agree with Peter Blake who stated that 'it seems reasonable to conclude, therefore, that the asymmetric modality distributions seen in many countries reflect an absence of true patient free choice. PD utilization rates over 40% and under 15% are both suggestive of such a situation [14]'.

One of the possible major medical barriers, still voiced in nephrology centers where PD is low is the perception that long-term results of PD, notably patient survival, are still inferior than on chronic hemodialysis. This perception is based on some studies that have raised concern of a higher long-term risk for death for PD patients [15, 16]. The fact that the results on comparative survival published also in the more recent literature are sometimes contradictory may indeed confuse the practicing nephrologist.

A number of various sources of bias threaten the interpretation of the results of the comparative studies on outcomes between both modalities: all these studies are observational in nature which may explain their seemingly conflicting results. These potential biasses (selection bias, bias by indication) have been discussed in the literature [17, 18]. It should also be realized that large center differences exist, notably with huge differences in PD experience, in propensity to start patients on PD.

Most of the previous studies comparing patient survival between chronic hemodialysis and chronic PD, mostly CAPD, have been summarized up till 2008 in two book chapters [19, 20].

With all the caveats for correct interpretation of the data taking into account, most of these earlier studies showed that at least over the first 1–2 years after initiation of dialysis, there were either no differences or even a better patient survival on PD compared to hemodialysis; these results were very similar in North America and in Europe [19, 20].

There was also compelling clinical/epidemiological evidence that PD showed advantages as the first RRT modality [21–23]. Perl et al. [24] recently hypothesized that some of the differences in early mortality might relate to the methods used in preparing patients for dialysis. Using data from the Canadian Organ Replacement Register (CORR), the survival differences between patients starting PD versus those starting hemodialysis with an arteriovenous (AV) fistula or graft were examined. Comparing unadjusted data, those starting dialysis with a cuffed catheter have a lower survival rate at all time points, and the major increase in 5-year mortality occurs in the first year. When the data were adjusted for age, race, gender, comorbidity, serum albumin, primary diagnosis, and late referral, the patients who started hemodialysis with an AV fistula or graft had better survival at 5 years. Separation of the two groups became clear at 2 years. These results shed some light on the puzzling question of why PD patients appear to have superior survival in the first year of dialysis when compared to all patients starting hemodialysis and they illustrate the point that patients who are prepared well for dialysis – whether PD or hemodialysis – will have better survival than patients who are less well prepared and start hemodialysis with a central venous catheter.

Some recent studies showed less-favorable results with PD compared to HD. A recent prospective analysis by Sens et al. [25] used data from the French Renal Epidemiology and Information Network (REIN) Registry to compare the survival of 4,401 incident dialysis patients with associated congestive heart failure who began PD (21%) and hemodialysis treatment (79%) between 2002 and 2008. Hemodialysis was associated with significantly better survival than PD. In this study, patients with an unplanned first dialysis session and patients who had undergone pre-emptive kidney transplantation were excluded to reduce bias, survival analysis was calculated from the day of the first dialysis session and data on switches in dialysis modality were not included in the primary analysis [25]. These results in fact confirm a previous study from the US, which showed that new patients with ESRD and congestive heart failure experienced worse survival when treated with PD than with hemodialysis [26]. In this study, as in many, if not all, US studies on survival, the start date was defined as day 90 of ESRD [26]. However, it should be stressed that the US study was conducted in the era when icodextrin was not available and the follow-up duration was only 2 years, whereas in the study by Sens et al. [25] >60% patients used icodextrin and the follow-up period was 5 years. Despite these differences, the results of these studies are essentially the same. Sens et al. [25] also performed a secondary analysis using day 90 as the study start date and censored patients who switched dialysis modality but the results were largely unchanged, with a higher risk of mortality in patients receiving PD than in those on HD.

By contrast, some recent observational studies suggest that patient outcomes are in fact similar with hemodialysis or PD [27–29].

In a propensity-matched comparison [29], the overall intention-to-treat mortality risk after initiation of dialysis was 8% lower with PD than with hemodialysis. Further sensitivity analysis of survival starting from day 90 after dialysis initiation showed no overall survival difference between PD and hemodialysis, but among subgroups of patients with cardiovascular disease and diabetes, hemodialysis was associated with improved outcomes. Another analysis based on the US Renal Data System found no significant difference in survival of patients treated with hemodialysis or PD at day 90 of ESRD over a 5-year follow-up period [27].

To exclude bias of differences in patient referrral, Quinn et al. [28] examined the relative risk for mortality for PD compared with hemodialysis among individuals who received at least 4 months of predialysis care and who started dialysis electively as outpatients. From a total of 32,285 individuals, 6,573 patients met the criteria for elective, outpatient initiation. After adjusting for relevant baseline characteristics, no difference in long-term (8 years) survival between PD and hemodialysis was found. In contrast, when definitions of chronic dialysis that have been traditionally used to study the effect of dialysis modality on mortality were used, the relative risk of death on PD compared with HD increased over time, which is consistent with previous studies. This association disappeared when patients who started dialysis therapy urgently were excluded, suggesting that the apparent increase in the relative risk of death over time on PD compared with HD is due to bias rather than a specific effect of dialysis modality. These findings do not support a strategy of electively switching patients to HD, as was suggested in previous studies recommending that PD should be the first dialysis modality to start in an 'integrated care' approach [15, 30, 31]. The results of Quinn et al. [28] strongly suggest thus that selection bias, rather than an effect of the treatment itself, likely explains the previously described change in the relative risk of death over time between hemodialysis and PD.

A growing group of patients that in the future will need renal replacement therapy are the elderly. As pointed out by Edwina Brown recently [32, 33], the number of 'old elderly' patients in need of dialysis is increasing. In the USA, the number of octogenarians and nonagenarians starting dialysis increased from 7,054 persons in 1996 to 13,577 persons in 2003; after allowing for population growth, this represents a 57% increase in the rate of dialysis starts in this age group [34]. In France in 2005, almost 40% of patients starting dialysis were over the age of 75 years [35]. Thus, the elderly are the largest and fastest growing patient group on dialysis. In France, where assisted PD using community nurses has been available for many years, PD is predominantly a treatment of the elderly, with 54% of men and 59% of women on PD in January 2006 being over 70 years of age [36]. The elderly are also successfully dialyzed on PD in Hong Kong, which has a PD-first policy: in March 2007, 80% of patients with a median age of 62.3 years were on PD [12]. These results suggest that the opinion that home dialysis, notably PD, is more difficult to realize in the elderly is wrong. In France, assisted PD using a nondisconnect CAPD with UV Flash (Baxter SAS, Maurepas, France) is the predominant method used, and is often the modality of choice for older patients [37] while in other countries automated PD (APD) is used as the PD modality for assisted patients. It was recently shown that assisted PD was associated with a lower risk for technique failure, i.e. lower risk for transfer to hemodialysis compared with patients undergoing self-care PD [38].

Health-related quality of life (QOL) is another important outcome for older people who are often on dialysis for life. A recent cross-sectional, multicentered study conducted QOL assessments in 140 people (aged 65 years or older) on PD and HD. Although this is obviously not a randomized trial it was found that overall, in two closely matched demographic groups of older dialysis patients, QOL was similar, if not better, in those on PD [39].

In conclusion, this short survey of the recent literature focusses on one of the most widely used medical barriers to PD as home dialysis treatment, i.e. patient survival. Most recent survival results show that even over a long follow-up time, PD at least in patients who are starting RRT in a planned way, has the same survival as patients starting on chronic hemodialysis. These recent results even more strongly emphasize the necessity of a careful follow up of CKD patients in order to prepare a timely start of RRT. PD can be a very successful home dialysis form and nephrologists should be further encouraged to promote it to their patients.

References

1 Lameire N, Van Biesen BW: Epidemiology of peritoneal dialysis: a story of believers and nonbelievers. Nat Rev Nephrol 2010;6:75–82.

2 Golper TA, Saxena AB, Piraino B, Teitelbaum I, Burkart J, Finkelstein FO, Abu-Alfa A: Systematic barriers to the effective delivery of home dialysis in the United States: a report from the Public Policy/Advocacy Committee of the North American Chapter of the International Society for Peritoneal Dialysis. Am J Kidney Dis 2011;58:879–885.

3 Bouvier N, Durand PY, Testa A, Albert C, Planquois V, Ryckelynck JP, Lobbedez T: Regional discrepancies in peritoneal dialysis utilization in France: the role of the nephrologist's opinion about peritoneal dialysis. Nephrol Dial Transplant 2009;24:1293–1297.

4 Mehrotra R, Boeschoten E: Current status of peritoneal dialysis; in Khanna R, Krediet R (eds): Nolph and Gokal's Textbook of Peritoneal Dialysis. Berlin, Springer, 2009, pp 19–37.

5 Mendelssohn DC, Mullaney SR, Jung B, Blake PG, Mehta RL: What do American nephologists think about dialysis modality selection? Am J Kidney Dis 2001;37:22–29.

6 Collins AJ, Foley RN, Chavers B, et al: United States Renal Data System 2011 Annual Data Report: Atlas of chronic kidney disease and end-stage renal disease in the United States. Am J Kidney Dis 2012;59:A7, e1-A7,420.

7 Mehrotra R, Marsh D, Vonesh E, Peters V, Nissenson A: Patient education and access of ESRD patients to renal replacement therapies beyond in-center hemodialysis. Kidney Int 2005;68:378–390.

8 Finkelstein FO, Story K, Firanek C, Barre P, Takano T, Soroka S, Mujais S, Rodd K, Mendelssohn D: Perceived knowledge among patients cared for by nephrologists about chronic kidney disease and end-stage renal disease therapies. Kidney Int 2008;74:1178–1184.

9 Goovaerts T, Jadoul M, Goffin E: Influence of a pre-dialysis education programme (PDEP) on the mode of renal replacement therapy. Nephrol Dial Transplant 2005;20:1842–1847.

10 Jassal SV, Krishna G, Mallick NP, Mendelssohn DC: Attitudes of British Isles nephrologists towards dialysis modality selection: a questionnaire study. Nephrol Dial Transplant 2002;17:474–477.

11 Van Biesen W: Peritoneal dialysis: how we can achieve improvement of PD penetration. Prilozi 2007;28:267–274.

12 Li PK, Szeto CC: Success of the peritoneal dialysis programme in Hong Kong. Nephrol Dial Transplant 2008;23:1475–1478.

13 Van Biesen W, Veys N, Lameire N, Vanholder R: Why less success of the peritoneal dialysis programmes in Europe? Nephrol Dial Transplant 2008;23:1478–1481.

14 Blake PG: Free modality choice: aspiration or illusion? Introduction. Perit Dial Int 2009;29:133–134.

15 Jaar BG, Coresh J, Plantinga LC, Fink NE, Klag MJ, Levey AS, Levin NW, Sadler JH, Kliger A, Powe NR: Comparing the risk for death with peritoneal dialysis and hemodialysis in a national cohort of patients with chronic kidney disease. Ann Intern Med 2005;143:174–183.

16 Termorshuizen F, Korevaar JC, Dekker FW, van Manen JG, Boeschoten EW, Krediet RT: Hemodialysis and peritoneal dialysis: comparison of adjusted mortality rates according to the duration of dialysis: analysis of The Netherlands Cooperative Study on the Adequacy of Dialysis 2. J Am Soc Nephrol 2003;14:2851–2860.

17 Lameire N, Van Biesen W: What can we learn from registry data on peritoneal dialysis outcomes? Contrib Nephrol. Basel, Karger, 2009, vol 163, pp 227–236.

18 Van Biesen W, Vanholder R, Debacquer D, De Backer G, Lameire N: Comparison of survival on CAPD and haemodialysis: statistical pitfalls. Nephrol Dial Transplant 2000;15:307–311.

19 Krediet RT: When to start dialysis and whether the first treatment should be extracorporeal therapy or peritoneal dialysis; in Molony D, Craig J (eds): Evidence-Based Nephrology. Chichester, Wiley-Blackwell, 2009, pp 403–409.

20 Lameire NH, Vanholder R, Van Biesen W: Selection of peritoneal dialysis as renal replacement therapy; in Molony D, Craig J (eds): Evidence-Based Nephrology. Chichester, Wiley-Blackwell, 2009, pp 471–477.

21 Lameire N, Van Biesen W, Vanholder R: The role of peritoneal dialysis as first modality in an integrative approach to patients with end-stage renal disease. Perit Dial Int 2000;20(suppl 2):S134–S141.

22 Van Biesen W, Vanholder RC, Veys N, Dhondt A, Lameire NH: An evaluation of an integrative care approach for end-stage renal disease patients. J Am Soc Nephrol 2000;11:116–125.

23 Van Biesen W, Davies S, Lameire N: An integrated approach to end-stage renal disease. Nephrol Dial Transplant 2001;16(suppl 6):7–9.
24 Perl J, Wald R, McFarlane P, Bargman JM, Vonesh E, Na Y, Jassal SV, Moist L: Hemodialysis vascular access modifies the association between dialysis modality and survival. J Am Soc Nephrol 2011;22:1113–1121.
25 Sens F, Schott-Pethelaz AM, Labeeuw M, Colin C, Villar E: Survival advantage of hemodialysis relative to peritoneal dialysis in patients with end-stage renal disease and congestive heart failure. Kidney Int 2011;80:970–977.
26 Stack AG, Molony DA, Rahman NS, Dosekun A, Murthy B: Impact of dialysis modality on survival of new ESRD patients with congestive heart failure in the United States. Kidney Int 2003;64:1071–1079.
27 Mehrotra R, Chiu YW, Kalantar-Zadeh K, Bargman J, Vonesh E: Similar outcomes with hemodialysis and peritoneal dialysis in patients with end-stage renal disease. Arch Intern Med 2011;171:110–118.
28 Quinn RR, Hux JE, Oliver MJ, Austin PC, Tonelli M, Laupacis A: Selection bias explains apparent differential mortality between dialysis modalities. J Am Soc Nephrol 2011;22:1534–1542.
29 Weinhandl ED, Foley RN, Gilbertson DT, Arneson TJ, Snyder JJ, Collins AJ: Propensity-matched mortality comparison of incident hemodialysis and peritoneal dialysis patients. J Am Soc Nephrol 2010;21:499–506.
30 Heaf JG, Lokkegaard H, Madsen M: Initial survival advantage of peritoneal dialysis relative to haemodialysis. Nephrol Dial Transplant 2002;17:112–117.
31 Van Biesen W, Vanholder RC, Veys N, Dhondt A, Lameire NH: An evaluation of an integrative care approach for end-stage renal disease patients. J Am Soc Nephrol 2000;11:116–125.
32 Brown EA: How to address barriers to peritoneal dialysis in the elderly. Perit Dial Int 2011;31 Suppl 2:S83–S85.
33 Brown EA, Johansson L: Epidemiology and management of end-stage renal disease in the elderly. Nat Rev Nephrol 2011;7:591–598.
34 Kurella M, Covinsky KE, Collins AJ, Chertow GM: Octogenarians and nonagenarians starting dialysis in the United States. Ann Intern Med 2007;146:177–183.
35 Couchoud C, Moranne O, Frimat L, Labeeuw M, Allot V, Stengel B: Associations between comorbidities, treatment choice and outcome in the elderly with end-stage renal disease. Nephrol Dial Transplant 2007;22:3246–3254.
36 Verger C, Ryckelynck JP, Duman M, Veniez G, Lobbedez T, Boulanger E, Moranne O: French peritoneal dialysis registry (RDPLF): outline and main results. Kidney Int Suppl 2006;S12–S20.
37 Lobbedez T, Moldovan R, Lecame M, de Ligny BH, El HW, Ryckelynck JP: Assisted peritoneal dialysis. Experience in a French renal department. Perit Dial Int 2006;26:671–676.
38 Lobbedez T, Verger C, Ryckelynck JP, Fabre E, Evans D: Is assisted peritoneal dialysis associated with technique survival when competing events are considered? Clin J Am Soc Nephrol 2012 Feb 16. [Epub ahead of print].
39 Brown EA, Johansson L, Farrington K, Gallagher H, Sensky T, Gordon F, Da Silva-Gane M, Beckett N, Hickson M: Broadening Options for Long-term Dialysis in the Elderly (BOLDE): differences in quality of life on peritoneal dialysis compared to haemodialysis for older patients. Nephrol Dial Transplant 2010;25:3755–3763.

Dr. Norbert Lameire
University Hospital
185, De Pintelaan
BE–9000 Ghent (Belgium)
E-Mail Norbert.Lameire@ugent.be

Ronco C, Rosner MH, Crepaldi C (eds): Peritoneal Dialysis – State-of-the-Art 2012.
Contrib Nephrol. Basel, Karger, 2012, vol 178, pp 53–57

How to Avoid Technique Failure in Peritoneal Dialysis Patients?

Thierry Lobbedez · Lucie Boissinot · Maxence Ficheux · Cindy Castrale · J.-P. Ryckelynck

Department of Nephrology, Dialysis and Renal Transplantation, University Hospital Center, Caen, France

Abstract

It is well established that technique failure is one of the main reasons for peritoneal dialysis cessation. Early PD failures occur during the first 6 months of PD and are mainly related to catheter dysfunction and psychosocial problems. Catheter malfunction should be treated by a video-laparoscopic procedure as this prolongs the catheter survival. Assisted peritoneal dialysis could help patients to cope with peritoneal dialysis. Preservation of residual renal function is of importance in peritoneal dialysis patients as it affects both patients and technique survival. Failure to obtain a sufficient ultrafiltration volume to maintain a euvolemic state without using large amount of hypertonic glucose solution can cause peritoneal dialysis failure. New approaches in the use of icodextrin to increase ultrafiltration and sodium removal are under investigation. A novel modality of prescribing automated peritoneal dialysis would improve ultrafiltration in peritoneal dialysis patients.

Although several reports have underlined the fact that peritoneal dialysis (PD) can be used for a long-term run, technique survival remains a main concern for nephrologists in charge of PD patients. In a report from the NECOSAD study group, the 2-year technique survival in Netherlands PD patients who started renal replacement therapy on peritoneal dialysis was 64% [1]. Data from the Australian and New Zealand registry (ANZDATA) showed that death-censored median technique survival was 3.7 years in incident PD patients [2]. In France, the median time on peritoneal dialysis of the patients transferred to hemodialysis in 2009 was 19 months [3]. Nephrologists in charge of end stage renal disease patients consider technique failure to be a barrier against PD utilization [4]. It has been demonstrated that center size is associated with technique failure [5]. PD patients treated in centers with greater number of PD patients have a lower risk of technique failure which could reflect the center experience and/or ability of these centers to select patients for PD. Lack of experience and training may affect technique survival. In support of this it has been shown that in the United States, the number of PD patients available for training fellows in teaching hospital is too small to allow training in peritoneal dialysis [6].

It is commonly admitted that early PD failure occurs during the first 6 months of PD. In a study from Switzerland, early failure accounted for 40% of technique failure [7]. In this report, catheter dysfunction and psychosocial problems were more often responsible for early than late failure. These findings are consistent with the results of a study from the Netherland regarding technique failure according to duration of treatment [8]. In contrast, late failures of PD are mainly related to peritonitis, ultrafiltration failure, malnutrition, and dialysis adequacy. In an attempt to avoid PD failure one should focus on the reasons for transfer to HD and on the option of preventing the causes of PD cessation [9].

Catheter Dysfunction

Clinical practice guidelines for peritoneal dialysis access are available and should be implemented to reduce the rate of catheter misplacement and early drainage failure [10]. However, peritoneal catheter malfunction may occur several months after PD initiation and can jeopardize technique survival. There is no clear explanation regarding the high rate of early PD failure due to catheter malfunction. Indeed, catheter malfunction results from occlusion by fibrin clot, tip migration, omental wrapping, or adhesions. Theoretically, these complications can be successfully managed with enema, catheter flushing, urokinase administration and fluoroscopic manipulation of the PD catheter. Failure to restore catheter function by conservative treatment can be countered by surgical replacement of the PD catheter. One may hypothesize that patients (and/or nephrologists) might be reluctant to replace the PD catheter by a surgical procedure and so that take the option of using HD instead of continuing PD when catheter replacement is necessary. Like others, we believe that, whenever possible, catheter malfunction should be treated by a video-laparoscopic procedure as this prolongs the catheter survival by treating the cause of the malfunction directly [11]. In addition, video-laparoscopy avoids catheter replacement. Furthermore, video-laparoscopy is associated with a reduced hospital stay and diminished postoperative pain compared with a surgical procedure. However, a laparoscopic procedure requires general anesthesia and patients may present side effects resulting from the pneumoperitoneum. Video-laparoscopy can be performed to visualize the abdominal cavity, to restore the catheter patency and for PD catheter repositioning, whilst at the same time allowing adhesiolysis during the procedure. Catheter fixation to the recto-vesical or recto-uterine pouch can be performed under direct vision during the laparoscopic procedure to prevent catheter tip migration Moreover, in one recent study it has been shown that systematic catheter fixation prevent catheter dislocation [12]. Prophylactic omentopexy or omentectomy can prevent omental wrapping. However, omentopexy alters the intra-abdominal anatomy and has the potential risk of internal small bowel herniation, omentectomy is a complicated procedure. It has been reported recently that omental folding can be performed during a laparoscopic procedure in case of catheter malfunction due to omental wrapping [13]. Catheter placement under a laparoscopic procedure is associated with a lower incidence of catheter migration and a higher cost but not with a longer technique survival compared with open surgery [11]. Therefore, systematic laparoscopy-assisted catheter placement is not recommended [14]. A randomized control study aiming to compare laparoscopic placement of the PD catheter with open surgery insertion is currently in progress [15].

Psychosocial Problems

Patient age and comorbidity are associated with PD failure. Older age and comorbidities are considered as contraindications for PD when assisted PD is not available. Chronic patient burnout, fatigue and loss of functional capacity may contribute to PD failure. Therefore, assisted PD could decrease the risk of transfer to hemodialysis. It has been suggested recently that providing social support on site decrease the incidence of technique failure [9]. Assisted PD is defined as a PD modality performed at the patients' home with the assistance of a health-care technician, a community nurse, a family member or a partner.

Assisted PD with community nurse assistance is fully covered by the national health care insurance in France. In addition, home visits by nurses from the dialysis center are funded by community or academic hospitals. Verger et al. [16] have reported that home visits were associated with a lower risk of peritonitis in assisted PD patients. Using the data of the French Language Peritoneal Dialysis Registry (RDPLF), we examined the association of assisted PD with all the possible outcomes on PD using methods developed for survival analysis in the presence of competing risks [17]. We found that compared with self-care peritoneal dialysis patients, assisted peritoneal dialysis patients had a lower risk of transfer to hemodialysis but a higher risk of death and a lower risk of transplantation. In view of the increasing age of the dialysis population, we believe that the funding of assisted PD should be evaluated and compared with the cost of in-center HD by the health care providers.

Dialysis Adequacy

Even though dialysis adequacy is one of the main causes of late technique failure there is no clear definition of the so-called 'inadequate dialysis'. Small solute clearance is commonly used to define dialysis adequacy. However, it is obvious that the kidney has many other functions than small solute removal. The ADEMEX study did not find any significant difference in term of survival between two groups receiving a different dialysis dose defined by small solutes removal. Nevertheless, in anuric patients, a negative effect of Kt/V on survival is apparent below 1.7. The EAPOS study has shown that peritoneal dialysis is feasible in anuric PD patients. However, it is admitted that residual renal function is the most important contributor to dialysis adequacy in PD patients. It can be hypothesized that renal function removes uremic toxins which are not, or are insufficiently, removed by peritoneal dialysis. Thus, preservation of residual renal function is of importance in peritoneal dialysis patients as it affects both patients and technique survival. Indeed, it has been shown that both residual renal function at dialysis start and decline in residual renal function under therapy are associated with patient drop out [18]. Two randomized control studies have shown that ACE inhibitor or ARB could preserve residual renal function in PD patients [19, 20]. Biocompatible dialysis fluid may also have an effect on the renal clearance. In the DIUREST study the decline of residual renal function was lower in the group of patients receiving biocompatible solution compared with conventional fluid [21]. In the Euro-Balance-Trial, it is suggested that lactate-buffered, low GDP fluid PD solution is associated with an improvement of residual renal function [22]. Free radicals may also influence residual renal function, and further studies are needed to evaluate whether if reducing oxidative stress in PD patients could improve renal function [23]. There are conflicting data regarding the effect of PD modality on residual renal function. However, one recent large scale study from the NECOSAD group shows that automated peritoneal dialysis is associated with a higher risk of losing residual renal function in the first year of dialysis [24]. Nephrotoxic drugs and radiocontrast agent must be avoided whenever possible as they are associated with acute renal dysfunction in PD patients [25]. One must also pay attention to dehydration in PD patients as it may cause acute kidney damage.

Ultrafiltration Failure

It is well established that ultrafiltration and sodium extraction are both associated with patient survival on peritoneal dialysis. Recommendations regarding targets for fluid removal have been proposed by the International Society of Peritoneal Dialysis. Failure to obtain a sufficient ultrafiltration volume to maintain a euvolemic state without using large amount of hypertonic glucose solution can cause peritoneal dialysis failure. High peritoneal permeability is no longer associated with technique failure in patients treated by automated peritoneal dialysis or by CAPD with icodextrin [26]. This finding could be explained by better fluid management in high transporter patients treated with APD. Icodextrin increases ultrafiltration volume compared with dextrose solution in both APD and CAPD patients. It had been suggested that icodextrin would increase technique survival in PD patients. Icodextrin is now widely used in peritoneal dialysis patients. Nowadays, new approaches in the use of icodextrin are under investigation. Performing two exchanges with icodextrin is associated with a reduction in glucose exposure in patients on APD [27]. In CAPD patients with ultrafiltration failure icodextrin administered twice daily improves blood pressure control and decreases left ventricular mass compared with icodextrin once a day [28]. In a prospective randomized control study Freida et al. [29] show that in high peritoneal permeability patients, a mixed colloid and crystalloid PD fluid increases ultrafiltration and sodium removal compared with icodextrin. These promising new strategies to use icodextrin need further investigation. Adapted APD, a novel modality of prescribing APD, results in a greater ultrafiltration volume compared with the standard APD prescription [30] The so-called adapted APD is based on a combination of short dwell time with low fill volume to promote ultrafiltration and longer dwell time with larger fill volume to promote uremic toxin removal.

Promoting a Real Transition

The term 'transition' has been used recently to refer to the movement between peritoneal dialysis and hemodialysis. Nevertheless, sudden peritoneal dialysis failure may jeopardize the gradual move to hemodialysis and affect patient outcome. In an attempt to prevent unplanned hemodialysis initiation, patients who are likely to fail peritoneal dialysis should be prepared for hemodialysis. The current concept of 'failure' of peritoneal dialysis leading to transfer to HD could become obsolete, to be replaced by the idea of a smooth transition from one dialysis modality to another as a normal stage in the trajectory of end-stage renal disease patients.

References

1 Jager KJ, Merkus MP, Dekker FW, et al: Mortality and technique failure in patients starting chronic peritoneal dialysis: results of the Netherlands Cooperative Study on the Adequacy of Dialysis. Kidney Int 1999;55:1476–1485.
2 ANZDATA Registry 2008 report chapter 6: Peritonal dialysis. Available at www.anzdata.org.
3 Available at http://www.rdplf.org/sorties/70-sortie-2009.html.
4 Troidle L, Kliger A, Finkelstein F: Barriers to utilization of chronic peritoneal dialysis in network # 1, New England. Perit Dial Int 2006;26:452–457.
5 Huisman RM, Nieuwenhuizen MGM, Th De Charro F: Patient-related and centre-related factors influencing technique survival of peritoneal dialysis in The Netherlands. Nephrol Dial Transplant 2002;17:1655–1660.
6 Mehrotra R, Blake P, Berman N, Nolph KD: An analysis of dialysis training in the United States and Canada. Am J Kidney Dis 2002;40:152–160.
7 Descoeudres B, Koller MT, Garzoni D, et al: Contribution of early failure to outcome on peritoneal dialysis. Perit Dial Int 2008;28:259–267.
8 Kolesnyk I, Dekker FW, Boeschoten EW, et al: Time-dependent reasons for peritoneal dialysis technique failure and mortality. Perit Dial Int 2010;30:170–177.
9 Chaudhary K, Sangha H, Khanna R: Peritoneal dialysis first: rationale. Clin J Am Soc Nephrol 2011;6:447–456.
10 Figueiredo A, Go BL, Jenkins S, Johnson DW, Mactier R, Ramalakshmi S, Shrestha B, Struijk D, Wilkie M: Clinical practice guidelines for peritoneal access. Perit Dial Int 2010;30:424–429.
11 Santarelli S, Zeiler M, Marinelli R, Monteburini T, Federico A, Ceraudo E: Videolaparoscopy as a rescue therapy and placement of peritoneal dialysis catheters: a thirty two cases single centre experience. Nephrol Dial Transplant 2006;21:1348–1354.
12 Kume H, Miyazaki H, Nagata M, Ishikawa A, Ishibashi Y, Jujita T, Homma Y: Peritoneal fixation prevents dislocation of Tenckoff catheter. Perit Dial Int 2011;31:694–697.
13 Goh YH: Omental folding: a novel laparoscopic technique for salvaging peritoneal dialysis catheters. Perit Dial Int 2008;28:626–631.
14 Jwo SC, Chen KS, Lee CC, Chen HY: Prospective randomized study of open surgery with laparoscopic assisted placement of Tenckoff peritoneal dialysis catheter. A single center experience and literature review. J Surg Res 2010;1:489–496.

15 Hagen SM, van Alphen AM, Ijzermans JN, Dor FJ: Laparoscopic versus open peritoneal dialysis catheter insertion, the LOCI-trial: a study protocol. BMC Surg 2011;20:11–35.
16 Verger C, Duman M, Durand PY, Veniez G, Fabre E, Ryckelynck JP: Influence of autonomy and type of assistance on the prevention of peritonitis in assisted automated peritoneal dialysis patients. An analysis of data from the French Language Peritoneal Dialysis Registry. Nephrol Dial Transplant 2007;22:1218–1223.
17 Lobbedez T, Verger C, Ryckelynck J-P, Evans D: Is assisted PD associated with technique survival when competings risks are considered? Clin J Am Soc Nephrol, in press.
18 Misra M, Vonesh E, Churchill DN, Moore HL, Van stone JC, Nolph KD: Preservation of glomerular filtration rate on dialysis when adjusted for patient drop out. Kidney Int 2000;57:691–696.
19 Li PK, Chow KM, Wong TY, Leung CB, Szeto CC: Effects of an angiotensin-converting enzyme inhibitor on residual renal function in patients receiving peritoneal dialysis. A randomized, controlled study. Ann Intern Med 2003;139:105–112.
20 Suzuki H, Kanno Y, Sugahara S, Okada H, Nakamoto H: Effects of an angiotensin II receptor blocker, valsartan, on residual renal function in patients on CAPD. Am J Kidney Dis 2004;43:1056–1064.
21 Haag-Weber M, Krämer R, Haake R, Islam MS, Prischl F, Haug U, Nabut JL, Deppisch R: Low GDP fluid attenuates decline of residual renal function in PD patients: a prospective randomized study. Nephrol Dial Transplant 2010;25:2288–2296.
22 Williams JD, Topley N, Craig KJ, Mackenzie RK, Pischetsrieder M, Lage C, Passlick-Deetjen J: The Euro-Balance Trial: the effect of a new biocompatible peritoneal dialysis fluid (balance) on the peritoneal membrane. Kidney Int 2004;66:408–418.
23 Morinaga H, Sugiyama H, Inoue T, Takiue K, Kikumoto Y, Kitagawa M, Akagi S, Nakao K, Maeshima Y, Miyazaki I, Asanuma M, Hiramatsu M, Makino H: Effluent free radicals are associated with residual renal function and predict technique failure in peritoneal dialysis patients. Perit Dial Int 2012 Jan 3. [Epub ahead of print].
24 Michel WM, Verdujin M, Groostendorst DC, le Cessie S, Boschoten EW, Dekker FW, Krediet RT: Decline in residual renal function in automated compared with continuous ambulatory peritoneal dialysis. Clin J Am Soc Nephrol 2011;6:537–542.
25 Herget-Rosenthal S, von Ostrowski M, Kribben A: Definition and risk factors of rapidly declining residual renal function in peritoneal dialysis: an observational study. Kidney Blood Press Res 2012;3:233–241.
26 Yang X, Fang W, Bargman JM, Oreopoulos DG: High peritoneal permeability is not associated with higher mortality or technique failure in patients on automated peritoneal dialysis. Perit Dial Int 2008;28:82–92.
27 Gobin J, Fernando S, Santacroce S, Finkelstein FO: The utility of two daytime icodextrin exchanges to reduce dextrose exposure in automated peritoneal dialysis patients: a pilot study of nine patients. Blood Purif 2008;26:279–283.
28 Sav T, Oymak O, Inanc M, Dogan A, Tokgoz B, Utas C: Effects of twice daily icodextrin administration on blood pressure and left ventricular mass in patients on continuous ambulatory peritoneal dialysis. Perit Dial Int 2009;29:443–449.
29 Freida P, Issad B, Dratwa M, Lobbedez T, Wu L, Leypoldt JK, Divino-Filho J: A combined crystalloid and colloid PD solution as a glucose sparing strategy for volume control in high transport APD patients: a prospective multicentre study. Perit Dial Int 2009;29:433–442.
30 Fischbach M, Issad B, Dubois V, Taamma R: The beneficial influence on the effectiveness of automated peritoneal dialysis of varying the dwell time (short/long) and fill volume (small/large): a randomized controlled trial. Perit Dial Int 2011;31:450–458.

Prof. J.-P. Ryckelynck
Nephrology, Dialyse and Transplantation, CHU Clemenceau
Avenue G. Clemenceau
FR–14033 Caen Cedex (France)
E-Mail ryckelynck-jp@chu-caen.fr

Ronco C, Rosner MH, Crepaldi C (eds): Peritoneal Dialysis – State-of-the-Art 2012.
Contrib Nephrol. Basel, Karger, 2012, vol 178, pp 58–67

Clinical Practice Guidelines: An Important Tool in Improving Dialysis Quality

Norbert Lameire · Wim Van Biesen

University Hospital, Ghent, Belgium

Abstract

Clinical practice guidelines (CPGs) are 'systematically developed statements to assist practitioner and patient decisions about appropriate health care for specific clinical circumstances'. Ideally they should provide a summary of the clinical evidence about a topic, based on relevant systematic reviews, well-performed meta-analyses or individual sufficiently powered randomized trials. CPGs can help physicians and their patients to incorporate the best evidence into their individual practice but also inform further research in the field by identifying flaws and trends in the literature. Guidelines complement but should not replace clinical judgment and are not intended to define a standard of care and should thus not be used as outcome performance measures. It should, however, be recognized that in nephrology and in dialysis most of the guidelines are based on weak evidence and are mostly expert or 'consensus' based. However, there is, albeit largely indirect, evidence that adhering to CPGs is associated with improvement in dialysis care and even patient outcomes.

Definitions of Clinical Practice Guidelines

Most guideline producing bodies aim at improving patient care and outcomes by developing clinical practice guidelines (CPGs). The Institute of Medicine defines CPGs as 'systematically developed statements to assist practitioner and patient decisions about appropriate health care for specific clinical circumstances' [1, 2]. Attributes of good guidelines include validity, reliability, reproducibility, clinical applicability, clinical flexibility, clarity, multidisciplinary process, review of evidence, and documentation [Institute of Medicine Committee to Advise the Public Health Service on Clinical Practice Guidelines, 1990].

Why Do We Need Clinical Practice Guidelines?

In the current internet era, information, i.e. valuable and relevant knowledge, is growing exponentially because the number of published clinical studies is dramatically high and cannot adequately be followed by even the most astute clinician. Citations in MEDLINE alone dramatically explode and include approximately 25,000 randomized, controlled trials (RCTs) per annum [3]. Although numbers are lower there has also been an ascending trend in the number of published RCTs in the field of nephrology [4].

By providing a summary of the clinical evidence about a topic, based on relevant systematic reviews, well-performed meta-analyses or individual sufficiently powered randomized trials, CPGs can help physicians and their patients to incorporate the best evidence into their individual practice but also inform further research in the field by identifying flaws and trends in the literature. In addition, CPGs by correct interpretation of meta-analyses can particularly be beneficial in disciplines, like nephrology where studies are often characterized by small sample size and with thus insufficient power to detect a statistical relationship between the predictors and outcomes. By combining multiple small trials, meta-analyses have the ability to show presence or absence of effects that were not seen in individual, smaller studies [5].

On the other hand, in parallel with this growing knowledge the 'noise', i.e. irrelevant or even incorrect information, is growing at an even much higher speed. Confronted with this overwhelming and often contradictory information, it is often stated that the guideline producing process is cumbersome and laborious, and that 'experts' could eventually come to the same conclusion based on their experience and knowledge of the literature. However, the human mind is not capable of digesting such an amount of information without introducing (emotional) choices on what is or is not relevant.

Characteristics of Good CPGs

The major advantage of a well-performed guideline process is its transparency. The retrieved information should be presented in 'extraction tables', where all relevant information is available. This also makes that, in fact and counterintuitively, keeping a well-produced guideline up to date is neither cumbersome nor time-consuming as is sometimes suggested: one has simply to add newly appearing evidence to the table and judge whether this changes the interpretation of the evidence. In contrast, in updating more 'eminence-based' guidance, the work has virtually to be restarted from zero, as it is unclear on which grounds the first interpretation was based so that new information cannot easily be 'plugged' in. Whereas it is true that writing a new guideline is initially time-consuming, making an update is rather easy, which counters the critique that guidelines tend to be outdated when they appear. In addition, the likelihood that the advice is going to change substantially with new emerging evidence is even incorporated in the appreciation of the 'evidence level' of the guideline in the GRADE (Grades of Recommendation Assessment, Development, and Evaluation) system [6, 7]. In GRADE, a level A means that it is very unlikely that additional evidence will change the recommendation, whereas level D means that it is very plausible that it will do so. The GRADE system is explicit, comprehensive, transparent, and pragmatic and is increasingly being adopted by guideline developing organizations worldwide. The GRADE approach appraises systematic reviews of benefits and harms of interventions to determine their health benefits. In grading the evidence it considers the design, quality, and the consistency and directness of findings in published studies. The problem of the categorization of evidence is in correct guideline production covered by the Patient/Intervention/Comparison/Outcome (PICO) strategy [8], which defines the patient group for whom the guideline is intended. In the data extraction table, information on the patient groups for whom this evidence is relevant should be mentioned. Moreover, it also defines the Outcome, making it clear from the beginning whether this outcome is relevant or hard (mortality, morbidity) or surrogate (e.g. decrease of serum phosphate levels). Furthermore, the GRADE system allows to judge the quality of the guideline separately for the 'rational' (evidence) and the 'emotional' ('would you like to do it or not') aspect. This allows the formulation of statements for which there is no evidence, but still recommending to follow them. In contrast, with 'eminence-based' guidance, in correctly produced guidelines, both 'rational' and 'emotional' decision making is allowed, but it should always be transparent in how far the statement is based on 'rational' versus 'emotional' arguments. 'Emotional' should in this context be seen as judgment on nonscientific grounds, thus for example including quality of life for the individual patient, and socio-economic aspects for the health care policy level. This distinction is key, as one will never be able to base his/her actions purely on rational knowledge, because this 'absolute' knowledge will rarely ever exist. The main argument in favor of these consensus recommendations is that patient care needs to be delivered and physicians may just need more guidance in making decisions when extensive evidence is lacking. Consensus might indeed increase the empirical expertise in these cases above personal clinical judgment. Because of this lack of 'hard' evidence in nephrology it is not surprising that many of the CPGs practice recommendations are based on expert opinion and/or consensus [9].

A last important aspect of correct guideline formulation is 'availability': the fact that a certain treatment or diagnostic test is available makes that people feel uncomfortable when it is not used, even if there is no evidence that it works. An epiphenomenon from this is the difficulty to get 'negative' trials published (i.e. publication bias). Industry sometimes takes advantage of this, by pointing to the positive impact of a product in surrogate or even meaningless outcomes, or by using terminology such as 'relative risk reduction' (RRR): a drug that results in a RRR of 100% sounds very impressive, but it can mean that the mortality goes from 2 in a million to 1 in a million.

The broad interest in clinical guidelines has its origin in issues that most healthcare systems actually face: rising healthcare costs, fueled by more expensive technologies, and an ageing population; variations in service delivery among providers, and the intrinsic desire of health care professionals to offer, and of patients to receive, the best care possible (the availability problem), whereby 'best' is unfortunately often mistaken as 'new and expensive'.

In order to tackle the 'availability problem', clinicians, policy makers and payers therefore correctly see guidelines as a tool for making care more efficient and for closing the gap between what patients expect, what clinicians do, and what scientific evidence really supports [10]. CPGs can also avoid the availability trap, by explicitly stating that certain interventions have no proven benefit, whereas the opinion of an individual or a group of experts might induce the use of spurious tests and interventions.

In conclusion so far, guidelines should alert physicians from the 'blind spots' in their decision making process, by providing them with the unbiased evidence. At the same time, they should allow some 'emotional' reasoning, and that, as defined above, as judgment on not strictly scientific grounds.

What CPGs Should Not Be

Guidelines as the term implies provide thus 'guidance or advice', rather than instructions, and are aids to and not substitutes for clinical judgment. Guidelines may be a valuable adjunct to traditional clinical decision making but as every patient is unique they must never become the 'Pied Piper' of physicians, leading each of us to write the same prescription for every patient. Guidelines complement but never should replace clinical judgment and are not intended to define a standard of care; they should therefore not be interpreted as prescribing an exclusive course of management. Variations in practice will inevitably and appropriately occur when clinicians take into account the needs or preferences of individual patients, and constraints, such as policies, community standards, and budgetary limitations. In addition, the recommendations for research contained within a guideline document are general and do not imply a specific protocol.

For all these reasons, most guideline developing bodies explicitly state that CPGs should not be used as outcome performance measures.

Notwithstanding this statement it should be recognized that audit and feedback can be effective in improving professional practice; however, the effects are usually modest and likely to be larger when baseline adherence to the recommended practice is low [11].

Clinicians, policy makers, and payers see guidelines as a tool for making care more consistent and efficient and for closing the gap between what clinicians do and what scientific evidence supports [10]. As summarized elsewhere [12, 13],

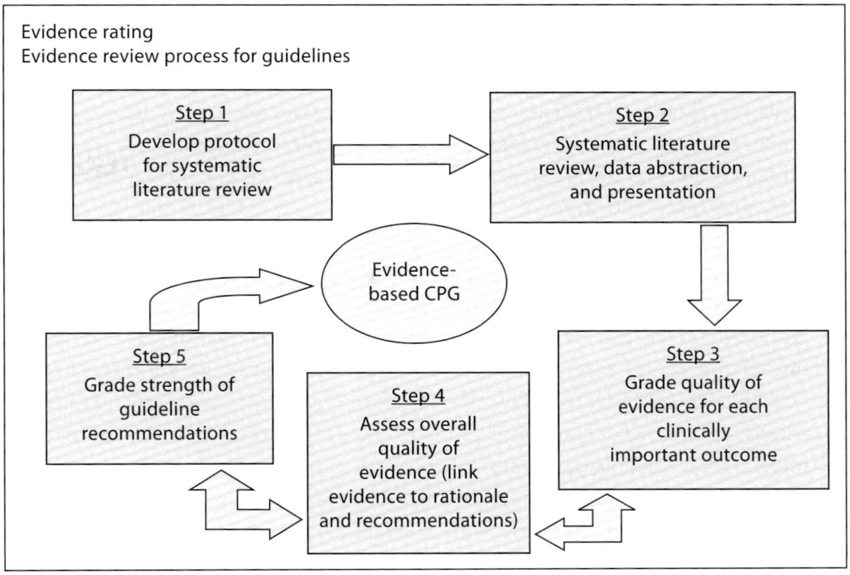

Fig. 1. Five-step methodology for formulating guidelines.

the practical specificity of well-defined guideline statements, which facilitates their translation into clinical practice, differentiates CPGs from the other important evidence-based approaches, like meta-analyses and systematic reviews, which distill and analyze the evidence in the literature ('rational') but do not make necessary practical recommendations for clinical practice.

Methodology of CPGs

The methodological challenges for correct guideline development, particularly in nephrology, have been described in detail elsewhere [14]. It should be emphasized that treatment targets, guidelines and clinical protocols as recommended in CPGs need to be revised continuously based on sound scientific data.

Figure 1 summarizes very broadly the 5-step methodology of formulating guidelines as used by, the international Kidney Disease Improving Global Outcome (KDIGO) group and by the US National Kidney Foundation (NKF). Most if not all CPGs in nephrology have been formulated by highly respected organizations. These organizations include the NKF in the USA, the European Renal Association/European Dialysis and Transplant Association (ERA/EDTA), the Canadian Society of Nephrology, the United Kingdom Renal Association, the Australian and New Zealand Society of Nephrology, the International Society of Peritoneal Dialysis (ISPD) and The Kidney Diseases: Improving Global Outcomes (KDIGO), a global extension of the NKF DOQI guideline formulating body.

Potential Benefits of CPGs in Nephrology

The principal benefit of guidelines should be an improvement of the quality of care received by patients and rigorous evaluations have shown that CPGs can indeed improve the quality of care in general practice [15]. The Dialysis Outcomes and Practice Patterns Study (DOPPS) describes variation in hemodialysis practice and monitors trends by following nationally representative samples of dialysis facilities. DOPPS identifies best practices to improve current care by analysis of the variations in practice and outcomes in hemodialysis. Many DOPPS reports have demonstrated relations between patient outcomes, including survival and variations in achieving anaemia and bone and mineral disease targets, choice of vascular access, referral patterns, treatment times, and many other parameters [16–24]. Although DOPPS is an observational registry, the results obtained can be useful and relevant because of the size of the samples and 'real-life' applicability. However, DOPPS describe the situation 'as is', and not what happens if CPG's would be implemented: there is observational evidence that dialysis patients with a normal hemoglobin have better outcomes than those with anemia; however, in several interventional trials, it has been demonstrated that trying to correct anemia to normal hemoglobin ranges in dialysis [25, 26] and CKD patients [27–29] does not improve outcomes. This difference between achieving threshold of parameters of interest in patients who are doing well, and aiming to achieve these thresholds by an intervention is key in interpreting other studies in this regard. Plantinga et al. [30] demonstrated that attaining the following accepted targets 6 months after study enrollment: albumin (≥4.0 g/dl), hemoglobin (≥11 g/dl), calcium-phosphate product (<55 mg^2/dl), dialysis dose (Kt/V ≥1.2), and vascular access type (fistula) was associated individually with decreased mortality, hospital admission rates, hospital days, and hospital costs. Increasing numbers of targets attained were also associated, in a graded fashion, with better outcomes.

Similar results were obtained by Rocco et al. [31] who analyzed the same targets in 15,287 patients. The main limitations of these studies are that it was not possible to determine the roles of severity of illness in the failure to meet performance measures. Finally, Tentori et al. [32] conducted a retrospective analysis of 13,792 incident HD patients who were treated at facilities operated by a not-for-profit dialysis provider. Cox proportional hazards models were used to assess the association between satisfying guidelines and mortality. Values within guidelines for single-pool Kt/V, hematocrit, serum albumin, calcium, phosphorus, and parathyroid hormone were associated with decreased mortality. Satisfying these six guidelines simultaneously was associated with an 89% reduction in mortality.

An interesting observation is the reporting of the inverse association, between blood pressure values satisfying the DOQI guideline and increased mortality. In commentaries, this result is explained by the fact that the blood pressure target values are largely extrapolated from the general population and thus do not apply to a dialysis population. An alternative explanation is that presence of low blood pressure in a hemodialysis patient reflects the presence of heart disease.

Although satisfying guidelines for multiple parameters presents a therapeutic challenge, significant increases in guideline adherence for single-pool Kt/V urea, haematocrit, and serum albumin were observed over time. This may reflect in part improved clinical practice patterns and in part survivor bias. Because results of models stratified by baseline values were identical, it is not likely that patient selection contributed to these findings.

Using targets of surrogate outcomes as quality indicator can even be detrimental if this is done at the expense of other, more relevant interventions.

For example, Spolter et al. [33] found only a weak correlation between anemia management and dialysis adequacy measures, but in a comment Wolfe and Port [34] remarked that this only confirms the fact that delivery of high quality care to dialysis patients is a multidimensional challenge.

Criticisms and Concerns on CPGs in Nephrology

Clinical practice guidelines in general and in nephrology in particular can and have sometimes appropriately been criticized [35–38].

A frequently voiced criticism is that despite the publication of CPGs in dialysis, the overall survival of chronic hemodialysis patients in the US has virtually not declined over the years, pointing to a rather weak contribution of the guidelines in improving the outcome of dialysis patients [37]. This criticism is in contradiction with the evolution of patient survival as revealed by the summary of the USRDS 2009 registry data [39]. In 1989, prevalent mortality rates per 1,000 patient-years hovered at approximately 275. By the mid-1990s, the rate had fallen to approximately 260 per 1,000 patient-years. The rate was relatively flat until the year 2000, when the overall prevalent mortality rate began to fall, reaching approximately 228 per 1,000 patient-years in 2006. During the 1990s, when the prevalent mortality rate was relatively flat, significant changes in mortality patterns occurred based on duration of dialysis therapy. Death rates fell continuously for patients on dialysis therapy for less than 2 years and for patients on dialysis therapy for 2 to 5 years. Between 1995 and 2001, these falling death rates coincided with rising death rates for patients on dialysis for 5 or more years. Since 2001, however, even prevalent death rates for patients on dialysis for 5 or more years have fallen by approximately 20% [39].

We believe that many of the criticisms can be explained by some misunderstanding of the guideline development process or by the lack of implementation of CPGs; in general, these criticisms reflect a rather negative attitude or even fear that imperfect guidelines will be 'abused' in audits and performance measures by authorities and policy makers.

In the discussion above, we have explained the correct definition and methodology of CPGs and recognized that certainly in nephrology most of the guidelines are indeed based on weak evidence and are mostly expert or 'consensus' based. We have also shown that there is, albeit indirect, evidence that adhering to CPGs is associated with improvement in dialysis care and even patient outcomes. Most of the concerns of both the clinical guideline proponents and critics are their use or abuse as clinical performance measures and that guidelines should form the foundation for auditing and regulation.

We believe it is appropriate to point to the quite substantial differences between CPGs and clinical performance measures (CPMs). Coupling performance with financial incentives has worried physicians who feel that being measured against collective benchmarks overrides their professional autonomy and acumen.

It should be recognized that performance measures in dialysis care are mostly surrogate markers and are often imperfect measures of health and outcomes, as explained above.

It will also in the future remain difficult to demonstrate that implementation of the CPGs in dialysis will result in better outcomes of the patient, like improved survival, less and/or shorter hospitalizations and better quality of life. As recently emphasized by Hegbrant et al. [40], many reasons can be invoked for these difficulties, chief among them the uncertain data on which several guideline statements rely, which is primarily due to the paucity of existing evidence. The failure to be able to directly attribute any specific guideline to a change in patient outcomes speaks to the complexity of CKD and ESRD patients, and the difficulty of measuring hard outcomes versus process outcomes [41].

The frequent lack of knowledge and hard evidence due to a shortage of RCTs in nephrology creates a problem for the production of new 'guidelines'. This has recently prompted the ERA-EDTA Guideline Advisory Board to offer expert guidance to clinicians in a format of 'position statements' that differs from 'traditional guidelines' [42].

In conclusion so far, in the discussion above we have explained the correct definition and methodology of CPGs and recognized that certainly in nephrology most of the guidelines are indeed based on weak evidence and are mostly expert or 'consensus' based. We have also shown that there is, albeit indirect, evidence that adhering to CPGs is associated with improvement in dialysis care and even patient outcomes. Most of the concerns of proponents as well as the opponents of CGPs are the use or abuse as clinical performance measures and that guidelines should form the foundation for auditing and regulation.

Implementation of Guidelines

Transfer of research evidence into clinical practice is often complex and incomplete and the availability of research evidence alone is usually insufficient to change physicians' practice.

For a variety of reasons, known and unknown, publication of clinical practice guidelines has had a limited effect in changing physician behavior [43]. In this respect, Pathman et al. [44] developed a four step model (1 awareness, 2 agreement, 3 adoption, 4 adherence) to look at the utilization of CPGs. To conform to guidelines, physicians must be aware of them, agree with them, decide to follow (adopt) them for some patients, and then actually follow (adhere to) them at appropriate times for all patients. The authors showed progressive drop off with a proportion dropping off at each step. This tendency was described as a 'pipeline', in which research evidence 'leaks' at various steps and reduces the extent to it is implemented in practice [45].

There is no lack of studies that have been devoted to the several implementation strategies of quality improvement in renal replacement therapy. A recent review [46] found a total of 96 papers describing 93 different quality improvement initiatives, all of which used at least one of the many strategies that are available to implement best practice.

We believe that the implementation of treatment guidelines in general and in dialysis in particular is therefore best performed as a part of a quality management system which effectively monitors that the prescription of the dialysis care and interventions are truly delivered. The final key step in a continuous quality improvement circle is represented by activities which include providing feedback and implementing action plans via medical initiatives and appropriate educational programmes and tools.

Furthermore, barriers in delivering care and interventions should be identified and actions to address them rapidly and consistently should be initiated.

In the field of dialysis a couple of studies have explored what the most important barriers to guideline adherence are. Allen et al. [47] assessed the use of evidence based medicine (EBM) and continuous quality indicators (CQI) of practioners in peritoneal dialysis (PD). EBM and CQI domains for assessment were selected based on commonalities in PD dialysis guidelines, formulated by KDOQI, CARI, the UK Renal Association and the ERBP guidelines. It appeared that the responses to the EBM portion of the questionnaire indicated that physicians generally follow guideline recommendations quite closely. Greater than 90% of the physicians indicated that they measured Kt/V, estimated GFR and residual renal function (RRF), and used dual antibiotics in empirically treating peritonitis. A slightly lower proportion of physicians used prophylactic antibiotics at the time of PD catheter insertion or antibiotic prophylaxis to prevent exit site infections and peritonitis (77 and 70%, respectively). The lowest proportion (64%) of physicians agreed to using angiotensin-converting enzyme inhibitors or angiotensin receptor blockers to preserve residual renal function.

Irving et al. [48] undertook semistructured face-to-face interviews with 19 nephrologists from a variety of clinical settings across Australia. Participants were asked about their views of CPGs in nephrology, both local (CARI) and international, and their opinions of other factors that shape their decision making.

First, the nephrologists interviewed trusted the CARI guideline process and output. Second, it was felt that guidelines served a variety of purposes, providing a good summary of evidence, a foundation for practice, an educational resource, and justification for funding requests to policy makers, as well as promoting patient adherence to treatment. Third, as expected, guidelines were only one input into decision making and other inputs included individual patient quality of life and circumstances, opinion leaders, peers, nephrologists' own experiences, the regulation and subsidy framework for drugs and devices, policies and work practices of the local unit, and other sources of evidence. Fourth, guideline uptake varied. Factors that favored the use of guidelines included having a strong evidence base, being current, including specific targets and an explicit treatment algorithm, being sent frequent reminders, and having local peer support for implementation and the necessary personnel and other resources for effective implementation.

Finally, the same authors [49] distributed a self-administered survey to all members of the Australasian professional organization for renal nurses in 2006. The results were compared with those from a similar survey in 2002 and an identical 2006 survey of Australian and New Zealand nephrologists. More than 95% considered the guidelines to be a good synthesis of the available evidence, 80% indicated that the guidelines had significantly influenced their practice and 86% considered that they had improved patient outcomes. Respondents were generally more positive about the CPGs in 2006 than in 2002. Although nephrologists were generally positive about the CARI guidelines, renal nurses were more positive, especially regarding the effect of the guidelines on practice and the improvement in health outcomes.

Conclusion

We tried to demonstrate that correct interpretation and implementation of clinical practice guidelines and achievement of multiple parameters that satisfy the current guidelines is associated with improved survival among hemodialysis patients. We believe that guidelines in nephrology, more particular in the field of hemodialysis, however imperfect they may be at present, may favorably impact on patient outcomes. Their role in education, research and health policy development should be emphasized such that there is an additional indirect benefit on dialysis practice and thus patient outcomes.

References

1 Field MJ, Lohr KN: Clinical Practice Guidelines: Directions for a new program. Washington, Institute of Medicine, 1990.
2 Woolf SH: Practice guidelines: a new reality in medicine. I. Recent developments. Arch Intern Med 1990;150:1811–1818.
3 Druss BG, Marcus SC: Growth and decentralization of the medical literature: implications for evidence-based medicine. J Med Libr Assoc 2005;93:499–501.
4 Strippoli GF, Craig JC, Schena FP: The number, quality, and coverage of randomized controlled trials in nephrology. J Am Soc Nephrol 2004;15:411–419.
5 Garg AX, Hackam D, Tonelli M: Systematic review and meta-analysis: when one study is just not enough. Clin J Am Soc Nephrol 2008;3:253–260.
6 Grade Working Group: Grading quality of evidence and strength of recommendations. BMJ 2004;328:1490–1494.
7 Guyatt GH, Oxman AD, Vist GE, Kunz R, Falck-Ytter Y, Onso-Coello P, Schunemann HJ: GRADE: an emerging consensus on rating quality of evidence and strength of recommendations. BMJ 2008;336:924–926.
8 Counsell C: Formulating questions and locating primary studies for inclusion in systematic reviews. Ann Intern Med 1997;127:380–387.
9 Tricoci P, Allen JM, Kramer JM, Califf RM, Smith SC Jr: Scientific evidence underlying the ACC/AHA clinical practice guidelines. JAMA 2009;301:831–841.
10 Woolf SH, Grol R, Hutchinson A, Eccles M, Grimshaw J: Clinical guidelines: potential benefits, limitations, and harms of clinical guidelines. BMJ 1999;318:527–530.
11 Jamtvedt G, Young JM, Kristoffersen DT, O'Brien MA, Oxman AD: Audit and feedback: effects on professional practice and health care outcomes. Cochrane Database Syst Rev 2006;CD000259.
12 Eknoyan G, Lameire N, Barsoum R, Eckardt KU, Levin A, Levin N, Locatelli F, Macleod A, Vanholder R, Walker R, Wang H: The burden of kidney disease: improving global outcomes. Kidney Int 2004;66:1310–1314.
13 Lameire N, Eknoyan G, Barsoum R, Eckardt KU, Levin A, Levin N, Locatelli F, Macleod A, Vanholder R, Walker R, Wang H: A new initiative in nephrology. 'Kidney disease: improving global outcomes'. Contrib Nephrol. Basel, Karger, 2005, vol 149, pp 90–99.
14 Uhlig K, Balk EM, Lau J, Levey AS: Clinical practice guidelines in nephrology – for worse or for better. Nephrol Dial Transplant 2006;21:1145–1153.
15 Grimshaw JM, Russell IT: Effect of clinical guidelines on medical practice: a systematic review of rigorous evaluations. Lancet 1993;342:1317–1322.

16 Couchoud C, Kooman J, Finne P, Leivestad T, Stojceva-Taneva O, Ponikvar JB, Collart F, Kramar R, de FA, Jager KJ: From registry data collection to international comparisons: examples of haemodialysis duration and frequency. Nephrol Dial Transplant 2009;24:217–224.
17 Ethier J, Mendelssohn DC, Elder SJ, Hasegawa T, Akizawa T, Akiba T, Canaud BJ, Pisoni RL: Vascular access use and outcomes: an international perspective from the Dialysis Outcomes and Practice Patterns Study. Nephrol Dial Transplant 2008;23:3219–3226.
18 Jadoul M, Lameire N, Bragg-Gresham JL, Eichleay MA, Pisoni RL, Port FK: Dopps estimate of patient life years attributable to modifiable haemodialysis practices in Belgium. Acta Clin Belg 2007;62:102–110.
19 Mendelssohn DC, Yeates KE, Ethier J, Trpeski L, Na Y, Bragg-Gresham JL, Eichleay MA, Pisoni RL, Port FK: DOPPS estimate of patient life years attributable to modifiable hemodialysis practices in Canada. Nephrol News Issues 2007;21:69–66.
20 Pisoni RL, Arrington CJ, Albert JM, Ethier J, Kimata N, Krishnan M, Rayner HC, Saito A, Sands JJ, Saran R, Gillespie B, Wolfe RA, Port FK: Facility hemodialysis vascular access use and mortality in countries participating in DOPPS: an instrumental variable analysis. Am J Kidney Dis 2009;53:475–491.
21 Pisoni RL, Bragg-Gresham JL, Fuller DS, Morgenstern H, Canaud B, Locatelli F, Li Y, Gillespie B, Wolfe RA, Port FK, Robinson BM: Facility-level interpatient hemoglobin variability in hemodialysis centers participating in the Dialysis Outcomes and Practice Patterns Study (DOPPS): associations with mortality, patient characteristics, and facility practices. Am J Kidney Dis 2011;57:266–275.
22 Port FK, Eknoyan G: The Dialysis Outcomes and Practice Patterns Study (DOPPS) and the Kidney Disease Outcomes Quality Initiative (K/DOQI): a cooperative initiative to improve outcomes for hemodialysis patients worldwide. Am J Kidney Dis 2004;44:1–6.
23 Port FK, Pisoni RL, Bommer J, Locatelli F, Jadoul M, Eknoyan G, Kurokawa K, Canaud BJ, Finley MP, Young EW: Improving outcomes for dialysis patients in the international Dialysis Outcomes and Practice Patterns Study. Clin J Am Soc Nephrol 2006;1:246–255.
24 Saran R, Bragg-Gresham JL, Rayner HC, Goodkin DA, Keen ML, Van Dijk PC, Kurokawa K, Piera L, Saito A, Fukuhara S, Young EW, Held PJ, Port FK: Nonadherence in hemodialysis: associations with mortality, hospitalization, and practice patterns in the DOPPS. Kidney Int 2003;64:254–262.
25 Besarab A, Bolton WK, Browne JK, Egrie JC, Nissenson AR, Okamoto DM, Schwab SJ, Goodkin DA: The effects of normal as compared with low hematocrit values in patients with cardiac disease who are receiving hemodialysis and epoetin. N Engl J Med 1998;339:584–590.
26 Parfrey PS, Foley RN, Wittreich BH, Sullivan DJ, Zagari MJ, Frei D: Double-blind comparison of full and partial anemia correction in incident hemodialysis patients without symptomatic heart disease. J Am Soc Nephrol 2005;16:2180–2189.
27 Drueke TB, Locatelli F, Clyne N, Eckardt KU, Macdougall IC, Tsakiris D, Burger HU, Scherhag A: Normalization of hemoglobin level in patients with chronic kidney disease and anemia. N Engl J Med 2006;355:2071–2084.
28 Pfeffer MA, Burdmann EA, Chen CY, Cooper ME, de ZD, Eckardt KU, Feyzi JM, Ivanovich P, Kewalramani R, Levey AS, Lewis EF, McGill JB, McMurray JJ, Parfrey P, Parving HH, Remuzzi G, Singh AK, Solomon SD, Toto R: A trial of darbepoetin alfa in type 2 diabetes and chronic kidney disease. N Engl J Med 2009;361:2019–2032.
29 Singh AK, Szczech L, Tang KL, Barnhart H, Sapp S, Wolfson M, Reddan D: Correction of anemia with epoetin alfa in chronic kidney disease. N Engl J Med 2006;355:2085–2098.
30 Plantinga LC, Fink NE, Jaar BG, Sadler JH, Levin NW, Coresh J, Klag MJ, Powe NR: Attainment of clinical performance targets and improvement in clinical outcomes and resource use in hemodialysis care: a prospective cohort study. BMC Health Serv Res 2007;7:5.
31 Rocco MV, Frankenfield DL, Hopson SD, McClellan WM: Relationship between clinical performance measures and outcomes among patients receiving long-term hemodialysis. Ann Intern Med 2006;145:512–519.
32 Tentori F, Hunt WC, Rohrscheib M, Zhu M, Stidley CA, Servilla K, Miskulin D, Meyer KB, Bedrick EJ, Johnson HK, Zager PG: Which targets in clinical practice guidelines are associated with improved survival in a large dialysis organization? J Am Soc Nephrol 2007;18:2377–2384.
33 Spolter YS, Seliger SL, Zhan M, Hsu VD, Walker LD, Fink JC: The relationship between dialysis performance measures: adequacy and anemia management. Am J Kidney Dis 2007;50:774–781.
34 Wolfe RA, Port FK: Evaluation of dialysis performance measures. Am J Kidney Dis 2008;51:867–868.
35 Amerling R: Practice guidelines: do we really need them? Perit Dial Int 2005;25:140–141.
36 Amerling R, Winchester JF: Comments on the guideline debate. Clin J Am Soc Nephrol 2007;2:208.
37 Amerling R, Winchester JF, Ronco C: Guidelines have done more harm than good. Blood Purif 2008;26:73–76.
38 Mendelssohn DC: Musings on guidelines and evidence: a pragmatic and nephrocentric view. Perit Dial Int 2007;27:31–34.
39 Collins AJ, Foley RN, Gilbertson DT, Chen SC: The state of chronic kidney disease, ESRD, and morbidity and mortality in the first year of dialysis. Clin J Am Soc Nephrol 2009;4(suppl 1):S5–S11.
40 Hegbrant J, Gentile G, Strippoli GF: The quest to standardize hemodialysis care. Contrib Nephrol 2011;171:39–49.

41 Levin A: Practice guidelines do improve patient outcomes: association or causation? Blood Purif 2008;26:67–72.
42 Vanholder R, Abramowicz D, Cannata-Andia JB, Cocchi V, Cochat P, Covic A, Eckardt K-U, Fouque D, Heimburger O, Jenkins S, Macleod A, Lindley E, Locatelli F, London G, i Monros AM, Spasovski G, Tattersall J, Van Biesen W, Wanner C, Wiecek A, Zoccali C: The future of European Nephrology 'Guidelines' – a declaration of intent by European Renal Best Practice (ERBP). NDT Plus 2009;2:213–221.
43 Cabana MD, Rand CS, Powe NR, Wu AW, Wilson MH, Abboud PA, Rubin HR: Why don't physicians follow clinical practice guidelines? A framework for improvement. JAMA 1999;282:1458–1465.
44 Pathman DE, Konrad TR, Freed GL, Freeman VA, Koch GG: The awareness-to-adherence model of the steps to clinical guideline compliance. The case of pediatric vaccine recommendations. Med Care 1996;34:873–889.
45 Mickan S, Burls A, Glasziou P: Patterns of 'leakage' in the utilization of clinical guidelines: a systematic review. Postgrad Med J 2011;87:670–679.
46 van der Veer SN, Jager KJ, Nache AM, Richardson D, Hegarty J, Couchoud C, de Keizer NF, Tomson CR: Translating knowledge on best practice into improving quality of RRT care: a systematic review of implementation strategies. Kidney Int 2011;80:1021–1034.
47 Allen N, Schwartz D, Sood AR, Mendelssohn D, Verrelli M, Tanna G, Schiff J, Komenda P, Rigatto C, Sood MM: Perceived barriers to guidelines in peritoneal dialysis. Nephrol Dial Transplant 2011;26:1683–1689.
48 Irving MJ, Tong A, Rychetnik L, Walker RG, Frommer MS, Craig JC: Nephrologists' perspectives on the effect of guidelines on clinical practice: a semistructured interview study. Am J Kidney Dis 2010;55:241–249.
49 Irving MJ, Johnson DW, McDonald S, Walker RG, Frommer MS, Fetherstonhaugh D, Deans P, Craig JC: Opinions on the content and effects of the Caring for Australasians with Renal Impairment (CARI) Guidelines: a survey of renal nurses and comparison with the opinions of nephrologists in Australasia. Nephrology (Carlton) 2010;15:48–53.

Dr. Norbert Lameire
University Hospital
185, De Pintelaan
BE–9000 Gent (Belgium)
E-Mail norbert.lameire@ugent.be

Ronco C, Rosner MH, Crepaldi C (eds): Peritoneal Dialysis – State-of-the-Art 2012.
Contrib Nephrol. Basel, Karger, 2012, vo 178, pp 68–73

Remote Monitoring for Continuous Peritoneal Dialysis

Mitchell H. Rosner[a] · Claudio Ronco[b]

[a]Division of Nephrology, University of Virginia Health System, Charlottesville, Va., USA; [b]Department of Nephrology, Dialysis and Transplantation, San Bortolo Hospital, Vicenza, Italy

Abstract

Peritoneal dialysis affords patients the luxury of independence and with this an improved quality of life. However, patients on peritoneal dialysis still require monthly visits with the care team to assess the quality of therapy (volume and blood pressure control, solute clearance, attainment of metabolic goals, and others). Furthermore, a critical aspect of therapy is that the patient must actively monitor their therapy with daily recordings of weight, blood pressure, and fluid removal. Remote monitoring of the patient on peritoneal dialysis offers the benefits of real-time monitoring and recording of the therapy as well as an interactive interface with the care team that may allow both acute 'trouble shooting' for problems as well as a means to interact with the patient for their monthly evaluation. This remote monitoring allows assurance of patient safety through surveillance of critical portions of the treatment as well as the ability to monitor compliance with prescribed therapy and automated collection of treatment data. Recent advances in telemedicine, telemonitoring, remote network access and sensor technologies have made such remote monitoring of peritoneal dialysis therapy feasible.

Peritoneal dialysis has a clear benefit of increasing patient independence as compared to in-center hemodialysis. However, with this independence comes a great responsibility that is placed upon the patient and their support system to manage the therapy at home without the benefit of direct thrice weekly nursing and physician oversight. Safe, easy-to-operate equipment and suitable training have allowed patients and their families to carry out treatments that have traditionally been restricted to medical staff. However, a medical support system for these peritoneal dialysis (either continuous ambulatory peritoneal dialysis, CAPD, or automated peritoneal dialysis, APD) patients is still necessary for backup. This usually involves monthly clinic visits with the care team where goals of therapy are reviewed, problems addressed and laboratory work obtained. In the United States, the Medicare End-Stage Renal Disease program mandates that monthly in-person visits occur [1]. Most patients performing peritoneal dialysis will also have either technical issues or medical concerns that require calls into the care center. These may include problems with catheter function, difficulties in managing fluid balance, uncertainties regarding the possibility of cloudy dialysate, concerns about the appearance of the catheter exit site, and many other medical problems. Often assessment of these concerns requires that patients either go to an emergency department or to the dialysis center, negatively impacting on their quality of life and independence. Recent advances in telecommunications, internet technology, and remote sensing can now be applied to the care of this patient group.

A telemedicine system (telemedicine is defined as the use of medical information exchanged from one site to another via electronic communications to improve patients' health status), especially one that includes a two-way video, is an effective way of monitoring patient data at home. Based upon individual needs, this could include the ability to communicate in real-time with the dialysis center to trouble-shoot problems, the ability of performing monthly assessments remotely, the ability to monitor treatment efficacy and compliance, and the ability to monitor the entire array of vital signs and laboratory data. A complete telemedicine program for the patient undergoing peritoneal dialysis would include: treatment monitoring, vital sign and laboratory monitoring and two-way real-time video communications. The ultimate goals of such a system are to increase functional independence, improve quality of life, increase acceptance and use of peritoneal dialysis and improve overall outcomes.

Treatment Monitoring

Benefits of Treatment Monitoring

First and foremost, monitoring of any complex and invasive therapy aims to ensure patient safety through surveillance of the critical portions of the treatment. For peritoneal dialysis which has a long history of safety, there is a less critical requirement for home monitoring. However, it would be very helpful to monitor those patients who have just initiated therapy or those patients with persistent or recurring problems such as peritonitis.

Monitoring of the treatment also allows assurance of patient compliance with the prescribed therapy. This is essential in allowing trouble-shooting of the procedure when clinical results appear to be out of the range from anticipated based on the prescription of the therapy. For example, in the diagnosis of a patient with a weekly Kt/V less than anticipated for the prescribed therapy understanding what therapy was actually performed or delivered is important.

Monitoring of therapy also allows for the automated collection of treatment data. This data can be used as part of a quality assessment and improvement program as well as to provide information for clinical trials. Finally, remote monitoring may be important in ensuring safety requirements that are part of obtaining regulatory approval for a new device.

Currently, several forms of home peritoneal dialysis monitoring are available. The Baxter PD Link™ software system (Baxter Healthcare, Deerfield, Ill., USA) as part of the HomeChoice PRO system® provides clinicians the ability to create patient prescriptions, collect and analyze therapy results (such as volume used, drain times, ultrafiltration amounts and more) and transmit these data to the dialysis center either though a modem or via a small electronic data card that can collect approximately 60 days of patient treatment data [2]. This card can also be used to change treatment settings. Several investigators have demonstrated that the use of the ProCard technology (an earlier version of the PD Link™ system) led to improved compliance with home therapy with improved outcomes [3–5]. Fresenius Medical Care (Waltham, Mass., USA) has also developed a similar system to use with their Liberty® cycler system, the IQSystem™ which is an integrated data management system that allows clinicians access to treatment data and alarm history [6]. Both of these systems are integrated into cycler technology and thus are not easily applicable to those patients utilizing CAPD.

These systems are limited to monitoring treatment variables that are dependent upon the cycler only and do not have the capability of monitoring patient-specific variables. Taking a step backward, it is helpful to define what the goals of a monitoring system for peritoneal dialysis should include to maximize the benefit and minimize the intrusiveness of the system.

What Are the Ideal Requirements for a Monitoring System?

A remote monitoring system for peritoneal dialysis should ideally have the following characteristics: (1) the ability to allow the user flexibility in movement and activities; (2) two-way communications including high-definition video; (3) simple and intuitive alarm systems with a high degree of specificity and sensitivity for alarms that are clinically appropriate; (4) modifiable and customizable (for instance, monitoring capability at the beginning of training and the first months of therapy may be more intensive and then scaled back as appropriate); (5) it should generate useful reports that can be used to monitor quality, and (6) should not be intrusive and maintain portability.

What Should Be Monitored?

Potentially, the number of variables that could be monitored during a peritoneal dialysis treatment is large (table 1). However, the vast experience with peritoneal dialysis has shown that this is a very safe therapy and that monitoring may have its greatest benefit in limited scenarios: (1) in the immediate post-training period to assess compliance with therapy, (2) in the monitoring of patients with unstable medical conditions, (3) in the monitoring of patients with a history of noncompliance, and (4) in monitoring patients with a history of peritoneal dialysis related complications such as ultrafiltration failure or peritonitis. Monitoring may also allow for changing of the dialysis prescription via remote access.

Perhaps, the greatest need for patients undergoing peritoneal dialysis is a real-time method for direct two-way communications. Having the ability to perform video conferencing would allow for troubleshooting of dialysis-related problems (such as visualizing an exit site for a catheter or viewing a dialysate to determine if it is cloudy). Such two-way communications could also be used for billing documentation and remove the necessity for on-site monthly visits.

Table 1. Parameters that can be monitored during a peritoneal dialysis session

Fill and drain volumes
Fill and drain times
Systolic and diastolic blood pressure
Pulse
Oxygen saturation
Weight or bioimpedance
Time/duration of treatment dwell
Number of exchanges
Prescription of dialysis
Symptoms during therapy
Alarms and patient response to alarms

Technology Needed for Remote Monitoring and Communications

The recent growth and technological advancement in the field of telemedicine provides a source of technological infrastructure for the development of remote peritoneal dialysis monitoring. Ideally, an integrated system for peritoneal dialysis would include: two-way videoconferencing, vital sign monitoring, a data management system, and the capability of monitoring the parameters of the treatment such as fill and drain times, volume of dialysate used, and ultrafiltration rates.

Within telemedicine, a wide range of systems are available; some are simple, such as special telephones with built-in computers that transmit still images and real-time audio; some are complex, transmitting images via broadband cable and linking users for computer-based, real-time videoconferences over statewide networks [7]. Internet-based technologies such as Skype® now allow for simple video calling or conferencing that is free of charge and requires only an internet connection and a high quality webcam [8]. Furthermore, remote monitoring of many chronic conditions such as congestive heart failure, hypertension and diabetes mellitus is now available and utilizes physiological sensors that can transmit data to central monitoring stations [8]. For example, Intel® has developed the Intel Health Guide® which is a comprehensive remote patient monitoring system that combines an in-home patient sensor device with a management suite of tools to enable clinicians to monitor patients and remotely manage care. Many of these patient sensors/monitors have the ability to communicate to computer networks through Bluetooth™ wireless technology. These systems may also include: multimedia educational content, vital sign devices and measurement capability, interactive patient health sessions, language translation services and two-way video conferencing [9]. Furthermore, the use of high speed broadband cable networks may allow for two-way communication through existing cable television technology. There are several commercially available two-way, high-definition telemedicine platforms already available (including: LifeSize® [10] and Vidyo® [11]) that provide 'out of the box' solutions to high quality two-way communications.

Even remote laboratory assessment of routine chemistries and blood counts could be obtained in the home setting using a portable device such as the i-STAT™ (Abbott Laboratories (Abbott Park, Ill., USA)) which allows for accurate and reliable laboratory data that can be transmitted back to the dialysis center [12].

Experience with Monitoring of Peritoneal Dialysis

Several centers have had experience with remote monitoring for peritoneal dialysis. Nakamoto and colleagues in Japan have reported on their experience over the past 10 years utilizing various telemedicine systems of varying complexity [13–16]. In the most recent version reported, they utilized transmission of vital sign and treatment data via data card technology to a computer server. This group has reported great patient satisfaction with this system. Gallar et al. [17] have also reported success with a telemedicine program for peritoneal dialysis patients. They reported that daily costs of the system were low, and there was significant savings in time and transportation experienced by the patients [17]. However, there have been no studies of direct two-way real-time video communications coupled with vital sign and treatment monitoring. Studies will have to focus on treatment outcomes, direct and indirect cost savings, patient satisfaction and patient quality of life.

Designing the Ideal System

Given the recent technological advances in telemedicine, an ideal system for monitoring the patient on peritoneal dialysis can be designed and implemented (fig. 1). It would include: (1) High-definition two-way video communication with an easily movable camera to allow for visualization of the patient to allow for documentation of important clinical data (such as the catheter exit-site, lower extremities for edema, etc.). (2) Remote sensors that would capture blood pressure, pulse, temperature, blood glucose and weight and transmit this data via Bluetooth™ technology to the dialysis center on a specified interval. Such a system would also allow direct patient access to this data as well as the ability to enter additional data such as urine output. (3) Treatment data collection similar to the pre-existing systems now available by Baxter and Fresenius. (4) Patient specific add-ons such as translation services, training videos, and other disease-specific monitoring if indicated. A more expensive add-on would be remote laboratory assessment. The ultimate goal of the system would be to increase patient autonomy, improve quality of life and improve outcomes.

Barriers to Implementation

While technology has advanced to the level that in-home monitoring of the patient on peritoneal dialysis can be accomplished there are significant hurdles before wide-spread implementation will occur. Cost-benefit analyses of such systems will have to occur as well as studies documenting clinical benefit. Regulatory agencies will have to grant approval for use in this setting and health insurers will have to agree to reimburse costs associated with the system as well as recognize and

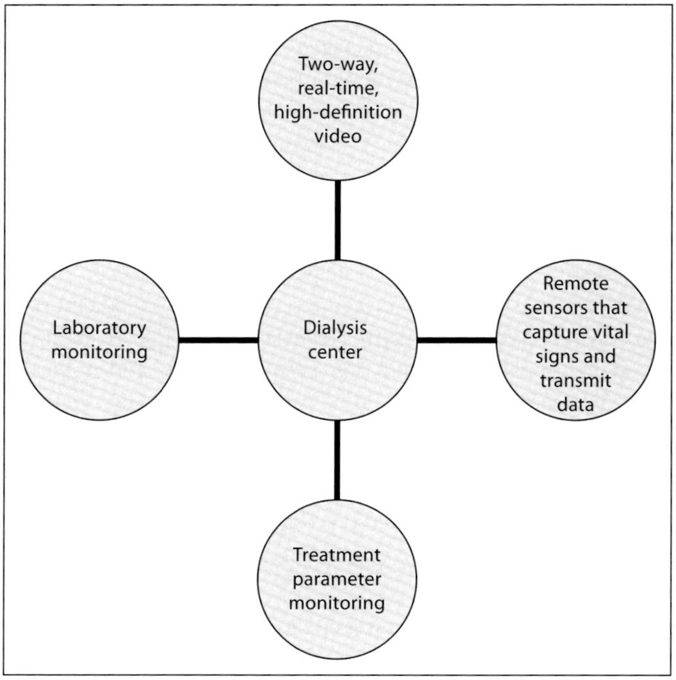

Fig. 1. The Ideal Telemedicine Platform for Peritoneal Dialysis. Several different data sources will feed into the dialysis center to give clinicians a complete picture of the patients' well-being as well as data regarding their dialysis therapy.

reimburse care given through this novel method. Finally, patients will have to accept home monitoring as not an intrusive entry into their home but as a technique that fosters independence and provides them with a greater degree of support.

Conclusion

Recent advances in technology now make home monitoring of the patient on peritoneal dialysis a reality. Implementing such advanced systems will require new payment models, development of technological expertise at dialysis centers and the willingness of both patients and clinicians to adopt a new model of care. The benefits of such a model may be an improved sense of patient independence, improved quality of life and improved health care outcomes. As these systems come into use, clinical studies will be required to document benefit.

References

1 https://www.cms.gov/manuals/downloads/bp102c11.pdf (accessed January 2, 2012).
2 http://www.baxter.com/health-care_professionals/products/renal/home_dialysis/pd_link.html (accessed January 2, 2012).
3 Juergensen PH, Gorban-Brennan N, Finkelstein FO: Compliance with the dialysis regimen in chronic peritoneal dialysis patients: utility of the Pro Card and impact of patient education. Adv Perit Dial 2004;20:90–92.
4 Neri L, Viglino G, Cappelletti A, Gandolfo C, Barbieri S: Compliance in automated peritoneal dialysis. Adv Perit Dial 2002;18:72–74.
5 Chand DH, Bednarz D: Daily remote peritoneal dialysis monitoring: An adjunct to enhance patient care. Perit Dial Int 2008;28:533–537.
6 http://fmcna-liberty.com/libertyTour.php (accessed January 2, 2012).

7 Doarn CR, Portilla LM, Sayre MH: NIH conference on the future of telehealth: essentials tools and technologies for clinical research and care – a summary. June 25–26, 2009 Bethesda, Maryland. Telemed J E Health 2010;16:89–92.
8 Adaji A, Schattner P, Jones K: The use of information technology to enhance diabetes management in primary care: a literature review. Inform Prim Care 2008;16:229–237.
9 http://www.intel.com/about/companyinfo/healthcare/products/healthguide.htm?id=239. Accessed on August 16, 2010.
10 http://www.lifesize.com/ (accessed January 2, 2012).
11 http://info.vidyo.com/VideoConferencingForMedical.html (accessed January 2, 2012).
12 http://www.abbottpointofcare.com (accessed January 2, 2012).
13 Nakamoto H, Hatta M, Tanaka A, et al: Telemedicine system for home automated peritoneal dialysis. Adv Perit Dial 2000;16:191–194.
14 Nakamoto H, Kawamoto A, Tanabe Y, et al: Telemedicine system using a cellular telephone for continuous ambulatory peritoneal dialysis patients. Adv Perit Dial 2003;19:124–129.
15 Nakamoto H, Nishida E, Ryuzaki M, Sone M, Yoshimoto M, Itagaki K: Blood pressure monitoring by cellular telephone in patients on continuous ambulatory peritoneal dialysis. Adv Perit Dial 2004;20:105–110.
16 Nakamoto H: Telemedicine system for patients on continuous ambulatory peritoneal dialysis. Perit Dial Int 2007;27(S2):S21–S26.
17 Gallar P, Gutierrez M, Ortega O, et al: Telemedicine and follow up of peritonealdialysis patients (in Spanish). Nefrologia 2006;26:365–371.

Mitchell H. Rosner, MD
Division of Nephrology, Box 800133
University of Virginia Health System
Charlottesville, VA 22908 (USA)
Tel. +1 434 924 2187, E-Mail mhr9r@virginia.edu

Ronco C, Rosner MH, Crepaldi C (eds): Peritoneal Dialysis – State-of-the-Art 2012.
Contrib Nephrol. Basel, Karger, 2012, vol 178, pp 74–78

e-Health: Remote Health Care Models in Peritoneal Dialysis

Dirk G. Struijk

Division of Nephrology, Department of Medicine, Academic Medical Centre, Amsterdam and Dianet, Amsterdam, The Netherlands

Abstract

A general review is given on advantages and disadvantages of the various forms of e-Health. The sparse available literature on e-Health and peritoneal dialysis is discussed. It is concluded that in general e-Health interventions lead to small but to moderate positive effects on primary health outcomes, although the evidence still is not fully convincing.

e-Health represents the use of information and communication technologies, with the emphasis on internet technology, to support health and health care. According the preliminary findings of a study conducted for the European Commission, the European Union is leading the world in the development of new technology in health care, such as electronic patient records and telemedicine, but serious political, legal, and practical obstacles to its wider use remain [1]. The necessity to develop e-Health from the perspective of national governments lies in the increasing aging of the population which eventually will lead to major capacity problems. In the Netherlands it is estimated that within 20 years 25% of the labor force will have to work in health care in order to satisfy the demands. E-Health offers according to these administrations many opportunities to solve these capacity problems by increased efficiency and effectiveness in health care [2].

Another important reason for the development of e-Health is that it offers opportunities to increase patient empowerment. The demands of the citizen are changing. They actively seek information, demand more autonomy, want to have a say in the various treatment options and participation in the treatment itself. This increased empowerment often leads to improved quality of care as well as improved quality of life. In this paper the currently known forms of e-Health will be discussed, with their possible benefits and disadvantages.

Literature Search Strategy

To obtain data specific for peritoneal dialysis, a literature search in the database PubMed was performed using MeSH main headings and subheadings of the National Library of Medicine's Medical Text Indexer as well as the appearance of keywords in the title or abstract. Peritoneal dialysis AND e-Health* OR eHealth* resulted in zero hits as well as dialysis AND e-Health* OR eHealth*. Then peritoneal dialysis was combined with remote OR telemedicine OR telemonitoring OR tele-monitoring OR telehealthcare OR tele-healthcare OR internet* OR web based* OR rural health services OR health services accessibility OR medically underserved area. This search strategy resulted in less than 10 peritoneal dialysis specific papers, all reporting studies on telemonitoring.

Forms of e-Health

Online Information

When internet became available for the public in the twentieth century, its information was unidirectional (Web 1.0). It has evolved to a major source of delivering on-demand health information, instruction and medical services into the homes. Nowadays the internet is bidirectional (Web 2.0) as users also ad data. In health care this medium can be used to increase patient empowerment. On the web site of our dialysis center (www.dianet.nl) as well as on many other web sites, information is given about renal replacement therapies using text, movies with lectures by professionals but also of personal stories of patients about their health en illness. Sometimes even decision-making tools are available. Advantages of online information are the large accessibility of information 24/7 and the possibility to serve large groups of patients with limited manpower. The patient can get his information within the privacy of his home and this information gives possibility to be better prepared for the conversation with the health care provider. However, there are also disadvantages. Due to the huge amount of information the patient could get lost, the information might be conflicting or even not complete or incorrect.

Social Media

The role of social media is rapidly increasing as a source of knowledge exchange and communication in health care. Forums and patient associations exist for various patient groups, including the patients with renal diseases. Patients also communicate through blogs and use media like Twitter or Hives. Again a great advantage is the accessibility, anonymity and the possibility for patients to exchange knowledge and their own experiences. A new expert has evolved, the POL or Patient Opinion Leader, patients or care takers of individuals with chronic diseases with extended experience who can advise fellow patients. Patients who have newly been diagnosed of similar disorders often tend to look at chronic sufferers for advice on treatment options. For the professional these media give an insight in the patient's perspective. A disadvantage could be the negative influence when confronted with the problems of others.

Telemedicine

Telemedicine is the use of telecommunication and information technologies in order to provide clinical health care at a distance. It helps eliminate distance barriers and can improve access to medical services that would often not be consistently available in distant rural communities.

In a Canadian study technique failure and death rate was investigated in relation to the distance the patients lived from the nephrologist [3]. Cox regression analysis showed that the adjusted likelihood of technique failure in people living 50.1–150, 150.1–300, and >300 km from the closest nephrologist was 0.86 (95% CI 0.75, 0.97), 0.78 (95% CI 0.65, 0.94), and 0.63 (95% CI 0.50, 0.79), respectively, compared with those residing within 50 km (p value for trend <0.0001). Compared to those living within 50 km of their nephrologist, the adjusted hazard ratio of death in people living 50.1–150, 150.1–300, and >300 km from the closest nephrologist was 1.17 (95% CI 1.07, 1.27), 1.07 (95% CI 0.95, 1.21), and 1.15 (95% CI 1.00, 1.32), respectively, as compared with those living within 50 km (p value for trend 0.03). Adjustment for physician supply did not influence their results, suggesting that reduced access to local primary care physicians or non-nephrologist specialists was not responsible for the increased risk of death among remote dwellers. It is not known if the use of telemedicine with closer follow-up may influence these outcomes.

Telemedicine use in peritoneal dialysis has been reported by several groups. Gallar et al. [4]

evaluated the use of videoconferencing in the long-term control of stable patients undergoing peritoneal dialysis at home in a randomly controlled study. 25 patients using videoconferencing were compared to 32 control patients during a mean of 8 months (range 3–24) with alternate months of teleconsultations and hospital visits. A total of 172 teleconsultations were conducted. A mean of 22 min was spent on each teleconsultation, significantly less than in hospital consultations, which took a mean of 33 min ($p < 0.01$). In 148 teleconsultations (89%) medical treatment was modified. In 4 cases (2%) patients needed a hospital visit. In all instances (100%) the condition of the catheter exit site and the presence of edema could be evaluated. In group A, the estimated cost of telemedicine was EUR 198 and that of a hospital visit was EUR 177. The mean hospitalization rate was 2.2 days/patient/year in group A and 5.7 days/patient/year in group B ($p < 0.05$). They concluded that home telemedicine appears to be clinically useful and the costs and savings encouraging. Another form of telemedicine is the remote monitoring of the peritoneal dialysis cycler [5]. Also the successful use of combining of videoconferencing and monitoring of the dialysis cycler has been reported [6].

More data are available from other areas in health care about the usefulness of telemedicine. In the Japanese town of Nishiaizu, an e-Health system has been used for several years since 1994 [7, 8]. The system monitors the health condition of elderly people at home. Health-related data, such as blood pressure, ECG and blood oxygen, are transmitted to a remote medical institution via a telecommunications network. e-Health users had a 21% lower medical expenditure on lifestyle-related illness than nonusers; long-time users of e-Health had lower medical expenditure than those who used it for a shorter time. Other studies showed that telemedicine can reduce the number of hospital admissions [9]. However, a recent systematic review of studies of the cost-effectiveness of telemedicine and telecare, undertaken from 1990 until September 2010, concluded that there still is no conclusive evidence that telemedicine and telecare interventions are cost-effective compared to conventional health care [10].

m-Health

This term is used for the practice of medicine and public health, supported by mobile devices. m-Health applications include the use of mobile devices in collecting community and clinical health data, delivery of health care information to practitioners, researchers, and patients, real-time monitoring of patient vital signs, and direct provision of care (via mobile telemedicine) [11, 12]. Especially the penetration of mobile phones is rapidly increasing. The number of global mobile phone subscribers is expected to reach 4.5 billion in 2012 [13].

In CAPD patients this technique was employed using a cellular telephone and an internet web site [14]. All data for the CAPD patients – blood pressure, heart rate, body weight, ultrafiltration volume, and urine volume – were collected and sent directly by cellular telephone to an internet data server. Anywhere, at any time, each patient could confirm changes in their data in graph form by using a cellular telephone or a computer connection to an internet web site. All data collected by cellular telephone were calculated and, in real time, sent directly to the treating physician's office over the Internet. Abnormal data were sent directly to the treating physician's office and shown in the host computer with an emergency signal (emergency alarm system). In addition, CAPD patients were able to easily contact the medical staff using the same telemedicine system. Unfortunately, their experiences are not described in detail.

E-Communication or E-Consultation

E-communication offers added value to patients as it decreases the threshold to contact the professional. The accessibility of the professional increases compared to contact by phone. The e-mail then can be read on a convenient time by both parties. It is a useful tool for patients to ask for results from investigations or repeat prescriptions. Especially in E-consultation an obvious disadvantage is the absence of personal contact.

Electronic Medical Record
An electronic health record can be defined as a systematic collection of electronic health information about individual patients or populations. Although these are operated by institutions, the data can be made available to the individual patients. Sometimes is it also possible for the patient to enter data such as blood pressure and body weight. Access to (parts) of his medical records might increase patient compliance, while additional health care data added by the patient could improve his treatment.

Patient Portals
A web-based personal health record, or PHR, is a health record where health data and information related to the care of a patient is entered by the patient [15]. An example of such a portal for managing health information is HealthVault from Microsoft. HealthVault can be connected using Apps with many databases (for example for prescriptions or laboratory results) and health tools. The intention of a PHR is to provide a complete and accurate summary of an individual's medical history which is accessible online. The health data on a PHR might include patient-reported outcome data, lab results, and data from devices such as wireless electronic weighing scales or collected passively from a smart phone.

Advantages of the use of a PHR are aiding patient self-management and reinforcement of the patient's role in making decisions about his disease. If necessary, the patient can provide access to (parts) of his PHR to his health care professionals.

Serious Gaming
Online gaming can be used either for learning purposes or as part of a treatment goal. For instance, In the Netherlands this is used with success to distract children with burns when the wounds are treated by the surgeon.

Policy Issues

A recent review of the literature identified many policy issues related to e-Health. These issues were grouped under the following themes: (1) networked care, (2) interjurisdictional practice, (3) diffusion of e-Health/digital divide, (4) e-Health integration with existing systems, (5) response to new initiatives, (6) goal-setting for e-Health policy, (7) evaluation and research, (8) investment, and (9) ethics in e-Health [16]. According to the authors, these themes should be addressed by policy makers at global, jurisdictional, and institutional levels, to facilitate smooth and reliable planning of e-Health programs.

Conclusions

The various applications of e-Health seem promising. They can be used to increase patient empowerment, which could result in improved quality of care as well as improved quality of life. In peritoneal dialysis only limited data are available on telemedicine using monitoring of the dialysis cycler, videoconferencing or a combination of both techniques. In general conclusive evidence is still lacking. It is encouraging that a recent systematic review in chronically ill patients on e-Health interventions concluded that they lead to small but to moderate positive effects on primary health outcomes, although the evidence was not fully convincing [17]. Further research is needed to confirm the cost-effectiveness of e-Health.

References

1 Watson R: European Union leads way on e-health, but obstacles remain. BMJ 2010;341:c5195.

2 Fortney JC, Burgess JF Jr, Bosworth HB, Booth BM, Kaboli PJ: A reconceptualization of access for 21st century healthcare. J Gen Intern Med 2011;26(suppl 2):639–647.

3 Tonelli M, Hemmelgarn B, Culleton B, Klarenbach S, Gill JS, Wiebe N, Manns B, Alberta Kidney Disease Network: Mortality of Canadians treated by peritoneal dialysis in remote locations. Kidney Int 2007;72:1023–1028.

4 Gallar P, Vigil A, Rodriguez I, Ortega O, Gutierrez M, Hurtado J, Oliet A, Ortiz M, Mon C, Herrero JC, Lentisco C: Two-year experience with telemedicine in the follow-up of patients in home peritoneal dialysis. J Telemedi Telecare 2007;13:288–292.
5 Chand DH, Bednarz D: Daily remote peritoneal dialysis monitoring: an adjunct to enhance patient care. Perit Dial Int 2008;28:533–537.
6 Ghio L, Boccola S, Andronio L, Adami D, Paglialonga F, Ardissino G, Edefonti A: A case study: telemedicine technology and peritoneal dialysis in children. Telemed J E Health 2002;8:355–359.
7 Akematsu Y, Tsuji M: An empirical analysis of the reduction in medical expenditure by e-health users. J Telemed Telecare 2009;15:109–111.
8 Minetaki K, Akematsu Y, Tsuji M: Effect of e-health on medical expenditures of outpatients with lifestyle-related diseases. Telemed J E Health 2011;17:591–595.
9 Darkins A, Ryan P, Kobb R, Foster L, Edmonson E, Wakefield B, Lancaster AE: Care Coordination/Home Telehealth: the systematic implementation of health informatics, home telehealth, and disease management to support the care of veteran patients with chronic conditions. Telemed J E Health 2008;14:1118–1126.
10 Mistry H: Systematic review of studies of the cost-effectiveness of telemedicine and telecare. Changes in the economic evidence over twenty years. Telemed Telecare 2012;18:1–6.
11 Tachakra S, Wang XH, Istepanian RS, Song YH: Mobile e-health: the unwired evolution of telemedicine. Telemed J E Health 2003;9:247–257.
12 Germanakos P, Mourlas C, Samaras G: A Mobile Agent Approach for Ubiquitous and Personalized eHealth Information Systems. Proc Workshop 'Personalization for e-Health', 10th International Conference on User Modelling (UM'05), Edinburgh, 2005, pp 67–70.
13 Global Mobile Phone Subscribers to Reach 4.5 Billion by 2012. Cellular-news.com. 4/1/2010 http://www.cellular-news.com/story/29824.php
14 Nakamoto H: Telemedicine system for patients on continuous ambulatory peritoneal dialysis. Perit Dial Int 2007;27(suppl 2):S21–S26.
15 Tang PC, Ash JS, Bates DW, Overhage JM, Sands DZ: Personal health records: definitions, benefits, and strategies for overcoming barriers to adoption. J Am Med Inform Assoc 2006;13:121–126.
16 Khoja S, Durrani H, Nayani P, Fahim A: Scope of policy issues in ehealth: results from a structured literature review. J Med Internet Res 2012;14:e34.
17 Eland-de Kok P, van Os-Medendorp H, Vergouwe-Meijer A, Bruijnzeel-Koomen C, Ros W: A systematic review of the effects of e-health on chronically ill patients. J Clin Nurs 2011;20:2997–3010.

Dr. Dirk G. Struijk
Division of Nephrology, Department of Medicine
Academic Medical Centre, Amsterdam and Dianet
Meibergdreef 9
NL–1105 AZ Amsterdam (The Netherlands)
Tel. +31 20 5669 111, E-Mail d.g.struijk@amc.uva.nl

Ronco C, Rosner MH, Crepaldi C (eds): Peritoneal Dialysis – State-of-the-Art 2012.
Contrib Nephrol. Basel, Karger, 2012, vol 178, pp 79–82

Remote Monitoring of Peritoneal Dialysis in Special Locations

Akash Nayak[a] · Sinoj Antony[b] · K.S. Nayak[b]

[a]Chemical Engineering and Economics, Birla Institute of Technology and Science, Pilani, Rajasthan, and
[b]Department of Nephrology and Renal Transplantation, Lazarus Hospitals, Hyderabad, India

Abstract

Peritoneal dialysis (PD) as a therapy with all its advantages has not grown as would have been expected except in certain pockets, notably in Asia. In our opinion, from patient and their family interviews, a perception among prospective PD patients of inaccessibility to the referral PD Unit (RPU), usually for patients from rural areas in far flung places, inaccessible due to difficult terrain or long distances, play a strong role against the choice of PD as their modality choice for end-stage renal disease. We decided to address this issue by adopting novel initiatives such as easy access to the RPU through usage of internet and mobile phones from the patient homes especially in addressing the more clinically relevant infectious complications such as peritonitis and exit site infections with immediate treatment management responses from the RPU. In addition, we found that inherently the rural PD patients had several advantages over their urban counterparts and also over their hemodialysis (HD) counterparts in many socioeconomic, emotional support and nutritional parameters. We enhanced these advantages with an intensive home visit program. This two pronged approach has paid dividends in that our rural PD patients do as well, if not better than the urban PD and the HD patients, contrary to prevailing international experience.

A major challenge affecting the acceptance and outcomes of peritoneal dialysis (PD) is the perceived 'inaccessibility' on the part of the patient to the nephrologist and the referral PD Unit (RPU) – more so in geographically large countries with remote and inaccessible habitations. Our PD unit has worked to innovate with practical and cost-effective solutions to overcome this barrier [1].

Rapid strides in communications connectivity have been made across the world: Internet and mobile phone technology now truly penetrate almost every geographic and socioeconomic boundary extant. We use the mobile phone Short Messaging Service, inexpensive digital cameras, and the World Wide Web to address specific patient accessibility needs (fig. 1). These technologies – coupled with a dedicated PD team, comprising medical and paramedical staff, and a regular home-visit protocol [2], have enabled us to develop a unique PD remote monitoring system. Patients are constantly in touch with their MU and nephrologist, communicating in real time, around the clock, with improved PD outcomes, especially in the rural patients [3, 4].

Home Visit Protocols

Well-structured home-visit protocols ensure patient compliance and rehabilitation, adherence to proper technique, monitoring of nutrition status, and early detection of evolving comorbidities

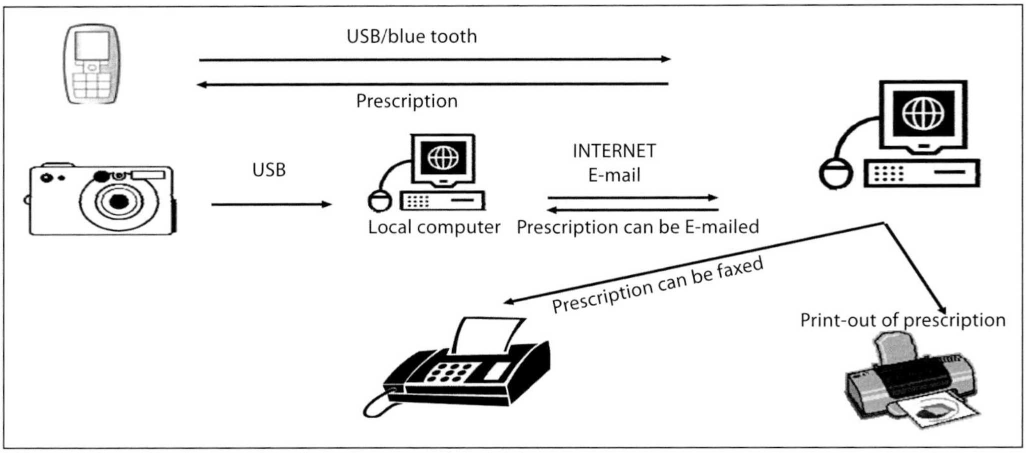

Fig. 1. Process overview of the PD remote monitoring system. SMS = Short messaging service; USB = universal serial bus connection technology.

and complications [2, 3]. Patients and their families are made aware that continuous support is available.

Home visits are scheduled by the Clinical Head and conducted by the CCs. The CCs are trained to follow a set protocol and are equipped with a standardized checklist for a step-by-step assessment of patient well-being during each visit. A detailed check of the patient's PD logbook and any conditions requiring the attention of the nephrologist are identified. All this information, together with a brief summary of the patient's most current laboratory results are conveyed to the nephrologist by Short Messaging Service from the patient's home. The CC is instructed to wait till he receives a response from the nephrologist (usually within 15 min) and then to counsel the patient accordingly. The CCs also assess and advise patients on nutrition, psychosocial well-being, and physical fitness and rehabilitation levels. Afterward, progress notes are entered into the RPU computer records.

Remote Monitoring System

The Internet-based remote monitoring system was created in our PD unit by our team to serve as a means of real-time interaction between the patient and the primary health care providers. It aims at integrating all services necessary for PD, making them easily accessible to the patient and the primary caregivers regardless of geographic distance from the RPU. These services include access to the nephrologist, clinical head, CC, urologist, and if needed, microbiologist, nutritionist, and so on. Each enrolled caregiver has a dedicated user name and password, through which they use the site for one-on-one communication with patients and with each other. Access to the technology is through the computer or the mobile phone using an android or iPhone based application. After signing into the website with a user name and password assigned at the end of the PD initiation period, the patients and caregivers are directed to a personalized home page from which they can navigate the site to access and enter/register all medical details, complaints and images.

Complaints made by patients using the site receive immediate responses. They are directed to a page where they are instructed to complete a basic description of their current concerns and answer certain pertinent questions. Patients are taught to check the condition of the exit site in terms of color, dryness, presence or absence of pain, swelling, leakage, and visibility of the external cuff, and to enter relevant information.

The two main infectious complications encountered being peritonitis and exit-site infections, patient and their caregiver or attendants are trained during their initial PD period to use their own mobile phone cameras or digital cameras to take relevant photographs of the PD effluent bag and exit site for uploading from their personal home computer or from a computer at the nearest Internet café along with their complaint. Most standard phones and computers are compatible with this technology. Generally, a 14- to 16-point typeface seen clearly through the effluent bag indicates clarity and no peritonitis. A 2MB image of the exit site with a zoom device application is adequate to assess any abnormality. Complaints about potential peritonitis are sent to the nephrologist and CC, who receive an alert both by e-mail and by cell phone. An immediate assessment and response is sent to the patient, and to the clinical head or CC, who schedules a home visit to follow-up. A horizontal and vertical image gallery of the exit site and PD bag is created and stored in each patient's electronic medical record (EMR). With every complaint, this gallery is updated, thus providing comprehensive and current information about the patient's clinical status [4].

Our Study

Studies comparing outcomes of chronic kidney disease patients have consistently shown poorer results in rural than in urban patients [4, 6], although there is paucity of data comparing these two groups on PD. Our center used remote monitoring strategies to target the major bottlenecks affecting penetrance and technique survival rates in rural patients: lack of connectivity and health awareness. Our system aims primarily to achieve early diagnosis and management of common infectious complications of PD (which has a far greater effect on PD technique survival), with integration of relevant health services and promotion of supervised autonomy unlike other researchers who focused on monitoring comorbid factors such as hypertension and cardiac events [7, 8].

We also feel that the PD Remote Monitoring significantly helped the PD patients especially the rural cohort in improving their social, emotional and due to this, their physical well-being leading to better rehabilitation and quality of life. Rural PD patients also spent less on their treatment every year than their urban counterparts. The rural PD patients did better than the urban PD patients and, the combined PD patients did significantly better than in-center hemodialysis (HD) patients on most socioeconomic and quality-of-life parameters. The assessments were done using the BDI (Beck Depression Inventory), SF-36 (Short Form Health Survey, 36) and administration of a specially designed financial questionnaire [9]. These benefits were assumed to be due to the benefits of the PD remote monitoring and additionally a well-structured home visit program leading to a complex interplay of multiple factors. Due to less therapy choice dilemma, agrarian lifestyle (much more active than an urban lifestyle), stronger family support and access to cheaper dairy and poultry products rural patients are in general healthier and more active than their urban counterparts and are hence are better at evading unnecessary hidden nonmedical expenses. We noticed similar results when we compared our group of PD patients to our group of HD patients. HD patients have a considerably higher requirement of erythropoietin. HD patients are also required to travel to clinics on a regular basis in addition to spending more time not working than PD patients. These factors contribute to an appreciable difference in the expenses towards hidden nonmedical costs for HD patients.

Conclusions

Despite the apparent odds, PD 'by choice and not default' should be the preferred therapy modality for ESRD patients in rural areas. The 'distance' between the patient and the PD Unit can be overcome by efficient usage of the internet, mobile phones and a strong home visit protocol.

References

1 Aditi NK, Sinoj AK, Prabhu MV: Improving peritoneal dialysis (PD) outcomes in rural patients compared to urban by employing novel and practical initiatives [Abstract]. Perit Dial Int 2010;30(suppl 2):S65.

2 Nayak KS, Sinoj KA, Subhramanyam SV, Mary B, Rao NV: Our experience of home visits in city and rural areas. Perit Dial Int 2007;27(suppl 2): S27–S31.

3 Nayak KS: Key success factors for a quality peritoneal dialysis program. Perit Dial Int 2007;27(suppl 2):S9–S15.

4 Aditi N, Akash K, Sinoj A, Subhramanyam S, Nayak KS: Use of a peritoneal dialysis remote monitoring system in India. Perit Dial Int 2012;32:2.

5 Zhang W, Gong Z, Peng X, Tang S, Bi M, Huang W: Clinical characteristics and outcomes of rural patients with ESRD in Guangxi, China: one dialysis center experience. Int Urol Nephrol 2010;42:195–204.

6 Tonelli M, Hemmelgarn B, Culleton B, et al: Mortality of Canadians treated by peritoneal dialysis in remote locations. Kidney Int 2007;72:1023–1028.

7 Nakamoto H: Telemedicine system for patients on continuous ambulatory peritoneal dialysis. Perit Dial Int 2007;27(suppl 2):S21–S26.

8 Gallar P, Vigil A, Rodriguez I, Ortega O, Gutierrez M, Hurtado J, et al: Two-year experience with telemedicine in the follow-up of patients in home peritoneal dialysis. J Telemed Telecare 2007;13:288–292.

9 Akash N, Sinoj A: Socio-economic factors also impact improved outcomes in rural PD patients. 32nd Annual Dialysis Conference, San Antonio, 2012.

Dr. K.S. Nayak
Department of Nephrology and Renal Transplantation
Lazarus Hospitals
Lakdikapul, Hyderabad, 500004 (India)
Tel. +91 98480 14555, E-Mail drksnayak@gmail.com

Ronco C, Rosner MH, Crepaldi C (eds): Peritoneal Dialysis – State-of-the-Art 2012.
Contrib Nephrol. Basel, Karger, 2012, vol 178, pp 83–88

Dialysis Modality Choice for the Elderly Patient with End-Stage Renal Disease

Mitchell H. Rosner[a] · Claudio Ronco[b]

[a]Division of Nephrology, University of Virginia Health System, Charlottesville, Va., USA; [b]Department of Nephrology, Dialysis and Transplantation, San Bortolo Hospital, Vicenza, Italy

Abstract

The number of elderly patients with stage 5 chronic kidney disease (CKD) is growing and leads to challenges in deciding the proper modality of treatment for these patients. The majority of these patients will not be candidates for transplantation and thus, the choice is between medical management, hemodialysis or peritoneal dialysis. Each of these choices had advantages and disadvantages and ultimately the decision to select a course of therapy must be individualized based upon the benefits and risks of the therapy, patient comorbidities, family and community resources and frank discussions regarding goals of care and end-of-life issues.

Over the past decade there has been tremendous growth in the number of elderly patients (here defined as aged <75 years) initiating dialysis therapy (either peritoneal dialysis or hemodialysis) (fig. 1). In fact, in the United States currently 1 in every 4 patients starting dialysis is >75 years of age [1]. Dialysis initiation among octogenarians and nonagenarians has also increased dramatically from 1996 to 2003, translating to a near doubling of the number of patients with incident end-stage renal disease (ESRD) who are older than 80 years of age [2]. The rising incidence of ESRD among the elderly can be explained by several factors: age-related changes in the incidence of chronic kidney disease (CKD); increasing prevalence of co-morbid conditions such as heart failure, hypertension, peripheral vascular disease and diabetes which are associated with increasing risk for ESRD; improved survival from cardiovascular disease; increased incidence of acute kidney injury (AKI) with either no or partial recovery of kidney function; broader access to ESRD care and earlier initiation of renal replacement therapy. Unfortunately, the survival after dialysis initiation for the elderly patient is quite poor: in the US, for those aged 80–84 years, the median survival is 15.6 months and for those greater than age 90 years, median survival is only 8.4 months [1]. The most common causes of death in those age ≥75 years are cardiac arrest, withdrawal from dialysis and sepsis [1]. Furthermore, the initiation of dialysis therapy is often met with a significant decline in functional ability and quality of life especially in the first months after starting dialysis [3]. This functional decline may lead to patients opting to withdraw from dialysis.

For those patients and their families facing the decision to initiate dialysis therapy, the choice can

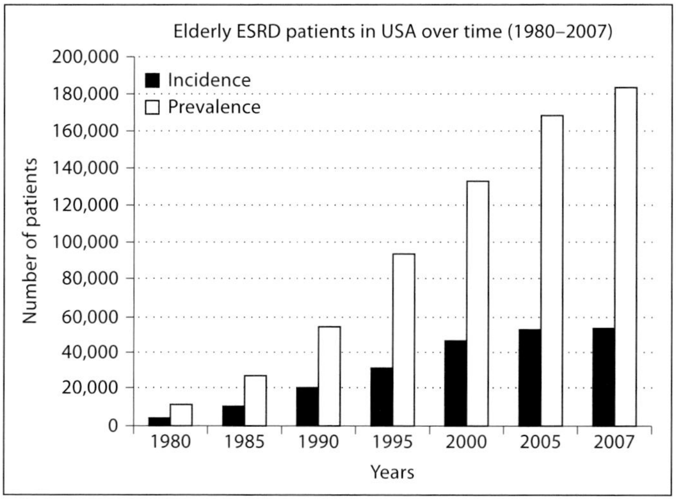

Fig. 1. The number of elderly (age >75 years) patients with ESRD over time.

be agonizing. For the majority of elderly patients, kidney transplantation may not be an option and the decision regarding renal replacement therapy centers on three choices: (1) hemodialysis – either in-center or at home; (2) peritoneal dialysis (assisted or not), and (3) conservative, nondialytic therapy. It is incumbent upon those caring for these patients to understand the benefits, complications, and limitations of these various options available for the treatment of ESRD in the elderly.

Conservative, Nondialytic Therapy

A growing number of nephrology programs in the United Kingdom are offering ongoing follow-up and multidisciplinary support to patients who have ESRD and choose not to start dialysis. It has been variously described as 'conservative management', 'maximum conservative management' (MCM), nondialysis treatment, and 'palliative renal care' [4]. In this care model, patients are followed in kidney clinics and receive active management of problems such as anemia, volume overload and other symptoms. In one study, Carson et al. [4] compared the clinical outcomes of a single-center cohort of 202 elderly patients who either chose MCM or a renal replacement therapy. In this cohort, they found that dialysis prolongs survival for elderly patients with significant comorbidity by approximately 2 years; however, patients who chose MCM survived for a substantial length of time, achieving similar numbers of hospital-free days to patients who choose hemodialysis. In fact, the increase in lifespan over MCM for those choosing dialysis was almost entirely accounted for by hospital-days. Other studies that have used a fixed glomerular filtration rate (GFR) as decision starting point (either dialysis or conservative management) have suggested that there is no significant difference in survival of elderly patients with multiple co-morbid conditions between MCM and dialysis [5, 6]. In fact, Chandna et al. [6] found that for the subgroup of female patients aged ≥75 years, MCM afforded better survival than dialysis.

While survival may not be markedly different between MCM and dialysis, it is critically important to understand any differences in quality of life. After all, with a limited life-span, most patients would likely opt for a therapy that maintains their quality of life for the longest period possible. Here the data is limited but suggests that patients receiving MCM can at least maintain their level of function until suffering a sharp decline immediately prior to dying [7]. This contrasts with the findings from Jassal et al. [3] where there was a steep functional decline at the time of dialysis initiation with a large percentage of patients losing their independence. This sharp loss of independence at the time of dialysis initiation may be due to several issues: (1) a consequence of hospitalization at or around the time of dialysis initiation; (2) the time spent on dialysis may deduct from time available to participate in physical activity, meals, and social interactions; (3) dialysis-related symptoms such as fatigue, dizziness, and cramping may be hard for the frail elderly patient to cope with, and (4) renal failure may be part of an inevitable decline in functional status that cannot be rescued with dialysis.

Thus, MCM should be considered a viable treatment modalilty for elderly patients with stage 5 CKD. Education of nephrologists is required so that this option can be discussed with patients as they approach this decision point. Furthermore, nephrologists must gain a new skill set to better manage issues such as pain, depression and symptoms associated with ESRD through conservative approaches.

Hemodialysis

The majority of elderly patients with stage 5 CKD who start dialysis do so with in-center, thrice weekly hemodialysis. However, this percentage is highly variable across different countries likely reflecting geographical differences in reimbursement, transportation access, family support networks, infrastructure and other reasons [8]. As discussed above, outcomes for the elderly patient on hemodialysis tend to be suboptimal. This is likely due to several issues beyond age alone. The interval between referrral to a nephrologist and the start of dialysis is substantially shorter in those patients age ≥75 years (3.5 weeks) versus those patients younger than 75 years (20.5 weeks) [9]. Importantly, those patients would had a referral to a nephrologist more than 8 weeks before starting dialysis had a threefold lower 1-year mortality rate [9]. Furthermore, in the US, only 23% of hemodialysis patients age ≥75 years undergo dialysis with an arteriovenous fistula [9]. Addressing these processes of care issues would likely have a significant positive impact on outcomes.

Survival on hemodialysis for the elderly patient is not uniform over time. Nearly 20% of patients (age ≥80 years) die within the first 3 months after dialysis initiation (twice the rate as patients aged 65–79 years) [10]. After this highly vulnerable period, the mortality rate decreases. Furthermore, data from Canada demonstrate that patients aged 75–80 years had 14% increase in life expectancy in the era 1995–1999 compared with those who started dialysis in 1990–1994, suggesting that care processes may have improved [11]. Several investigators have developed clinical scoring systems to predict outcomes in elderly patients initiating dialysis in an effort to better inform decision making and family discussions. For example, Cohen et al. [12] developed a short-term prognostic model in 512 patients that identified 5 variables associated with poor outcomes [including older age, dementia, peripheral vascular disease, decreased albumin and a 'no' answer to the surprise question (meaning, would you be surprised if this patient died in the next year?)]. The area under the curve for predicting 6-month mortality was 0.80–0.87 in this study. This simple clinical score effectively predicts short-term prognosis among elderly patients starting dialysis. It should help to illuminate clinical decision making, but should not, in itself, be used to withhold dialysis. It ought to only be used by nephrologists to facilitate the discussion with the patients and their families and provide realistic expectations.

Quality of life for elderly patients on hemodialysis has not been well studied but in the HEMO trial there was a comparison of health-related quality of life (HRQOL) between patients ≥70 years and those aged 55–69 and 18–54 years [13]. Not surprisingly, elderly hemodialysis patients had lower physical quality-of-life scores but had similar mental quality-of-life scores as compared to the younger cohorts. Over 3 years of follow-up there were small declines in these parameters and there was no substantial relationship between age and average decline in HRQOL score [13]. This suggests that quality of life can be maintained in the elderly dialysis patient. Further work in this area is warranted to determine how best to maintain quality of life in a group of patients with limited longevity.

Other important issues for the elderly patient on hemodialysis include: frailty, falls and cognitive decline. Frailty has been defined as having three of the following criteria: unintentional weight loss, self-reported exhaustion, slow gait speed, weakness and low physical activity [14]. In the Dialysis Morbidity and Mortality Study Wave II, the prevalence of frailty was 78.8% in those age ≥80 [14]. Frail patients have less physiological reserve and may not tolerate the dramatic and rapid changes in internal milieu that are typical of thrice-weekly hemodialysis treatments. This may translate into dialysis-related hypotension, an increased rate of falls and bone fractures, cognitive decline, longer time to functional recovery after a dialysis session and overall failure to thrive with an associated increase in mortality. Attention to these critical issues may improve outcomes in this vulnerable group and may require a change in the paradigm of dialysis care to emphasize functional assessment over laboratory values.

Recently, Cornelis et al. [15] proposed that more intensive dialysis provided by either nocturnal or short-daily hemodialysis could improve outcomes for elderly patients with ESRD. They present two illustrative cases to make the point that many of the complications experienced by elderly dialysis patients could be improved with longer and/or more frequent dialysis. This possibility will require further study. There would be considerable obstacles to providing this therapy to many elderly patients but an individualized approach for modality selection may make this feasible for some patients.

Peritoneal Dialysis

Peritoneal dialysis has several potential advantages for the elderly patient such as promoting greater independence with a more active social life, more stable hemodynamics with less dramatic shifts in fluid balance and uremic solutes and less disruption of their schedule with more time to participate in beneficial activities of daily life. Despite these clear benefits, the utilization of peritoneal dialysis for elderly patients across countries varies tremendously. For example, in the United Kingdom in 2007 an analysis of dialysis modality showed that peritoneal dialysis was utilized by 30% in those age <65 years and only 17% in those ≥65 years [16]. However, in France where community-based nursing assistance for peritoneal dialysis is available, over 50% of elderly patients utilize peritoneal dialysis [16]. These variations in utilization rates likely reflect numerous factors. However, it does beg the question as to whether some countries may have bias against utilizing peritoneal dialysis in older patients, or may lack the infrastructure needed to support this modality. Furthermore, while it is true that older patients suffer from greater levels of cognitive and physical impairment as well as more social isolation, some countries are able to overcome these barriers to a greater extent than others.

There are two longitudinal studies that examine quality of life for elderly patients on peritoneal dialysis [17]. In the North Thames Dialysis Study, there were no differences in survival and quality of life in patients ≥70 years between hemodialysis and peritoneal dialysis [17]. In the more recent Broadening Options for Long-term Dialysis in the Elderly (BOLDE) study, there once again was no difference in quality of life measure between elderly patients on hemodialysis and peritoneal dialysis [18]. In fact, patients felt that hemodialysis was more intrusive to their daily activities. Examining the quality of life for caregivers of the elderly patient on dialysis is also critical. Belasco et al. [19] examined the status of the caregivers of elderly patients either undergoing hemodialysis or peritoneal dialysis. They found that 78% of the caregivers were female and 32% have signs of depression. For those caregivers for patients on peritoneal dialysis, there were higher levels of adverse effects on their quality of life (more anxiety, fatigue, social isolation, and deterioration in relationships). This highlights the critical need for educational, social and psychological support for caregivers of elderly patients undergoing dialysis.

Understanding the mortality differences between hemodialysis and peritoneal dialysis is complex given the bias in modality selection and the differences in comorbidities between these groups of patients. Thus, while several studies have shown an increased mortality rate in elderly patients undergoing peritoneal dialysis, other studies have shown a similar rate of mortality between hemodialysis and peritoneal dialysis and some have shown improved mortality with peritoneal dialysis [11, 17, 20, 21]. For example, Winkelmayer et al. [20] used a propensity score-adjusted model to examine the mortality rates of patients aged ≥65 initiating dialysis. Those patients on peritoneal dialysis had a 16% higher rate of death during the first 90 days of dialysis as compared with hemodialysis patients. Mortality did not differ between day 91 and day 180, but after day 180, the hazard rate for mortality in the elderly group undergoing peritoneal dialysis was 1.45 as compared to hemodialysis. Not surprisingly, mortality for those with diabetes mellitus undergoing peritoneal dialysis was more pronounced. A Canadian study showed no differences in mortality between dialysis modalities and a study from the Netherlands showed a time- and comorbidity-dependent change in mortality between modalities with an initial benefit from peritoneal dialysis that decreased with time and in diabetic patients [11, 21]. Clearly, more data are needed in this area but it is clear that mortality is driven by comorbid factors emphasizing the need for an individualized approach to dialysis modality selection.

Assisted peritoneal dialysis (where a nurse or other caregiver provides in-home assistance with exchanges) has demonstrated positive benefits. In France, a community nurse is available to provide assistance to elderly patients many of whom have significant comorbid conditions [22]. Patients undergoing such care demonstrated good quality of life and improved mortality [23]. Overall, the cost of such programs is less than in-center hemodialysis and has the added benefits of limiting travel costs and maximizing time for rehabilitation and social interactions. Either CAPD or APD can be utilized but each requires specific models of nursing assistance. This modality deserved more attention and offers great promise for improving outcomes.

Conclusions

The number of elderly patients with stage V CKD is growing and will lead to challenges for the health care provider, family and patient in determining the best course of treatment as the need for renal replacement therapy approaches. It is imperative that the limits of dialysis are discussed as well as the potential impact of dialysis on functional and cognitive ability. A goal should be to distinguish which patients are good dialysis candidates and who would do poorly. Unfortunately, this is often difficult and requires a multi-disciplinary assessment of the patient. This will require a new skill set for the nephrologist that includes: geriatric assessment, improved symptom (depression, pain, anorexia, etc.) management and a willingness to consider all treatment modalities on an individual basis. It is not acceptable to default to hemodialysis as a modality choice simply for convenience or based upon preconceived notions of a patient's or families abilities to provide in-home dialysis. A thoughtful, individualized approach to modality selection is needed.

References

1 US Renal Data System, USRDS 2011 Annual Data Report: Atlas of Chronic Kidney Disease and End-Stage Renal Disease in the United States. Bethesda, National Institutes of Health, National Institute of Diabetes and Digestive and Kidney Diseases, 2011.
2 Kurella M, Covinsky KE, Collins AJ, Chertow GM: Octogenarians and nonagenarians starting dialysis in the United States. Ann Intern Med 2007;146:177–183.
3 Jassal SV, Chiu E, Hladunewich M: Loss of independence in patients starting dialysis at 80 years of age or older. N Engl J Med 2009;361:1612–1613.
4 Carson RC, Juszczak M, Davenoirt A, Burns A: Is maximum conservative management an equivalent treatment option to dialysis for elderly patients with significant comorbid disease? Clin J Am Soc Nephrol 2009;4:1611–1619.
5 Murtagh FE, Marsh JE, Donohoe P, et al: Dialysis or not? A comparative survival study of patients over 75 years with chronic kidney disease stage 5. Nephrol Dial Transplant 2007;22:1955–1962.
6 Chandna SM, Da Silva-Gane M, Marshall C, et al: Survival of elderly patients with stage 5 CKD: comparison of conservative management and renal replacement therapy. Nephrol Dial Transplant 2011;26:1608–1611.
7 Murtagh FE, Addington-Hall JM, Higginson IJ: End-stage renal disease: a new trajectory of functional decline in the last year of life. J Am Geriatr Soc 2011;59:304–308.
8 Brown EA, Johansson L: Dialysis options for end-stage renal disease in older people. Nephron Clin Pract 2011;119(suppl 1):c10–c13.
9 Xue JL, Dahl D, Ebben JP, Collins AJ: The association of initial hemodialysis access type with mortality outcomes in elderly Medicare ESRD patients. Am J Kidney Dis 2003;42:1013–1019.
10 Chauveau P, Combe C, Laville M, et al: for the French Study Group for Nutrition in Dialysis. Factors influencing survival in hemodialysis patients aged older than 75 years: 2.5-year outcome study. Am J Kidney Dis 2001;37:997–1003.
11 Jassal SV, Trpeski L, Zhu N, Fenton S, Hemmelgarn B: Changes in survival among elderly patients initiating dialysis from 1990 to 1999. CMAJ 2007;177:1033–1038.
12 Cohen LM, Ruthazer R, Moss AH, Germain MJ: Predicting six-month mortality for patients who are on maintenance hemodialysis. Clin J Am Soc Nephrol 2010;5:72–79.
13 Unruh ML, Newman AB, Larive B, et al: The influence of age on changes in health-related quality of life over three years in a cohort undergoing hemodialysis. J Am Geriatr Soc 2008;56:1608–1617.
14 Anand S, Kurella Tamura M, Chertow GM: The elderly patients on hemodialysis. Minerva Urol Nefrol 2010;62:87–101.
15 Cornelis T, Kotanko P, Goffin E, et al: Can intensive hemodialysis prevent loss of functionality in the elderly ESRD patient? Semin Dial 2011;24:645–652.
16 Brown EA: How to address barriers to peritoneal dialysis in the elderly. Perit Dial Int 2011;31(suppl 2):S83–S85.
17 Lamping DL, Constantinovici N, Roderick P, et al: Clinical outcomes, quality of life and costs in the North Thames Dialysis Study of elderly people on dialysis: a prospective cohort study. Lancet 2000;356:1543–1550.
18 Brown EA, Johansson L, Farrington K, et al: Broadening options for long-term dialysis in the elderly (BOLDE): differences in quality of life on peritoneal dialysis compared to haemodialysis patients. Nephrol Dial Transplant 2010;25:3755–3763.
19 Belasco A, Barbosa D, Bettencourt AR, Diccinie S, Sesso R: Quality of life of family caregivers of elderly patients on hemodialysis and peritoneal dialysis. Am J Kidney Dis 2006;48:955–963.
20 Winkelmayer WC, Glynn RJ, Mittleman MA, et al: Comparing mortality of elderly patients on hemodialysis versus peritoneal dialysis: a propensity score approach. J Am Soc Nephrol 2002;13:2353–2362.
21 Liem YS, Wong JB, Hunink MG, de Charro FT, Winkelmayer WC: Comparison of hemodialysis and peritoneal dialysis survival in The Netherlands. Kidney Int 2007;71:153–158.
22 Lobbedez T, Moldovan R, Lecame M, et al: Assisted peritoneal dialysis. Experience in a French renal department. Perit Dial Int 2006;26:671–676.
23 Povlsen JV, Ivarsen P: Assisted automated peritoneal dialysis (AAPD) for the functionally dependent and elderly patient. Perit Dial Int 2005;25(suppl 3):S60–S63.

Mitchell H. Rosner, MD
Division of Nephrology, Box 800133, University of Virginia Health System
Charlottesville, VA 22908 (USA)
Tel. +1 434 924 2187, E-Mail mhr9r@virginia.edu

Ronco C, Rosner MH, Crepaldi C (eds): Peritoneal Dialysis – State-of-the-Art 2012.
Contrib Nephrol. Basel, Karger, 2012, vol 178, pp 89–94

Anemia Management in Patients on Peritoneal Dialysis

Lucia Del Vecchio · Andrea Cavalli · Francesco Locatelli

Department of Nephrology, Dialysis and Renal Transplant, Ospedale A. Manzoni, Lecco, Italy

Abstract

Anemia is a common complication of patients receiving peritoneal dialysis (PD) but has been little studied compared to other chronic kidney disease (CKD) populations. A number of factors can affect its severity or response to erythropoiesis-stimulating agents (ESA). Some, such as iron deficiency, occult blood loss, infection, inflammation, oxidative stress, inadequate dialysis dose, and hyperparathyroidism are common to all dialysis patients but they may be more or less important depending on dialysis modality. The net balance of their contribution explains the fact that on average PD patients require less ESA doses compared to hemodialysis patients to correct anemia and maintain stable Hb levels. As in other CKD patients, low hemoglobin levels have been associated with increased mortality in PD patients. Unfortunately, no clinical trials have been carried out specifically in this population whether aiming at different Hb targets with ESAs may modify patient outcome. Given the lack of a vascular access, it is advisable to give PD patients ESA therapy subcutaneously. Long-acting molecules may be of advantage, especially when the drug is administered at the dialysis center.

Anemia is a common complication of chronic kidney disease (CKD) that develops early in the course of the disease and affects nearly all patients with CKD stage 5. It is characterized by a reduced ability of the damaged kidney to produce erythropoietin (EPO). Left untreated, it may significantly impair quality of life and may reduce long-term survival. In the 1970s and 1980s, treatment options were essentially limited to blood transfusions, exposing patients to infections and iron overload, or androgen therapy. This allowed only slight improvement of anemia that largely contributed to the poor quality of life patients experienced in those days. Since the late 1980s, the availability of erythropoiesis-stimulating agents (ESA) has revolutionized the management of anemia in CKD patients. Today, these drugs, together with either oral or intravenous iron, are the main tool for anemia correction in CKD patients.

Compared to other CKD patients, the role of anemia in patients treated with peritoneal dialysis (PD) has been little studied. The same holds true for the optimal hemoglobin (Hb) target to aim at with ESAs. In this paper, we summarize the main factors contributing to anemia in PD patients, together with the main aspects of its management in this particular setting.

Contributing Factors to Anemia in Patients Receiving Peritoneal Dialysis

Anemia in CKD patients is a complex syndrome in which many factors other than absolute or relative EPO deficiency may contribute towards causing anemia. In this setting, a number of factors can affect the severity of anemia or ESA response. Some of them, such as iron deficiency, occult blood loss, infection, inflammation, oxidative stress, inadequate dialysis dose, hyperparathyroidism are common to all dialysis patients. However, they may be more or less important depending on dialysis modality and account for differences in ESA dose needs. Indeed, it is well established that on average PD patients require less ESA doses compared to hemodialysis patients to correct anemia and maintain stable Hb levels. According to data from the United Kingdom Renal Registry, despite similar median Hb values, PD patients received nearly one third less rHuEPO dose (6,212 vs. 9,507 IU/week) [1]. The average dose difference was even higher in a large cohort of PD and hemodialysis patients from the United States [2]. This is mainly explained by the fact that hemodialysis patients experience frequent treatment-related blood losses together with occult blood losses enhanced by anticoagulation. PD patients are also more likely to receive ESAs subcutaneously, further reducing dose needs in the case of short-acting rHuEPO. Moreover, a higher percentage of PD patients have residual renal function and thus a certain degree of endogenous EPO synthesis. Iron deficiency is common to all dialysis patients, but the reason of this is different in hemodialysis compared to PD. In hemodialysis, blood losses are more frequent but intravenous iron can be easily administered; conversely, in PD patients despite lower blood losses, iron stores are often insufficient, mainly because inadequate iron therapy due to the lack of a vascular access. It is also well known that the chronic exposure of the blood to the hemodialysis membrane and lines has a pro-inflammatory effect leading to a chronic inflammatory state. This may also enhance oxidative stress. Even if this is not the case of PD, the fact that the peritoneum is chronically exposed to very high concentrations of glucose and its degradation products (GDPs) may contribute to the formation of advanced glycation end-products (AGEs) and to a chronic inflammatory state. It has been suggested that the use of more biocompatible PD solutions may influence the inflammatory status of PD patients [3] and possibly the severity of anemia [4]. However, this is to be confirmed by well-designed and controlled studies. Interestingly, it has been reported that erythrocytes of PD patients have a lower erythrocyte susceptibility to oxidative stress compared to hemodialysis patients [5]. Moreover, the index of rigidity of erythrocytes is significantly higher in hemodialysis than in PD patients [6]. Recurrent peritonitis episodes may also contribute to chronic inflammation in PD patients and influence anemia severity. Conversely, they are not exposed to vascular access thrombosis with consequent hospitalizations and surgical procedures, as it is the case for hemodialysis patients. Finally, it should be considered that PD patients have a higher degree of salt-water retention compared to hemodialysis patients, and thus have a certain degree of hemodilution leading in general to an underestimation of their true Hb levels. Moreover, differing from hemodialysis patients, PD patients do not experience Hb fluctuations following ultrafiltration during the dialysis session.

Anemia and Increased Mortality: Is It Also True for Peritoneal Dialysis Patients?

A number of observational studies have described a clear relationship between anemia and mortality in CKD patients [7–9]. This is probably due to the impact of severe chronic anemia on cardiac function, as it causes vasodilatation, cardiac dilation and increased cardiac output, leading to left ventricular dilation and compensatory hypertrophy.

In the 1990s this association was found to be linear: the lower the Hb value, the higher the mortality risk. However, in those days only a few patients had near-to-normal Hb values. More recent studies suggested that this relationship is not linear: hematocrit (Ht)/Hb values exceeding the reference value of 33 to <36% were not clearly associated with further reduction in the mortality risk [7, 3]. Interestingly, those patients who have normal Hb levels without ESA treatment have the best survival [10].

The relationship between anemia and mortality has not been investigated a lot in PD patients.

Some years ago, Li et al. [11] studied this association in in a large cohort of PD patients. They collected data about 13,974 ESA-treated Medicare patients who initiated PD between 1991 and 1998. Using a Hb value between 11 and 11.9 g/dl as the reference group, they found that after adjustment for demographic characteristics and comorbid conditions, associations were similar in nondiabetic and diabetic patients, with Hb values of <10 g/dl and 10–10.9 g/dl associated with higher mortality; Hb values of ≥12 g/dl had similar mortality associations than the reference value. Hb values of <11 g/dl were also associated with higher adjusted hospitalization rates compared with the same reference value used for the analysis about mortality. While the hazard ratio reached a plateau at 11–11.9 g/dl in the nondiabetic population, Hb levels of ≥12 g/dl were associated with a further reduction in first-hospitalization rate in the diabetic population.

More recently, Molnar et al. [12] analyzed data from 9,269 ESA-treated PD patients from DaVita dialysis clinics in the United States from July 2001 through June 2006. They confirmed that patients having Hb values below 11 g/dl had a higher mortality risk compared to values between 11 and 12 g/dl. Similar to Li et al. [11], they were not able to demonstrate an increased all-cause or cardiovascular mortality in those PD patients achieving high Hb values with ESAs.

Unfortunately, by definition these association studies cannot demonstrate a causative role of anemia on negative outcome. Following the disappointing results of randomized clinical trials testing the effect of complete anemia correction with ESA on cardiovascular mortality, these somehow overemphasized relationships have been downsized. In particular, the possibility that anemia may be the consequence of a higher burden of comorbidities influencing both survival and ESA dose needs has been put under more consideration, in the light of the fact that the majority of these studies did not take into account the ESA dose needed to achieve a given Hb value. Indeed, very recently it has been demonstrated that, as in hemodialysis patients, ESA-hyporesponsive patients on PD have reduced survival [13].

The Hemoglobin Target Approach: Is It Still Actual?

One major question concerning ESA use in CKD patients is the Hb target. Over the last 15 years, a number of clinical trials have tested whether correcting anemia decreases mortality as well as reducing transfusion requirement and improving the quality of life. Unfortunately, none of them has been done specifically in the PD population.

On the basis of the assumption that complete anemia correction would lead to the best results, these have compared lower and higher Hb targets. Unfortunately, the experience has been disappointing in hemodialysis patients [14], while no data are available for PD patients. Aiming at near-to-normal Hb values with ESAs may even increase cardiovascular risk in patients not on dialysis [15]. Recently, the Trial to Reduce Cardiovascular Events with Aranesp® Therapy (TREAT) [16] found a similar risk of reaching the two primary cardiovascular and renal endpoints in two groups of diabetic patients with CKD stage III–IV randomized to either darbepoetin-alfa with an Hb target level of 13 g/dl or to placebo (with rescue darbepoetin-alfa for Hb levels of <9.0 g/dl). However, the secondary analyses showed a higher risk of stroke, death due to cancer in patients with a history of malignancies, and venous and arterial thromboembolic events, with the risk of stroke seeming to be particularly higher in the patients with a baseline history of stroke [17]. Following these findings, the most recent position paper of the European Renal Best Practice (ERBP) [18] did not modify the Hb target to be generally sought in the CKD population (i.e. 11–12 g/dl without intentionally exceeding 13 g/dl), but suggested a risk-benefit evaluation and avoiding high doses in hyporesponsive patients. In June 2011, the Food and Drug Administration suggested to not use anymore the Hb target approach during ESA therapy that should be aimed at reducing the transfusion need, balancing benefit and risks in the single patients [19]. For dialysis patients, without specifying whether receiving PD or hemodialysis, it was suggested to start ESA therapy when Hb levels are below

10 g/dl, aiming at maintaining Hb values below 11 g/dl. The international guidelines by Kidney Disease: Improving Global Outcomes' (KDIGO), which will be published in mid-2012, seem to go in the same direction, i.e. towards lower Hb values for both dialysis or nondialysis patients. However, suggestions are somehow conflicting: on the one hand, treatment is to be individualized while forgetting the Hb target approach and on the other, Hb values are still there.

Clinical Management of Peritoneal Dialysis Patients with Erythropoiesis-Stimulating Agents

All ESAs are effective in correcting renal anemia and increasing Hb levels, but their different molecular characteristics affect their half-lives and biological activity, and consequently their clinical use. Less-frequent dosing is more likely in the case of long-acting molecules. The administration route needs to be chosen on the basis of the characteristics of the individual ESA, economic considerations, and the stage of CKD. Given the lack of a vascular access, it is advisable to give PD patients ESA therapy subcutaneously. Long-acting ESA may be convenient since they allow in-center administration when the patient comes from the monthly visit. This may be of importance in the light that adherence to both dialysis procedure [20] and drug treatment [21] is often suboptimal. In this setting, a number of studies have evaluated the efficacy of different ESA molecules in maintaining adequate Hb levels [22, 23]. Recently, Feriani et al. [24] published the data analysis of the ALTERNATE (A Long-term Non-Interventional Study to Evaluate the Effectiveness of Aranesp® in Dialysis Patients when Administered Once Every Two Weeks), a large multicenter observational trial made in Europe and Australia. Of 742 PD patients, 640 (ESA naïve or shifted from another ESA) finished the study. The primary endpoint was Hb concentration 12 months after conversion to darbepoetin-alfa every 2 weeks. At the end of the follow-up, Hb values were maintained above 11 g/dl, without the need of increasing the ESA dose. At month 12, 73% had Hb concentrations >11.0 g/dl. While the majority of the patients (70%) were receiving darbepoetin-alfa every 2 other weeks, only a small percentage (5.5%) were treated with darbepoetin-alfa once a month. The results of this large observational study are in line with those reported in a pooled analysis of eight trials, evaluating the shift from epoetin-alfa or epoetin-beta to darbepoetin-alfa administered once every other week [25]. The continuous erythropoietin receptor activator (CERA, methoxy polyethylene glycol-epoetin-beta) became available some years ago for the treatment of CKD-related anemia with extended administration intervals (every 2 or 4 weeks). Sixteen ESA-naïve PD patients, who were given either intravenous (0.4 μg/kg) or subcutaneous (0.8 μg/kg) doses of CERA, were evaluated in a small, open-label, randomized, multicenter, crossover study [26]. Also, in this population it was found that the drug has a comparable half-life when given intravenously or subcutaneously (nearly 130 h). A large, open-label, multicenter, randomized, parallel-group, phase 3 study evaluated the efficacy of CERA in ESA-naïve dialysis (hemodialysis and PD) patients administered every 2 weeks in comparison with epoetin three times weekly [27]. The intravenous administration of CERA once every 2 weeks was safe and effective in the correction of CKD anemia. However, the number of PD patients was quite small. CERA proved to be effective also in children receiving PD who were converted from twice-a-week epoetin to subcutaneous CERA every 2 weeks and up to once monthly. As expected in a pediatric population, dose needs were higher compared to adult patients.

Conclusions

As in other CKD patients, anemia is a complex syndrome in PD patients. Some of the factors influencing its development and severity are common to all CKD patients, others are peculiar to the PD population. Unfortunately, this population has largely been neglected by both large observational and interventional studies. For this reason, clinical practice about anemia management, especially about the optimal Hb target to be obtained with ESA, is not driven by ad hoc studies but by data coming from nondialysis CKD patients or those receiving hemodialysis. However, it is unlikely that this gap in the knowledge will be filled in the future considering that, in general, PD patients are not willing to come to the dialysis center more often than needed.

References

1 Gilg J, Webb L, Feest T, Fogarty D: UK Renal Registry 13th Annual Report (December 2010): chapter 9. Haemoglobin, ferritin and erythropoietin amongst UK adult dialysis patients in 2009: national and centre-specific analyses. Nephron Clin Pract 2011;119(suppl 2):c149–c177.

2 Snyder JJ, Foley RN, Gilbertson DT, Vonesh EF, Collins AJ: Hemoglobin levels and erythropoietin doses in hemodialysis and peritoneal dialysis patients in the United States. J Am Soc Nephrol 2004;15:174–179.

3 Stankovic-Popovic V, Nesic V, Popovic D, et al: Effects of conventional versus biocompatible peritoneal dialysis solutions on peritoneal and systemic inflammation, malnutrition and atherosclerosis in CAPD patients. Clin Nephrol 2011;76:314–322.

4 Adachi Y, Nakagawa Y, Nishio A: In patients treated with peritoneal dialysis, icodextrin improves erythropoietin-resistant anemia through blockade of asialo receptors on hepatocytes. Adv Perit Dial 2006;22:41–44.

5 Lucchi L, Bergamini S, Iannone A, et al: Erythrocyte susceptibility to oxidative stress in chronic renal failure patients under different substitutive treatments. Artif Organs 2005;29:67–72.

6 Sotirakopoulos N, Tsitsios T, Stambolidou M, et al: The red blood cell deformability in patients suffering from end stage renal failure on hemodialysis or continuous ambulatory peritoneal dialysis. Ren Fail 2004;26:179–183.

7 Collins AJ, Li S, St Peter W, et al: Death, hospitalization, and economic associations among incident hemodialysis patients with hematocrit values of 36 to 39%. J Am Soc Nephrol 2001;12:2465–2473.

8 Locatelli F, Pisoni RL, Combe C, et al: Anaemia in haemodialysis patients of five European countries: association with morbidity and mortality in the Dialysis Outcomes and Practice Patterns Study (DOPPS). Nephrol Dial Transplant 2004;19:121–132.

9 Volkova N, Arab L: Evidence-based systematic literature review of hemoglobin/hematocrit and all-cause mortality in dialysis patients. Am J Kidney Dis 2006;47:24–36.

10 Harford AM, Zager PG: Mortality risk in dialysis patients with naturally higher hemoglobins. J Am Soc Nephrol 2011;22:205–206.

11 Li S, Foley RN, Collins AJ: Anemia, hospitalization, and mortality in patients receiving peritoneal dialysis in the United States. Kidney Int 2004;65:1864–1869.

12 Molnar MZ, Mehrotra R, Duong U, Kovesdy CP, Kalantar-Zadeh K: Association of hemoglobin and survival in peritoneal dialysis patients. Clin J Am Soc Nephrol 2011;6:1973–1981.

13 Duong U, Kalantar-Zadeh K, Molnar MZ, et al: Mortality associated with dose response of erythropoiesis-stimulating agents in hemodialysis versus peritoneal dialysis patients. Am J Nephrol 2012;35:198–208.

14 Besarab A, Bolton WK, Browne JK, et al: The effects of normal as compared with low hematocrit values in patients with cardiac disease who are receiving hemodialysis and epoetin. N Engl J Med 1998;339:584–590.

15 KDOQI Clinical Practice Guideline and Clinical Practice Recommendations for Anemia in Chronic Kidney Disease, 2007 Update of Hemoglobin Target. Am J Kidney Dis 2007;50:471–530.

16 Pfeffer MA, Burdmann EA, Chen CY, et al: TREAT investigators: a trial of darbepoetin alfa in type 2 diabetes and chronic kidney disease. N Engl J Med 2009;361:2019–2032.

17 Skali H, Parving HH, Parfrey PS, et al: Stroke in patients with type 2 diabetes mellitus, chronic kidney disease, and anemia treated with darbepoetin Alfa: the trial to reduce cardiovascular events with Aranesp therapy (TREAT) experience. Circulation 2011;124:2903–2908.

18 Locatelli F, Aljama P, Canaud B, et al: Anaemia Working Group of European Renal Best Practice (ERBP). Target haemoglobin to aim for with erythropoiesis-stimulating agents: a position statement by ERBP following publication of the Trial to reduce cardiovascular events with Aranesp therapy (TREAT) study. Nephrol Dial Transplant 2010;25:2846–2850.

19 Available at: http://www.fda.gov/NewsEvents/Newsroom/PressAnnouncements/ucm260670.htm; last visited on the 29th of February, 2012.

20 Hollis J, Harman W, Goovearts T, et al: Managing peritoneal dialysis (PD)–factors that influence patients' modification of their recommended dialysis regimen. A European study of 376 patients. J Ren Care 2006;32:202–207.

21 Holley JL, DeVore CC: Why all prescribed medications are not taken: results from a survey of chronic dialysis patients. Adv Perit Dial 2006;22:162–166.

22 Fang YW, Chang CH: Subcutaneous administration of darbepoetin alfa effectively maintains hemoglobin concentrations at extended dose intervals in peritoneal dialysis patients. Perit Dial Int 2009;29:199–203.

23 Li WY, Chu TS, Huang JW, Wu MS, Wu KD: Randomized study of darbepoetin alfa and recombinant human erythropoietin for treatment of renal anemia in chronic renal failure patients receiving peritoneal dialysis. J Formos Med Assoc 2008;107:843–850.
24 Feriani M, De Meester JM, McMahon LP, et al: Extended dosing of darbepoetin alfa in peritoneal dialysis patients. BMC Nephrol 2011;12:13.
25 Mann J, Kessler M, Villa G, et al: Darbepoetin alfa once every 2 weeks for treatment of anemia in dialysis patients: a combined analysis of eight multicenter trials. Clin Nephrol 2007;67:140–148.
26 Macdougall IC, Robson R, Opatrna S, et al: Pharmacokinetics and pharmacodynamics of intravenous and subcutaneous continuous erythropoietin receptor activator (C.E.R.A.) in patients with chronic kidney disease. Clin J Am Soc Nephrol 2006;1:1211–1215.
27 Klinger M, Arias M, Vargemezis V, et al: Efficacy of intravenous methoxy polyethylene glycol-epoetin beta administered every 2 weeks compared with epoetin administered 3 times weekly in patients treated by hemodialysis or peritoneal dialysis: a randomized trial. Am J Kidney Dis 2007;50:989–1000.

Prof. Francesco Locatelli
Department of Nephrology, Dialysis and Renal Transplant
Ospedale A. Manzoni
Via dell'Eremo 9
IT–23900 Lecco (Italy)
Tel. +39 0 341489862, E-Mail nefrologia@spedale.lecco.it

Ronco C, Rosner MH, Crepaldi C (eds): Peritoneal Dialysis – State-of-the-Art 2012.
Contrib Nephrol. Basel, Karger, 2012, vol 178, pp 95–99

Maximizing the Erythropoietin Response: Iron Strategies

Mayoor V. Prabhu[a] · Aditi Nayak[b] · G. Sridhar[a] · S.V. Subhramanyam[b] · K.S. Nayak[b]

[a]Department of Nephrology, Global Hospital and [b]Department of Nephrology and Renal Transplantation, Lazarus Hospitals, Hyderabad, India

Abstract

Anemia is a significant cause of morbidity and lowers the quality of life of patients suffering from chronic kidney disease (CKD). Iron deficiency is the most important cause of erythropoietin (EPO) hyporesponsiveness in CKD. EPO administration significantly increases the costs of CKD management. It follows that paramount importance must be given to enhancing responsiveness to EPO thereby ensuring that the patient derives maximum benefit. Intravenous iron (IVI) administration has been used for decades to replenish body iron stores. Multiple preparations of Iron are available in the market. However, IVI administration is fraught with dangers like adverse drug reactions, susceptibility to infection, and, as recently postulated, direct cellular toxicity. Traditional approaches to IVI administration have focused on multiple administrations of lower doses for fear of adverse reactions. However, recent studies have demonstrated that higher doses can be safely administered in a single infusion, thereby reducing hospitalization costs and patient inconvenience. Newer preparations of IVI are relatively safer, easier to administer and efficacious. Preparations like Iron sucrose, ferumoxytol, ferric carboxymaltose and iron isomaltoside do not require test doses and allow higher doses to be administered at a time with cost and effect benefits

Anemia of chronic kidney disease (CKD) is multifactorial and significantly reduces the quality of life of patients with this condition. Anemia contributes to morbidity associated with CKD and its attendant costs. The introduction of recombinant human erythropoietin (EPO) has revolutionized the management of anemia of CKD. However, many patients show suboptimal response to EPO therapy. Iron deficiency is considered to be the most important cause of hyporesponsiveness to EPO and it is well documented that restoring iron stores reduces EPO requirement and improves efficiency in dialysis patients [1]. Iron deficiency in CKD is due to a combination of factors such as reduced iron intake (anorexia of renal failure, low animal protein diet with low iron content), low gastrointestinal (GI) iron absorption (GI dysmotility of renal failure, phosphate binders, H2 blockers or PPI usage), GI bleeding (uremic gastro-enteropathy, platelet dysfunction, prophylactic aspirin usage), urinary loss of iron in nephrotics, and reduced utilization of oral iron. It follows that replenishment of body iron stores can enhance EPO

Table 1. Causes of EPO hyporesponsiveness

Iron deficiency (total/functional)
Infection
Chronic blood loss
Non infectious chronic inflammatory states
Hyperparathyroidism
Inadequate dialysis
Aluminium toxicity
Vit B 12/folic acid deficiency
Vit C deficiency
Malignancy

responsiveness and lead to clinically significant improvements in patient satisfaction and quality of life. Other causes of EPO hyporesponsiveness are enumerated in table 1.

Iron replacement can be through administration of oral preparations of iron, or by IVI administration. Optimizing anemia management with the resultant cost effectiveness of EPO response is a strong indication for IV iron therapy in CKD [2]. This review looks at the various regimens available and suggested for iron replacement, evidence available in support of such regimens, and newer IVI preparations.

Iron Deficiency in Chronic Kidney Disease

Iron deficiency in CKD may be absolute or functional. Iron deficiency is considered absolute in case of depleted body stores (ferritin <20 mg/l) or functional in cases where body stores are adequate; however, there is increased requirement of iron to match the demands of erythropoiesis [3]. Iron deficiency may be manifest both in predialysis CKD and in patients of CKD on hemodialysis (HD) or peritoneal dialysis (PD). The NKF-KDOQI workgroup in its guidelines recommends that patients of CKD maintain a Hb of 11–12 g/dl (hematocrit 33–36%), and that to maintain such Hb levels patients should be administered sufficient iron to maintain serum transferrin saturation (TSAT) of >20% and serum ferritin of >100 ng/ml [4]. It is important to analyze iron status through the interpretation of laboratory investigations before tailoring appropriate route of administration (oral/IV), and dose of iron administration. The NKF-KDOQI guidelines recommend testing for iron status every 1–3 months, depending on the patients Hb level and the likelihood of blood loss [4]. Approaches to IVI treatment include: (a) periodic iron repletion, consisting of a series of IV iron doses administered episodically to replenish iron stores whenever iron status tests decrease to less than target range, or (b) continuous maintenance treatment, consisting of smaller doses administered at regular intervals to maintain iron status tests stable within target. No evidence exists to compare the efficacy and safety of these 2 approaches. Evidence exists to support the view that the preferred route of administration of iron administration is the IV route [5–7]. These studies demonstrated that IV iron showed a greater Hb level, lower EPO dose, or both compared with oral iron administration. However, with regard to predialysis CKD or PD, the evidence is not strong enough as to recommend one route over the other and hence the NKF-KDOQI workgroup states that the route can be either IV or oral [4]. One study did, however, demonstrate the superiority of IVI over oral iron supplementation in predialysis CKD [8]. In this study, the group randomized to receive IVI showed correction of anemia with replenishment of iron stores as assessed by Hb and ferritin response. This held true particularly in cases where EPO was used and the GFR was lower. The weight of currently available evidence, however, is still not conclusively in favor of the use of IVI over oral iron in predialysis CKD and PD, and the NKF-KDOQI guidelines permit the usage of either strategy. Where used, oral iron is supplemented in the form of 200 mg of elemental iron/day and if found insufficient to maintain response after 2–3 months of therapy, a switch is made to IVI therapy. Issues with oral iron therapy include poor oral bioavailability, GI symptoms due to iron intolerance and added pill burden. Advantages include ease of administration, avoiding need for hospitalization and freedom from the potentially serious adverse effects of IVI.

Intravenous Iron Therapy

Preparations of iron that have been administered by the IV route include iron dextran, iron polymaltose, iron sucrose, and ferric gluconate. Newer IV preparations of iron include ferric carboxymaltose, ferumoxytol and iron isomaltoside. Initially, the introduction of parenteral iron in humans, which was administered as an iron oxyhydroxide complex, was thought to be responsible for the toxicity associated with the administration of IVI. This problem was overcome when the toxic iron was incorporated into a carbohydrate shell consisting of dextran, sucrose or gluconate. It is advised that resuscitative medications and trained personnel be available in the event of the use of iron dextran preparations [2]. In India, with cheaper, excellent quality generics of iron sucrose available, which we have been using (QRON, La Renon Healthcare, Ahmedabad, India), it has become our preferred IVI preparation. The FDA black box warnings for iron sucrose have been removed and test doses are no longer recommended. Apart from the usual concerns about adverse effects with the administration of IVI, concerns have been raised about the association of IVI with oxidative stress/infection and cardiovascular disease. However, analyses of available data reveal that judicious use of IVI does not lead to increased morbidity or mortality, infection, or risk of cardiovascular disease [9–11]. Most concern exists regarding the relation with infection. In vivo, transfusion iron overload in patients is associated with infection by specific iron-related organisms. Evidence linking IVI to dialysis-related infections is lacking. Organisms that thrive on IVI in vitro or afflict patients with spontaneous iron overload in vivo are uncommon among iron-treated dialysis patients [10, 11].

Table 2. An effective IV iron sucrose protocol in PD patients from our center

Repletion regimen
TSAT<20% and serum ferritin <200 ng/ml
Administer 500 mg of Iron Sucrose over 4 h
Repeat 500 mg of Iron Sucrose after 1 week
Draw labs 2 weeks post-iron course completion
If still TSAT <20% and serum ferritin <200 ng/ml, then repeat repletion regimen
Maintenance regimen
If iron replete, recheck labs after 12 weeks and follow above course once again

Dosage Regimens and Adverse Reactions

Recommended dosage for iron dextran and iron sucrose is an IV push or infusion of 100 mg. Ferric gluconate is administered as a 125 mg IV push or infusion. Iron dextran is accompanied by a black box warning of the risk of serious adverse effects. Anaphylactic reactions are seen almost exclusively with iron dextran and mandate the use of a test dose. Anaphylactic reactions are not dose dependent. Mechanisms of hypersensitivity reactions are unknown but may include anti-dextran antibody-mediated mast cell activation, alternate pathway complement activation and direct stimulation of mast cell degranulation. Other adverse effects attributed to IVI preparations include dizziness, hypotension, nausea, diarrhea and back pain. Administration of 500–1,000 mg of IVI, which is usually required to correct deficiency and replenish tissue stores in CKD patients, hence requires multiple infusions or injections which significantly increases costs and morbidity besides being inconvenient to the patient especially in those on PD. Chandler et al. [12] observed that the incidence of adverse reactions increased with the higher doses of around 500 mg in a single infusion and that adverse effects were infrequent in doses lesser than 300 mg.

Our Experience

Our own experience has been that doses of up to 500 mg of iron sucrose can be administered safely as a single infusion over 3–4 h, in patients on PD [13].

89 patients on PD received this regimen over a period of 2 years (211 doses) as per our IVI infusion protocol (table 2), whereby we administered 2 separate infusions of 500 mg each of iron sucrose with an interim period of 1 week between the two 500-mg doses. Adverse reactions were very infrequent and none were life-threatening. We were able to achieve significant cost savings and ensure compliance with our center-specific protocol.

Newer Preparations-Ferric Carboxymaltose, Ferumoxytol and Iron Isomaltoside

Ferric carboxymaltose was the first agent to be approved in the search for newer IVI preparations that could be administered in larger single doses. It is approved in Europe, Asia and Australia. Doses of up to 1,000 mg can be administered in a 15-min infusion. It has been shown to be effective and safe in a trial on predialysis CKD patients [14]. The results of ongoing, adequately powered safety trials with this agent are awaited. Ferumoxytol was approved for use in CKD by the FDA in 2009. The drug is available for intravenous injection in single-use vials. Each vial contains 510 mg of elemental iron in 17 ml (30 mg/ml of elemental iron and 44 mg/ml of mannitol). It has been compared and found superior to oral iron; however, it has not yet been compared to other IVI preparations [15]. Singh et al. [16] administered 510 mg of ferumoxytol or placebo in 17 s twice in 1 week to 711 patients versus placebo to 713 patients. One episode of nonfatal anaphylaxis was observed in the treatment arm in a patient with a history of multiple drug allergies. The authors concluded that ferumoxytol is well tolerated and has a safety profile similar to placebo in anemic patients with CKD. The Ferumoxytol Compared to Iron Sucrose Trial (FIRST) is a multicenter randomized trial of ferumoxytol compared with iron sucrose for the treatment of iron deficiency anemia in adult subjects with CKD, where intravenous ferumoxytol is being compared with other IVI to evaluate the safety of ferumoxytol and assess changes in hemoglobin level. Iron isomaltoside contains strongly bound iron that enables a controlled and slow release of bioavailable iron to iron-binding proteins with minimal free iron release. No test dose is required and is approved for administration in doses up to 20 mg/kg. Wikstrom et al. [17] used iron isomaltoside in a trial of 182 patients of CKD with iron deficiency anemia of CKD. A total of 584 injections were given as a 100- to 200-mg bolus or TDI in doses ranging from 462 to 1,800 mg in 30–60 min. No serious AEs were observed. Efficacy was consistent with established guidelines for CKD. This agent is currently undergoing further evaluation.

Conclusions

IVI is the preferred means of iron administration in CKD patients receiving HD or PD and in predialysis CKD patients. Overall, it is safe and with increasing experience, larger doses are safely being administered. Concerns of increased incidence of infections, inflammation, and long-term oxidative stress have not been proven beyond reasonable doubt. Safety concerns still persist; however, serious adverse effects are very uncommon especially with time tested iron sucrose and relatively less used newer formulations. In our center, we have safely administered two doses of 500 mg of iron sucrose in a single 3- to 4-hour infusion each time with a gap of 1 week between the two infusions with virtually no serious adverse effects. Newer compounds are available in the market which largely circumvent the needs for multiple injections and the attendant inconvenience to the patients. In our experience, our IVI protocol of iron sucrose infusion is probably the most cost effective and safe regimen for regular usage in PD patients.

Disclosure Statement

None declared.

References

1 Drueke T: Hyporesponsiveness to recombinant human erythropoietin. Nephrol Dial Transplant 2001;16:25–28.
2 Aronoff GR: Safety of intravenous iron in clinical practice: implications for anemia management protocols. J Am Soc Nephrol 2004;15:S99–S106.
3 Horl WH, Jacobs C, McDougall IC, et al: European Best Practice Guidelines: inadequate response to epoietin. Nephrol Dial Transplant 2000;15:43–50.
4 K/DOQI Clinical Practice Guidelines and Clinical Practice Recommendations for Anemia in Chronic Kidney Disease. Am J Kidney Dis 2006;47(5 suppl 3):S11–S145.
5 Fishbane S, Frei GL, Maesaka J: Reduction in recombinant human erythropoietin doses by the use of chronic intravenous iron supplementation. Am J Kidney Dis 1995;26:41–46.
6 Macdougall IC, Tucker B, Thompson J, Tomson CR, Baker LR, Raine AE: A randomized controlled study of iron supplementation in patients treated with erythropoietin. Kidney Int 1996;50:1694–1699.
7 Fudin R, Jaichenko J, Shostak A, Bennett M, Gotloib L: Correction of uremic iron deficiency anemia in hemodialyzed patients: a prospective study. Nephron 1998;79:299–305.
8 Van Wyck DB, Roppolo M, Martinez CO, Mazey RM, McMurray S: A randomized, controlled trial comparing IV iron sucrose to oral iron in anemic patients with nondialysis-dependent CKD. Kidney Int 2005;68:2846–2856.
9 Feldman HI, Joffe M, Robinson B, Knauss J, Cizman B, Guo W, Franklin-Becker E, Faich G: Administration of parenteral iron and mortality among hemodialysis patients. J Am Soc Nephrol 2004;15:1623–1632.
10 Harford A, Stidley C, Hunt C, Paine S, Pai A, Scavini S, Brown R, Zager P: Iron dose and survival in hemodialysis patients (abstract). J Am Soc Nephrol 2003;14:266A.
11 Hoen B, Paul-Dauphin A, Hestin D, Kessler M: EPIBACDIAL: a multicenter prospective study of risk factors for bacteremia in chronic hemodialysis patients. J Am Soc Nephrol 1998;9:869–876.
12 Chandler G, Harchowal J, MacDougall IC: Intravenous iron sucrose: establishing a safe dose. Am J Kidney Dis 2001;38:988–991.
13 Sridhar G: High dose intravenous iron therapy in CAPD – a safe, convenient and cost effective alternative (abstract). Perit Dial Int 2009;29:5.
14 Qunibi WY, Martinez C, Smith M, Benjamin J, Mangione A, Roger SD: A randomized controlled trial comparing intravenous ferric carboxymaltose with oral iron for treatment of iron deficiency anaemia of non-dialysis-dependent chronic kidney disease patients. Nephrol Dial Transplant 2011;26:1599–1607.
15 Provenzano R, Schiller S, Rao M, Coyone D, Brenner L, Pereira BJ: Ferumoxytol as an intravenous iron replacement therapy in hemodialysis patients. Clin J Am Soc Nephrol 2009;4:389–393.
16 Singh AJ, Patel T, Hertel J, et al: Safety of ferumoxytol in patients with anemia and CKD. Am J Kidney Dis 2008:52:907–915.
17 Wikstrom B, Bhandari S, Barany P, et al: Monofer, a novel intravenous iron oligosaccharide for treatment of iron deficiency in patients with chronic kidney disease (CKD). World Congress of Nephrology, Milan, 2009.

Dr. K.S. Nayak
Department of Nephrology and Renal Transplantation
Lazarus Hospitals
Lakdikapul, Hyderabad, 500004 (India)
Tel. +91 98480 14555, E-Mail drksnayak@gmail.com

Ronco C, Rosner MH, Crepaldi C (eds): Peritoneal Dialysis – State-of-the-Art 2012.
Contrib Nephrol. Basel, Karger, 2012, vol 178, pp 100–105

Lipid Disorders in Uremia and Dialysis

George L. Bakris

ASH Comprehensive Hypertension Centre, University of Chicago Medicine, Chicago, Ill., USA

Abstract

Treatment of cholesterol in people with advanced stage chronic kidney disease (CKD) clearly reduces cardiovascular risk; however, it does not significantly slow nephropathy progression. Moreover, cholesterol reduction does not reduce mortality in people on dialysis. In general, cholesterol reduction is very important for reducing cardiovascular risk in people with GFR values >15 ml/min who are not on dialysis. There are many reasons for the lack cardiovascular risk reduction with cholesterol lowering in dialysis patients including a defective HDL and higher than usual oxidation rates of LDL. The reviews some of the biochemistry of lipids in uremia and discusses the randomized trial data that support these statements and provides greater detail regarding use of statin in patients with stages 4 and 5 CKD. Caution should be used in dosing statins in stage 3b or higher CKD. Specifically, all statins except for atorvastatin and pravastatin need dose reductions due to safety issues. Given the more 'metabolic syndrome like' profile of lipids in stage 5 CKD adjunctive methods such as fibrates and omega-3 is discussed, however no good data are available in this group on outcomes with these agents.

Importance of Lipid Control in Chronic Kidney Disease

The general philosophy when reducing cardiovascular risk is that absolute risk determines absolute benefit. The greater the absolute risk, the greater the absolute benefit that can be obtained by its reduction. Low-density lipoprotein (LDL) reduction has been clearly associated with cardiovascular risk reduction in the general population. However, a close examination of the baseline lipid levels in advanced nephropathy demonstrated a profile much more like metabolic syndrome with high triglycerides (TGs) and low high-density lipoproteins (HDL) rather than a high LDL [1, 2]. Stage 5 chronic kidney disease (CKD) patients on dialysis are at very high absolute risk for heart disease. Therefore, it was assumed that the greatest absolute benefit could be obtained by LDL-cholesterol lowering treatment in these patients.

To explore this premise, subgroup analyses were performed on data from patients with various stages of CKD enrolled in several statin studies [1, 2].The analyses, however, were predominantly in stages 2 and 3a nephropathy and not stage 4 and 5. These analyses demonstrated reduction in cardiovascular events with stain therapy. Nevertheless a meta-analysis by the Cochrane Group and the Oxford group demonstrated clear benefit of statin therapy in early nephropathy but little to no data in advanced nephropathy [3, 4].

Lipid disorders in advanced kidney disease consist of clear difference from early stage CKD or the general population. Alterations both in the levels of the differing lipoprotein classes as well as alteration in their structures exist. Triglycerides

(TGs) are increased, and both HDL and LDL levels are reduced. HDL fails to mature normally primarily as a consequence of decreased activity of lecithin cholesterol ester transfer protein (LCAT), and HDL levels are reduced because of increase clearance. The HDL that is present consist of small pre-β discoid HDL that fails to function as an antioxidant. All of the apo B-containing lipoproteins exhibit decreased clearance in part because of increased levels of the lipoprotein lipase inhibitory apolipoproteins apo CI and apo CIII [5]. The concentration of oxidized LDL, an atherogenic risk factor, is increased, in part because of the inability of the HDL to reduce oxidized LDL and in part because of the increased LDL residence time effected by decreased clearance. Other factors that also contribute to this lipid profile include relative physical inactivity and high carbohydrate diet [6]. These biochemical issues could not be expected to be corrected by statin therapy alone. Unfortunately much of this information was not known at the time statin trials in dialysis patients were being designed.

Three prospective randomized controlled trials, the German Diabetes Dialysis (4D), the Prevention of REnal and Vascular ENdstage Disease Intervention (PREVEND-IT), and a study to evaluate the use of rosuvastatin in subjects on regular hemodialysis: an assessment of survival and cardiovascular events (AURORA) trials were performed. Two studies in patients with ESRD and the third at an earlier stage of nephropathy. All three studies, however, failed to show a benefit [7–9].

In the PREVEND-IT trial, subjects with microalbuminuria were treated with pravastatin 40 mg daily for a mean follow-up of 3.8 years. No effect on the rate of cardiovascular events as compared to placebo treatment was observed [10]. The longer-term follow-up also failed to show a major cardiovascular risk reduction with pravastatin [9]. However, the trial was underpowered to show a difference between treatments and the event rate was lower than expected.

The two main trials, however, the engendered scepticism regarding statin associated reductions I cardiovascular events in dialysis patients came first from the 4D study and then about two years later from AURORA.

The 4D study evaluated the effect of atorvastatin 20 mg daily versus placebo for 4 years in 1,255 patients with type 2 diabetes undergoing hemodialysis. Surprisingly, the treatments did not differ in the resultant rates of cardiovascular events. Although there was a reduction in all cardiac events seen with the atorvastatin treatment, there was also an increase in fatal stroke. This raised the question of whether the participants in this trial had passed a 'point of no return', whereby lipid treatment was no longer beneficial [7].

The AURORA trial came on the heels of 4D and included 2,776 patients followed for a mean of 3.8 years. This study also failed to show a reduced rate of death from cardiovascular causes, nonfatal myocardial infarction, or nonfatal stroke in patients on hemodialysis, approximately half of whom had coronary heart disease (CHD). This failure to achieve cardiovascular risk reduction by rosuvastatin (10 mg daily) was in spite of significant lowering of LDL levels in comparison to a placebo [8]. More recently, a post hoc analysis in the dialysis subgroup of AURORA (n = 731) sought to determine whether rosuvastatin might reduce the risk of cardiac events. In this analysis only baseline age and high-sensitivity C-reactive protein were independent risk factors for cardiac events with a 16.2% nonsignificant reduction in the primary cardiovascular endpoint [11].

In both 4D and AURORA, patients in the statin group had similar outcomes compared to those in the placebo group for the composite primary end point of cardiovascular death, nonfatal MI, and stroke. Hence, it was suggested by many that since both trials were adequately powered reduction of LDL cholesterol would not benefit dialysis patients. Moreover, the results of these trials prompted some practitioners to totally discontinue statin therapy in these patients.

While AURORA and 4D trials were both powered to evaluate cardiovascular events, the results indicated a higher incidence of events that are not normally affected by statin therapy. Incidences of MI and hemorrhagic stroke, in fact, were greater than what typically occurs in patients on dialysis.

To better understand these trial results a more carefully examination was undertaken of the AURORA trial along with a cardiovascular trial Justification for the Use of Statins in Prevention: an Intervention Trial Evaluating Rosuvastatin (JUPITER) [12]. This analysis examined the effect of statins in two specific patient populations who currently do not meet the guidelines for statin treatment, but nonetheless, are at high cardiovascular risk. One of the major points made was that the lipid profile in dialysis patients may be more responsive to triglyceride lowering therapy in concert with statin therapy. Moreover, it is clear that based on the lipid profile initiating statin therapy in patients at this final stage of CKD may, in fact, be too late to provide a benefit.

More Recent CKD Statin Trials: The SHARP Study

The Study of Heart and Renal Protection (SHARP) trial addressed a very important clinical question – whether lipid-lowering medication – specifically ezetimibe/simvastatin – impacts the risk of atherosclerotic and/or vascular events in patients with advanced CKD in comparison to placebo. The trial was performed largely because of the dearth of data regarding CV outcomes and lipid lowering in stages 3b and 4 nephropathy. The SHARP study was a randomized double-blind trial designed to test the effect of lowering LDL cholesterol on major vascular events as well as on the rate of progression of CKD [13]. The trial was performed in patients with moderate-to-severe CKD, in contrast to the more restrictive enrolment criteria and disease stage requirements in other studies. The trial included both predialysis and dialysis patients.

A total of 9,438 patients were enrolled and randomized to ezetimibe/simvastatin, simvastatin monotherapy or placebo for a 4-year follow-up. The randomization of 1,054 of these patients to simvastatin monotherapy allowed for a comparison of the safety and efficacy of ezetimibe/simvastatin in comparison to simvastatin alone for the initial year of SHARP.

The primary outcome was a composite endpoint of major atherosclerotic events including coronary death, MI, nonhemorrhagic stroke, or any revascularization. Secondary outcomes considered individually included major vascular events (cardiac death, MI, any stroke, or any revascularization) and components of major atherosclerotic events. The main renal outcome among predialysis patients was ESRD requiring long-term dialysis or transplantation.

The mean age of participants was 62 years, and 63% were men. The blood pressure of the participants was fairly controlled (139/79 mm Hg). The mean BMI was 27, 13% were smokers, 23% had diabetes, and 15% had a history of vascular disease (angina, stroke, or peripheral vascular disease). Baseline characteristics of the 6,247 nondialysis patients who were enrolled in the study included a mean GFR of 27 ± 13 ml/min/1.73 m^2, and 80% had albuminuria. This was a high-risk cohort, therefore, for which there was unproven benefit regarding cholesterol-lowering treatment.

After a median follow-up of 4.9 years, there was a significant 17% risk reduction for the primary outcome of a major atherosclerotic event in treatment compared with placebo group patients. These risk reductions were observed across all composite events. This 17% risk reduction was achieved with a mean LDL-cholesterol difference between groups of 32 mg/dl, with the mean LDL cholesterol in the active group being 71 mg/dl. Of 3,023 study patients on dialysis, there were no differences between active therapy and placebo, although there was a trend for benefit, hence, consistent with previous studies.

Dosing of Statins in CKD

Statins are primarily metabolized by the liver, while the amount of renal elimination varies among the statins. There is a risk of adverse events with high-dose statins, particularly those that undergo more renal elimination, in patients with eGFR values <45 ml/min (ref.). The Study of the Effectiveness of Additional Reductions in Cholesterol and Homocysteine (SEARCH) trial explored intensive lowering of LDL-cholesterol with simvastatin 80 mg compared with simvastatin 20 mg in patients post-MI during a mean follow-up of 6.7 years, and showed increased myopathy in the high-dose group [14]. Other statins, i.e. rosuvastatin have been evaluated for safety in patients on peritoneal dialysis and noted that lower maximal doses should be used in such patients [15, 16]. Moreover, some statins like simvastatin infer with drug metabolism of various classes commonly used in conjunction with these agents and hence, make them less attractive than atorvastatin or rosuvastatin [17]. Thus, if administered to dialysis patients, all commonly used statins except atorvastatin and pravastatin [18] should be given in lower than maximal doses due to safety issues.

Additional Lipid Control Considerations in CKD

To reduce the risk for cardiovascular events in dialysis patients current guidelines, published in 2003, suggest a goal for LDL-cholesterol reduction of <100 mg/dl [19]. More recent studies such as data from the SHARP trial support a lower level since the mean LDL achieved was 71 mg/dl [13]. However, since no study has shown a clear reduction in mortality with statin therapy among dialysis patients and the fact that the biochemistry is different than CKD stages 1–4, achieving a target LDL-cholesterol concentrations is not sufficient.

Recent data from Kaysen [20] suggest that HDL cholesterol level is low in dialysis patients and the HDL that is present is dysfunctional. As a result there is a failure to protect LDL from oxidation; thus, there is a disproportionately high amount of oxidized LDL. Addition of the orally absorbable amphipathic peptide 4-F to LDL obtained from dialysis patients protects LDL from oxidation in vitro and reduces the capacity of oxidized LDL to induce expression of monocyte chemoattractant protein-1 (MCP-1) by vascular endothelial function in culture. This may prove to be a useful tool to reduce cardiovascular risk in dialysis patients. Additionally, reducing carbohydrate intake and increasing exercise may also help although no direct data are available on this intervention.

Treating High Triglycerides

As a result of alterations in diet and overall physiology, patients with advanced CKD manifest a mixed dyslipidemia; that is, they have high triglycerides and low HDL. Treating triglycerides and low HDL in patients with decreased renal filtration requires careful attention to the safety and effectiveness profiles of the compounds available. Fibrates are an option but neither has been tested in outcome trials and there major safety issues in the dialysis cohort.

The National Kidney Foundation guidelines (2003), with an update in development, recommend gemfibrozil as the fibrate of choice [16]. Unfortunately, gemfibrozil is associated with many drug interactions, especially with statins. Fenofibrate is not useful as it increases urinary creatinine excretion and elevates homocysteine levels. A recent post-hoc analysis of the FIELD trial, however, suggests it is safe to use down to a eGFR of 30 ml/min [21]. The current Food and Drug Administration labeling, however, precludes use of fenofibrate in in patients with GFR <30 ml/min/1.73 m^2.

Niacin is unfortunately not an option as it worsens diabetes control and is cleared renally, and hence could prove dangerous in dialysis patients. Omega-3 fatty acids can also lower triglycerides. They are metabolized in the liver, therefore renal clearance is not an issue, and they may represent an acceptable add-on therapy. A review of clinical trial database information up to 2009 demonstrates that trials evaluating omega-3 fatty acids did not show significant reductions in LDL or cardiovascular events in this population [22]. In a more recent pilot study, 15 adult peritoneal dialysis patients all on low-dose statin therapy were treated with daily oral 2.4 g docosahexaenoic acid and 1 g eicosapentaenoic acid supplementation in three divided doses with meals for 8 weeks. After 2 months of treatment, triglyceride levels were decreased significantly while total, HDL and LDL cholesterol levels were not affected. Other inflammatory markers such as, CRP, IL-6 and TNF-alpha were not reduced [23]. Taken together with other studies omega-3 fatty acids are well tolerated and are useful to lower triglycerides but do not affect inflammatory markers and have not been tested in an outcome trial.

In summary, data from two randomized placebo-controlled trials and one large substudy in dialysis patients make it clear that once someone starts and requires dialysis for life there is no significant reduction of cardiovascular events with statin treatment. However, the data are quite clear that proper intervention with a statin is of benefit down to stage 4 CKD and must be considered as part of the management of such patients. It is also clear that defects in HDL clearance of LDL particles and a failure to protect LDL against oxidation is a major contributor to increased atherogenicity in the dialysis cohort. The diet of stage 5 CKD patients is a high-carbohydrate, low-protein diet, exactly what will yield a metabolic syndrome lipid profile with low HDL and high triglycerides. Thus, combination therapy using agents with complementary mechanisms must be examined is stage 5 CKD patients since adding ezetimibe did little to improve outcomes in this group. Omega-3 oils or gemfibrozil or dietary adjustments should all be examined.

References

1 Tonelli M, Isles C, Curhan GC, et al: Effect of pravastatin on cardiovascular events in people with chronic kidney disease. Circulation 2004;110:1557–1563.
2 Landray MJ, Thambyrajah J, McGlynn FJ, et al: Epidemiological evaluation of known and suspected cardiovascular risk factors in chronic renal impairment. Am J Kidney Dis 2001;38:537–546.
3 Baigent C, Blackwell L, Emberson J, et al: Efficacy and safety of more intensive lowering of LDL cholesterol: a meta-analysis of data from 170,000 participants in 26 randomised trials. Lancet 2010;376:1670–1681.
4 Strippoli GF, Navaneethan SD, Johnson DW, et al: Effects of statins in patients with chronic kidney disease: meta-analysis and meta-regression of randomised controlled trials. BMJ 2008;336:645–651.
5 Kaysen GA: New insights into lipid metabolism in chronic kidney disease. J Ren Nutr 2011;21:120–123.
6 Johansen KL, Chertow GM, Kutner NG, Dalrymple LS, Grimes BA, Kaysen GA: Low level of self-reported physical activity in ambulatory patients new to dialysis. Kidney Int 2010;78:1164–1170.
7 Wanner C, Krane V, Marz W, et al: Atorvastatin in patients with type 2 diabetes mellitus undergoing hemodialysis. N Engl J Med 2005;353:238–248.
8 Fellstrom BC, Jardine AG, Schmieder RE, et al: Rosuvastatin and cardiovascular events in patients undergoing hemodialysis. N Engl J Med 2009;360:1395–1407.
9 Brouwers FP, Asselbergs FW, Hillege HL, et al: Long-term effects of fosinopril and pravastatin on cardiovascular events in subjects with microalbuminuria: ten years of follow-up of Prevention of Renal and Vascular End-stage Disease Intervention Trial (PREVEND IT). Am Heart J 2011;161:1171–1178.
10 Asselbergs FW, Diercks GF, Hillege HL, et al: Effects of fosinopril and pravastatin on cardiovascular events in subjects with microalbuminuria. Circulation 2004;110:2809–2816.
11 Holdaas H, Holme I, Schmieder RE, et al: Rosuvastatin in diabetic hemodialysis patients. J Am Soc Nephrol 2011;22:1335–1341.
12 Narla V, Blaha MJ, Blumenthal RS, Michos ED: The JUPITER and AURORA clinical trials for rosuvastatin in special primary prevention populations: perspectives, outcomes, and consequences. Vasc Health Risk Manag 2009;5:1033–1042.
13 Baigent C, Landray MJ, Reith C, et al: The effects of lowering LDL cholesterol with simvastatin plus ezetimibe in patients with chronic kidney disease (Study of Heart and Renal Protection): a randomised placebo-controlled trial. Lancet 2011;377:2181–2192.
14 Bowman L, Armitage J, Bulbulia R, Parish S, Collins R: Study of the effectiveness of additional reductions in cholesterol and homocysteine (SEARCH): characteristics of a randomized trial among 12064 myocardial infarction survivors. Am Heart J 2007;154:815–823.
15 Bologa R, Levine D, Parker T, et al: Pharmacokinetics of rosuvastatin in patients with end-stage kidney disease undergoing peritoneal dialysis. Clin Nephrol 2009;72:437–441.
16 Stern RH, Yang BB, Horton M, Moore S, Abel RB, Olson SC: Renal dysfunction does not alter the pharmacokinetics or LDL-cholesterol reduction of atorvastatin. J Clin Pharmacol 1997;37:816–819.
17 Launay-Vacher V, Izzedine H, Deray G: Statins' dosage in patients with renal failure and cyclosporine drug-drug interactions in transplant recipient patients. Int J Cardiol 2005;101:9–17.

18 Gehr TW, Sica DA, Slugg PH, Hammett JL, Raymond R, Ford NF: The pharmacokinetics of pravastatin in patients on chronic hemodialysis. Eur J Clin Pharmacol 1997;53:117–121.
19 K/DOQI clinical practice guidelines for management of dyslipidemias in patients with kidney disease. Am J Kidney Dis 2003;41:I–91.
20 Kaysen GA: Potential restoration of HDL function with apolipoprotein A-I mimetic peptide in end-stage renal disease. Kidney Int 2009;76:359–361.
21 Ting RD, Keech AC, Drury PL, et al: Benefits and safety of long-term fenofibrate therapy in people with type 2 diabetes and renal impairment: the FIELD study. Diabetes Care 2012;35:218–225.
22 Marrs JC, Saseen JJ: Effects of lipid-lowering therapy on reduction of cardiovascular events in patients with end-stage renal disease requiring hemodialysis. Pharmacotherapy 2010;30:823–829.
23 Hassan KS, Hassan SK, Hijazi EG, Khazim KO: Effects of omega-3 on lipid profile and inflammation markers in peritoneal dialysis patients. Ren Fail 2010;32:1031–1035.

Prof. George L. Bakris, MD
Section of Endocrinology, Diabetes and Metabolism, University of Chicago
5841 South Maryland Ave.
Chicago, IL 60637 (USA)
Tel. +1 773 702 7930, E-Mail gbakris@gmail.com

Ronco C, Rosner MH, Crepaldi C (eds): Peritoneal Dialysis – State-of-the-Art 2012.
Contrib Nephrol. Basel, Karger, 2012, vol 178, pp 106–110

Statins and Lipid-Lowering Strategies in PD

Olof Heimbürger

Division of Renal Medicine, Department of Clinical Science, Intervention and Technology, Karolinska Institutet, Karolinska University Hospital, Stockholm, Sweden

Abstract

Both traditional and nontraditional cardiovascular risk factors are considered to contribute to the high prevalence of cardiovascular disease (CVD) in peritoneal dialysis (PD) patients, and CVD is a major cause of both morbidity and mortality in this patient population. Among traditional risk factors, lipid disturbances are very common in patients with chronic renal failure and PD patients have in general, compared to hemodialysis (HD) and nondialyzed patients, an even more atherogenic lipid profile. The pathogenesis of the lipid disturbances in PD patients is not completely understood, but both the protein loss in the dialysate, and the glucose absorption from the dialysate may contribute to these alterations. Hydroxymethylglutaryl coenzyme A reductase inhibitors, more commonly known as statins, are effective to reduce low density cholesterol levels in PD patients and have few side effects. The use of statins is associated with reduced mortality in PD patients, but so far no large randomized controlled trial has been performed concerning the effects on clinical outcome in PD patients (except for the fact that 496 patients in the SHARP trial were treated with PD). In addition, except from their lipid lowering effects, statins also have pleiotropic effects, independent of their lipid lowering effect, that theoretically have beneficial effects on the peritoneal membrane remodeling. Use of alternative osmotic agents as well as nutritional interventions has also been reported to improve the lipid profile in PD patients.

In patients with renal failure both traditional cardiovascular risk factors such as diabetes, smoking, hypertension and hyperlipidemia, as well as nontraditional risk factors such as vascular calcification, inflammation, oxidative stress and endothelial dysfunction, are considered to contribute to the high prevalence of cardiovascular disease (CVD) in peritoneal dialysis (PD) patients, and CVD is a major cause of both morbidity and mortality among these patients.

Dyslipidemia in PD Patients

Among traditional risk factors, lipid disturbances are very common in patients with chronic renal failure and PD patients have in general an even more atherogenic lipid profile [1, 2] (table 1). Compared to nondialyzed patients with chronic kidney disease (CKD) stage 5 and hemodialysis (HD) patients, PD patients usually have higher low-density lipoprotein (LDL)-cholesterol, apolipoprotein B levels, and markedly increased triglyceride and lipoprotein(a) levels. It may be advisable to measure apolipoprotein B level in PD patients as the LDL-cholesterol level cannot always be calculated using the Fridewald equation because of marked hypertriglyceridemia in some patients. In addition, PD patients have been reported to have increased levels of the small dense LDL particles that are particularly atherogenic [1]. The high-density lipoprotein (HDL) cholesterol and apolipoprotein A1 levels are usually low in PD patients.

Table 1. Typical pattern of dyslipidemia in patients with chronic kidney disease stage 5

	Nondialyzed patients	Hemo-dialysis patients	Peritoneal dialysis patients
LDL cholesterol	= or ↑	= or ↑	↑
HDL cholesterol	↓	↓	↓↓
Triglycerides	↑	↑	↑↑
Lipoprotein (a)	↑	↑	↑↑
Apolipoprotein B	= or ↑	= or ↑	↑↑
Apolipoprotein A1	↓	↓	↓↓
Oxidized LDL	↑	↑	↑ or ↑↑

The pathogenetic mechanisms behind the lipid disturbances in PD patients are not completely understood, but both the peritoneal protein loss (about 5–10 g/day) and the resulting slight hypoalbuminemia are considered to contribute to increased hepatic synthesis of albumin and cholesterol enriched lipoproteins resulting in increased levels of LDL cholesterol and lipoprotein(a) similar to in patients with nephrotic syndrome [1, 2]. The hypertriglyceridemia is a result of increased hepatic production of VLDL and lipoprotein lipase deficiency. In addition, the glucose absorption from the dialysate and the resulting increase in insulin levels may contribute to the lipid disturbances in general, and to the hypertriglyceridemia and the increase in lipoprotein(a) in particular [1–3]. The low HDL cholesterol may at least partly be due to loss of HDL in the dialysate.

The association between lipid disturbances and cardiovascular outcome in patients with CKD is also complicated by the so-called reverse epidemiology phenomenon, i.e. the well-known association between established risk factors in the general population, such as hypercholesterolemia, and obesity appear to be reversed in patients with advanced CKD [4]. Part of the explanation for this is likely that there are different time profiles for different risk factors in the different populations, as premature deaths in CKD patients preclude the impact of complications, which are more important for long-term mortality [4]. Furthermore, persistent inflammation and/or protein-energy wasting which both are common in advanced CKD (and both associated with low cholesterol as well as with increased mortality), seems to a large extent account for the seemingly paradoxical association between hypercholesterolemia and improved cardiovascular outcome among these patients [4, 5]. In summary, in spite of the reverse epidemiology between lipid levels and clinical outcome in patients with advanced CKD, hyperlipidemia is still considered to be harmful and to contribute to atherosclerosis and cardiovascular disease in the longer perspective.

Use of Statins to Treat Lipid Disorders in PD Patients

In the population without renal disease, there is strong evidence that hydroxymethylglutaryl coenzyme A reductase inhibitors, more commonly known as statins, reduces the progression of coronary atherosclerosis and reduces mortality from cardiovascular disease. Several studies have demonstrated that statins are similarly effective to reduce LDL-cholesterol as well as apolipoprotein B levels in dialysis patients (in both PD and HD), and that most of these drugs are well tolerated in dialysis patients [1, 2, 6–10].

Three relatively large, randomized controlled trials have been published concerning the benefit of statin therapy in dialysis patients, the 4D [7, 8], the AURORA [9] and the SHARP studies [10] (table 2), However, only the SHARP study included PD patients.

The 4D study [7], which included 1,255 prevalent HD patients with diabetes that were randomized to receive 20 mg atorvastatin or placebo, showed no effect of statin treatment on the composite primary end point of cardiovascular death, nonfatal myocardial infarction, and stroke. However, there was a positive effect of atorvastatin on all cardiac events combined (which was a secondary end-point) [7]. Furthermore, in 2011 a post-hoc analysis of

Table 2. Large placebo-controlled randomized trials of statin therapy in dialysis patients

Study	Number of patients	Therapy used	Decrease in LDL-cholesterol	Median follow-up years	Result
4D [7, 8]	1,255 HD	atorvastatin (20 mg)	42%	4	no significant difference in the composite primary end-point (subgroup analysis suggests effect in patients with LDL-cholesterol in the highest quartile)
Aurora [9]	2,773 HD	rosuvastatin (10 mg)	43%	3.8	no significant difference in the composite primary end-point
SHARP [10]	9,270 (6,247 CKD 5, 2,527 HD, 496 PD)	simvastatin (20 mg) + ezetimibe (10 mg)	39%	4.9	17% reduction in the primary end-point (no significant effect in subgroup analysis of the dialysis patients)

the 4D trial was published. It was conducted to investigate whether LDL-cholesterol at baseline was predictive of cardiovascular events and if the effect of atorvastatin on outcome was dependent on the LDL-cholesterol level [8]. The analysis demonstrated that high LDL-cholesterol levels tended to increase the risks and that atorvastatin significantly reduced the rates of adverse outcomes in the patients in the highest quartile of LDL-cholesterol (>3.76 mmol/l, >145 mg/dl), whereas no effects were seen in the other three quartiles.

In the AURORA study, the effect of 10 mg daily rosuvastatin versus placebo on cardiovascular morbidity and mortality was tested in 2,773 hemodialysis patients (age 50–80 years) [9]. Similar to the 4D study, a marked reduction of LDL-cholesterol was seen but there was no difference in the primary endpoint (death from cardiovascular causes, nonfatal myocardial infarction, or nonfatal stroke; 9.2 vs. 9.5 events per 100 patient-years in patients treated with rosuvastatin and placebo, respectively). In addition, there were no differences in the individual components of the primary endpoint or in total mortality.

The SHARP study included 9,270 CKD patients, that were randomized to placebo or 20 mg simvastatin in combination with 10 mg ezetimibe (which blocks the absorption of cholesterol in the small intestine) and the median follow-up was 4.9 years [10]. There was a significant 17% decrease in the primary end-point of major atherosclerotic events (11.3 vs. 13.4%, $p = 0.0021$). After weighting for subgroups differences in decrease in LDL-cholesterol, there 'was no good evidence that the proportional effect on major atherosclerotic events differed from the summary rate ration in any subgroup examined' including in dialysis patients [9]. In the dialysis patients, the event rates were 15 vs. 16.5% in patients with active treatment and placebo, respectively, a difference that was not significant. However, the risk ratio (treatment/placebo) was higher in HD patients (0.95; 95% CI 0.78–1.15) compared to PD patients (0.70; 95% CI 0.46–1.08), but none of these subgroup analyses was statistically significant [10]. One might speculate that the treatment had better effect in PD patients due to the more atherogenic lipid profile in PD patients, but the SHARP study was clearly not powered to analyze differences between PD and HD patients or even between nondialyzed and dialyzed CKD patients.

Thus, there are no adequately powered randomized trials of lipid-lowering therapy in PD patients. However, results from observational studies suggest a beneficial effect of statin treatment in PD patients. Goldfarb-Rumyantzev et al. [11] made a retrospective analysis of the effect of lipid lowering therapy on clinical outcome in 1,053 incident PD patients from the USRDS prospective dialysis morbidity and mortality wave 2 study, and found that use of lipid lowering therapy (mainly statins) was associated with decreased all-cause mortality (HR 0.74; 95% CI 0.56–0.95) as well as cardiovascular mortality (HR 0.67; 95% CI 0.47–0.95). In a recent retrospective cohort in study in 1,024 incident PD patients from Korea (using a propensity score-matched comparison to reduce potential confounding), statin use (in 38% of the patients) was associated with a 41% lower adjusted hazard ratio for death ($p = 0.002$) [12]. Together these data suggest that statin therapy is indicated in PD patients with hyperlipidemia, at least in patients with elevated LDL-cholesterol and a high cardiovascular risk. However, as the evidence supporting use of lipid lowering therapy in PD patients is based on relatively poor evidence, it is not possible to define a clear treatment target for the LDL-cholesterol level in PD patients. Guidelines for the general population may be used for guidance [13], but their relevance for PD patients is not well documented.

In addition, except from their lipid lowering effects, statins also have pleiotropic effects, independent of their lipid lowering effect, that have theoretically beneficial effects on the peritoneal membrane remodeling, as they might positively affect some of the pathogenetic pathways behind the long-term changes in peritoneal structure and function [14]. Further studies in PD patients are needed concerning the potentially beneficial effects of statins on the peritoneal membrane.

Additional Therapeutic Strategies

Apart from statins and ezetimibe, there are several other drugs that may be considered in PD patients. Fibrates, however, are rarely used in CKD patients as they are eliminated by the kidney and dose adjustment is required [1, 2]. In addition, there is a risk of rhabdomyolyis in particular with the combination of statins and fibrates and this combination should be avoided in dialysis patients. Sevelamer, a non-calcium phosphate binder, also reduces LDL-cholesterol levels as much as 20% in HD patients and is also well tolerated in PD patients, though it is not licensed for treatment of hyperlipidemia [1].

Use of alternative osmotic agents such as amino acid- and icodextrin-based PD solutions may also have favorable effects on the lipid profile, though the effects on lipid levels are not dramatic, and conflicting results have been published. However, particularly the use of icodextrin in PD patients with high glucose load may dramatically reduce the glucose absorption resulting in less weight gain and reduced triglyceride levels in PD patients [15]. Small pilot studies suggest that supplements with omega-3 may reduce triglyceride levels [16], and that supplementation with 14 g soy protein daily, may reduce the lipoprotein(a) levels [17]. In addition, weight reduction strategies including dietary interventions and exercise have positive effects on the lipid profile in the general population, but are difficult to maintain in the long run and to achieve sustained effects. These strategies are even more cumbersome to implement in PD patients due to other diet restrictions and comorbidity, but some preliminary reports show that these strategies may at least be used in some patients. However, for the majority of PD patients with marked lipid disturbances, statin therapy is the therapy of choice as it in general is well tolerated, effective to reduce LDL-cholesterol levels, and has the best documented effect in PD patients.

In summary, lipid abnormalities are more common in PD patients than in HD and nondialyzed CKD 5 patients and the lipid abnormalities in PD patients are considered to be particularly atherogenic. Therefore, lipid-lowering therapy is often warranted in PD patients though no large randomized outcome study has been performed in PD patients. Statins are well tolerated and have similar effects on the lipid levels in PD patients as in other patients groups. In addition, the role of exercise, dietary interventions and other pharmacological therapy need to be better evaluated in PD patients.

References

1 Prichard SS: Management of hyperlipidemia in patients on peritoneal dialysis: current approaches. Kidney Int 2006;(suppl 103):S115–S117.

2 Epstein M, Vaziri ND: Statins in the management of dyslipidemia associated with chronic kidney disease. Nat Rev Nephrol 2012 Feb 21. doi: 10.1038/nrneph.2012.33. [Epub ahead of print].

3 Heimbürger O, Stenvinkel P, Berglund L, Tranoeus A, Lindholm B: Increased plasma lipoprotein(a) in continuous ambulatory peritoneal dialysis is related to peritoneal transport of proteins and glucose. Nephron 1996;72:135–144.

4 Kalantar-Zadeh K, Block G, Humphreys MH, Kopple JD: Reverse epidemiology of cardiovascular risk factors in maintenance dialysis patients. Kidney Int 2003;63:793–808.

5 Liu Y, Coresh J, Eustace JA, Longnecker JC, Jaar B, Fink NE, Tracy RP, Powe NR, Klag MJ: Association between cholesterol level and mortality in dialysis patients. Role of inflammation and malnutrition. JAMA 2004;291:451–459.

6 Navaneethan SD, Nigwekar SU, Perkovic V, Johnson DW, Craig JC, Strippoli GF: HMG CoA reductase inhibitors (statins) for dialysis patients. Cochrane Database Syst Rev 2009;2:CD004289.

7 Wanner C, Krane V, März W, Olschewski M, Mann J, Ruf G, Ritz E, German Diabetes and Dialysis Study Investigators: Atorvastatin in patients with type 2 diabetes mellitus undergoing hemodialysis. N Engl J Med 2005;353:238–248.

8 März W, Genser B, Drechsler C, Krane V, Grammer TB, Ritz E, Stojakovic T, Scharnagl H, Winkler K, Holme I, Holdaas H, Wanner C, German Diabetes and Dialysis Study Investigators: Atorvastatin and low-density lipoprotein cholesterol in type 2 diabetes mellitus patients on hemodialysis. Clin J Am Soc Nephrol 2011;6:1316–1325.

9 Fellström BC, Jardine AG, Schmieder RE, et al: Rosuvastatin and cardiovascular events in patients undergoing hemodialysis. N Engl J Med 2009;360:1395–1407.

10 Baigent C, Landray MJ, Reith C, et al: The effects of lowering LDL cholesterol with simvastatin plus ezetimibe in patients with chronic kidney disease (Study of Heart and Renal Protection): a randomised placebo-controlled trial. Lancet 2011;377:2181–2192.

11 Goldfarb-Rumyantzev AS, Habib AN, Baird BC, Barenbaum LL, Cheung AK: The association of lipid-modifying medications with mortality in patients on long-term peritoneal dialysis. Am J Kidney Dis 2007;50:791–802.

12 Lee JE, Oh K-H, Choi KH, Kim SB, Kim Y-S, Do J-Y, Kim Y-L, Kim DJ: Statin therapy is associated with improved survival in incident peritoneal dialysis patients: propensity-matched comparison. Nephrol Dial Transplant 2011;26:4090–4094.

13 Catapano AL, Reiner Z, De Backer G, Graham I, Taskinen MR, Wiklund O, Agewall S, Alegria E, Chapman MJ, Durrington P, Erdine S, Halcox J, Hobbs R, Kjekshus J, Perrone Filardi P, Riccardi G, Storey RF, Wood D, ESC Committee for Practice Guidelines 2008–2010 and 2010–2012 Committees: ESC/EAS Guidelines for the management of dyslipidaemias: The Task Force for the management of dyslipidaemias of the European Society of Cardiology (ESC) and the European Atherosclerosis Society (EAS). Atherosclerosis 2011;217(suppl 1):S1–S44.

14 Heimburger O: Lipid disorders, statins and the peritoneal membrane. Contrib Nephrol. Basel, Karger, 2009, vol 163, pp 177–182.

15 Paniagua R, Ventura MD, Avila-Díaz M, Cisneros A, Vicenté-Martínez M, Furlong MD, García-González Z, Villanueva D, Orihuela O, Prado-Uribe MD, Alcántara G, Amato D: Icodextrin improves metabolic and fluid management in high and high-average transport diabetic patients. Perit Dial Int 2009;29:422–432.

16 Hassan KS, Hassan SK, Hijazi EG, Khazim KO: Effects of omega-3 on lipid profile and inflammation markers in peritoneal dialysis patients. Ren Fail 2010;32:1031–1035.

17 Tabibi H, Imani H, Hedayati M, Atabak S, Rahmani L: Effects of soy consumption on serum lipids and apoproteins in peritoneal dialysis patients: a randomized controlled trial. Perit Dial Int 2010;30:611–618.

Olof Heimbürger, MD, PhD
Department of Renal Medicine, K56, Karolinska University Hospital, Huddinge
SE–141 86 Stockholm (Sweden)
Tel. +46 8 5858 2530, E-Mail olof.heimburger@ki.se

Ronco C, Rosner MH, Crepaldi C (eds): Peritoneal Dialysis – State-of-the-Art 2012.
Contrib Nephrol. Basel, Karger, 2012, vol 178, pp 111–115

Statin Therapy Is Associated with Decreased Small, Dense Low-Density Lipoprotein Levels in Patients Undergoing Peritoneal Dialysis

Anna Clementi[a–c] · Jeong Chul Kim[a,b,f] · Matteo Floris[a,b,d] · Dinna N. Cruz[a,b] · Francesco Garzotto[a,b] · Monica Zanella[a,b] · Federico Nalesso[a,b] · Alessandra Brendolan[a,b] · Davide Giavarina[e] · Giuliano Soffiati[e] · Claudio Ronco[a,b]

[a]Department of Nephrology, Dialysis and Transplantation, San Bortolo Hospital and [b]International Renal Research Institute (IRRIV), Vicenza, and [c]Department of Nephrology and Dialysis, University of Catania, [d]Department of Nephrology, San Michele Hospital, Cagliari, and [e]Clinical Chemistry Laboratory, San Bortolo Hospital, Vicenza, Italy, [f]Institute of Medical and Biological Engineering, Medical Research Center, Seoul National University, Seoul, Korea

Abstract

Cardiovascular disease is a major cause of morbidity and mortality among hemodialysis (HD) and peritoneal dialysis (PD) patients, and dyslipidemia plays an important role in its pathogenesis. In particular, small, dense LDL (sd-LDL) particles have been recently highlighted as an emerging cardiovascular risk factor. PD patients exhibit a more overtly abnormal lipid profile than HD patients, probably due to the metabolic interference of the peritoneal dialysis fluid. Statins are the main drugs for the treatment of dyslipidemia and they are able to decrease all LDL subclasses levels, but it remains unclear whether they can influence the proportion of sd-LDL. Only few studies regarding the effect of statins on the proportion of these particles have been performed in HD patients and, to our knowledge, no trials have been carried out in PD patients. Therefore, we compared the lipid profile and the proportion of sd-LDL in two populations of HD and PD patients. Our study suggests that statin therapy may be effective in reducing both the absolute amount and the proportion of sd-LDL in patients with a more overtly abnormal lipid profile, such as patients undergoing peritoneal dialysis. Statins do not seem to be effective in altering sd-LDL levels in patients undergoing hemodialysis with other factors that can influence LDL subfractions generation, such as hypertension and diabetes mellitus. If and when our results prove to be reproducible in large-scale studies, such studies should provide new insights into sd-LDL and its actual role in atherogenesis in patients undergoing hemodialysis or peritoneal dialysis.

Cardiovascular (CV) disease is a major cause of morbidity and mortality among hemodialysis (HD) and peritoneal dialysis (PD) patients. Dyslipidemia is considered to be an important CV risk factor both in the general population and in patients with end-stage renal disease (ESRD). HD patients usually present with an atherogenic profile characterized by relatively normal total cholesterol (TC) and LDL-cholesterol (LDL-C) accompanied by high triglyceride (TG), low HDL-cholesterol (HDL-C), moderately increased apoprotein B and E (Apo B and Apo E), significantly increased apoprotein C-III (Apo C-III), and depressed apoprotein A-I and A-II (Apo

A-I and Apo A-II). PD patients exhibit a more overtly abnormal lipid profile than HD patients probably due to the metabolic interference of the peritoneal dialysis fluid. Different studies have, indeed, demonstrated higher levels of TC, LDL-C, Apo-B, TG and small, dense low-density lipoprotein (sd-LDL) with lower levels of HDL-C in PD patients compared to HD patients [1, 2]. Statins are the main drugs used in the treatment of dyslipidemia and they are very effective in the prevention of cardiovascular events. The recent Study of Heart and Renal Protection (SHARP), which enrolled both dialysis-dependent and nondialysis-dependent patients, showed a significant decrease in major atherosclerotic events with simvastatin plus ezetimibe [3]. Sd-LDL particles have been recently highlighted as an emerging cardiovascular risk factor by the National Cholesterol Education Program Adult Treatment Panel III. Since statins are able to decrease all LDL subclasses levels, their net effect on LDL particle size might be null or only moderate and it remains unclear whether they can influence the proportion of sd-LDL [4]. Only few studies regarding the effect of statins on the proportion of these particles have been performed in HD patients and, to our knowledge, no trials have been carried out in PD patients. Therefore, we compared the lipid profile and the proportion of sd-LDL in two populations of HD and PD patients. We also evaluated the effect of statins on LDL subfractions and on the proportion of sd-LDL both in HD and PD patients.

Study Population

The study was conducted at the Department of Nephrology, Dialysis and Transplantation of St. Bortolo Hospital in Vicenza, Italy and was approved by the institutional review board.

We enrolled all the patients who were undergoing HD and PD in our center. The study population included 180 patients: 101 undergoing HD and 79 undergoing PD. The mean age of HD and PD patients was 66 ± 13.9 and 58 ± 15.9 years, respectively. Men were 67.3 and 59.5% in the two groups. 84 HD patients and 64 PD patients had hypertension (83.2 and 81%, respectively). 28 HD patients and 15 PD patients had diabetes mellitus (27.7 and 19%, respectively).

We divided HD and PD patients into 2 subgroups on the basis of the presence or not of statin therapy. The statin-treated group among HD and PD patients included, respectively, 27 and 54 individuals who had been prescribed statins for at least 6 weeks before sampling their blood for lipid profile determination and small, dense LDL measurement. These patients had taken atorvastatin, simvastatin, pravastatin, fluvastatin or rosuvastatin. We compared the lipid profile in HD patients to PD patients. We also evaluated the effect of statins on the proportion of sd-LDL both in HD and PD patients and in the selected subgroups.

Materials and Methods

Small dense LDL cholesterol was measured by LDL-EX 'SEIKEN' homogeneous Assay, (Denka Seiken Co., Ltd., Chuo-Ku, Tokyo, Japan) on ADVIA 2400 Clinical Chemistry System (Siemens Healthcare Diagnostic Inc., Deerfield, Ill., USA). The assay consists of two steps, using surfactants and enzymes that selectively react with certain groups of lipoproteins. In the first step, non-sd-LDL lipoproteins (chylomicrons, VLDL, IDL, LDL and HDL) are decomposed by a surfactant (polyoxyethylene benzylphenyl ether derivative) and sphingomyelinase. The cholesterol released from such non sd-LDL lipoproteins is then degraded to water and oxygen by the action of enzymes. Cholesterol ester is hydrolyzed by the cholesterol esterase and then oxidized by the cholesterol oxidase. Produced hydrogen peroxides are finally decomposed to water and oxygen by the catalase. In the second step, another surfactant (polyoxyethylene styrenephenyl ether derivative) releases cholesterol only from sd-LDL particles and cholesterol released from sd-LDL then undergoes the standard cholesterol assay.

Statistical Analysis

Statistical analysis was performed with the use of SPSS software version 17 (SPSS Inc., Chicago, Ill.,

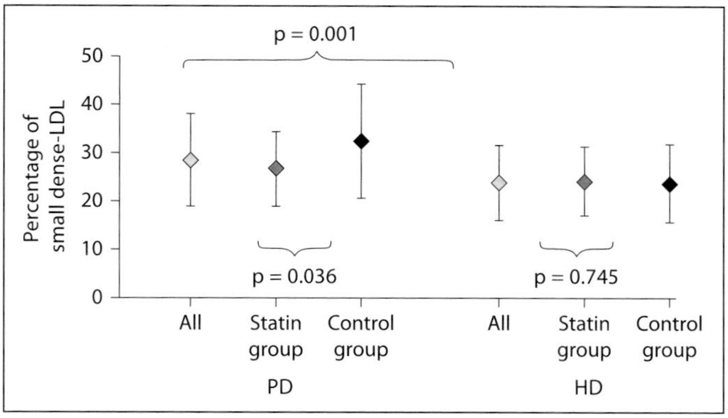

Fig. 1. Small dense-LDL percentage in HD and PD patients.

USA). Continuous variables were expressed as mean ± SD and compared between any two groups using Student's t test. Categorical variables were expressed as proportions and compared with the χ^2 test or Fisher's exact test. Two-tailed probability values of <0.05 were considered statistically significant.

Results

HD patients presented significantly lower levels of TC (p = 0.001), TG (p = 0.007), LDL-C (p = 0.001) and Apo-B (p = 0.001). Both the absolute amount of sd-LDL and their proportion were significantly higher in PD than HD patients (p = 0.001) (fig. 1). No significant differences were found between the two groups in terms of HDL-C (0.602), although Apo-AI level was significantly higher among PD patients (p = 0.003). Among HD patients, the statin group presented significantly lower levels of TC (p = 0.002), LDL-C (p = 0.002), HDL-C (p = 0.001), Apo-A I (p = 0.009), Apo-B (p = 0.006). No significant differences were found between the two groups in terms of sd-LDL and their proportion (p = 0.058 and p = 0.745, respectively) (fig. 1). Among PD patients, the statin group presented significantly lower levels of TC (p = 0.011), LDL-C (p = 0.01), Apo-B (p = 0.001). No significant differences were found between the two groups in terms of TG (p = 0.18), HDL-C (p = 0.618) and Apo-A I (p = 0.956). Both the absolute amount of sd-LDL and their proportion were significantly lower in the treated group than in the control group (p = 0.013 and p = 0.036, respectively) (fig. 1).

Discussion

In this study, we found that statin therapy might be associated with a lower absolute amount and lower proportion of sd-LDL in PD patients, but not in HD patients. Many factors can influence the lipid profile, thus altering LDL subfractions, such as age, male sex, hypertension and diabetes mellitus. For this reason, we decided to calculate the mean age, the percentage of males and the percentage of patients with hypertension or diabetes mellitus for each group of patients.

In our study, we compared the lipid profile of HD patients to that of PD patients. The two studied populations possessed similar characteristics in terms of percentages of male patients (p = 0.348), patients with diabetes mellitus (p = 0.218), and hypertension (p = 0.845). In spite of a higher percentage of patients taking statins (p = 0.001) and a significant younger age (p = 0.001), PD patients presented a more overtly abnormal lipid profile than HD patients with higher levels of TC, LDL-C, TG, Apo-B, and small, dense LDL, both the absolute amount and the proportion. This is in accordance with previous studies regarding lipid profile in PD patients [1, 2]. Further data supporting the concept of a more atherogenic lipid profile in PD patients were provided by a large multicenter cross-sectional study that compared 564 HD patients with 168 PD patients [5]. Several mechanisms have been proposed to explain the pathogenesis of a more atherogenic profile in patients who undergo PD rather than HD. One of these is the absorbtion of glucose from the dialysate solution which can stimulate hepatic lipoprotein synthesis or increase insulin levels, and thus TG synthesis. This is supported by the observation that the lipid profile improves when the overnight dwell is switched from a dextrose-based solution to icodextrin [6]. The daily loss of protein in the dialysate solution may also promote dyslipidemia by mechanisms similar to those relating to protein loss in the nephrotic syndrome. Finally, smaller sized proteins, including different lipoproteins, are lost due to peritoneal sieving. All of these mechanisms might be responsible for a more atherogenic lipid profile in PD patients than in HD patients.

In the present study, we also compared the lipid profile of patients treated with statins and patients without therapy undergoing HD and PD. In HD patients statins did not seem to be effective in decreasing the absolute amount and the proportion of sd-LDL, in spite of a significant reduction of TC, LDL-C and Apo-B. This might be due to the significant higher proportion of patients with hypertension ($p = 0.005$) and diabetes mellitus ($p = 0.002$) in the statin group. The absolute amount and the proportion of sd-LDL can be affected by different conditions, such as metabolic syndrome, diabetes mellitus and hypertension. Anyway, the real efficacy of statin therapy on LDL subfractions is still debated. One of the first studies performed on HD patients was carried out in 2003 by van den Akker et al. [7] who stated that atorvastatin and simvastatin might reduce LDL cholesterol in all LDL subfractions, without altering the overall LDL particle density. Lins et al. [8] have then demonstrated that atorvastatin may be able to shift LDL-C from the small dense to the larger, buoyant, less atherogenic form in HD patients. In a systematic review performed in 2009 by Rizzo et al. [9], rosuvastatin was demonstrated to modulate significantly LDL size and subclasses towards less atherogenic particles as well as the LDL particle number. On the other hand, Choi et al. have recently shown that statins do not decrease the proportion of small dense LDL levels in patients with normal renal function [10].

To our knowledge, this is the first study to demonstrate the association of statin therapy with decreased levels of sd-LDL in PD patients. There were no significant differences between the statin and the control group in terms of age ($p = 0.632$), number of males ($p = 0.461$) and percentage of patients with hypertension ($p = 0.365$) and diabetes mellitus ($p = 0.365$). Our data suggest that statins might be effective in reducing both the absolute amount and the proportion of sd-LDL in patients undergoing PD. TC, LDL-C and Apo-B levels were significantly higher among patients without therapy. There are several possible reasons to explain the different effect of statin therapy on sd-LDL levels between HD and PD patients. First, HD groups were not so homogenous as PD ones, since a higher number of patients with hypertension or diabetes mellitus was found in the statin group. Second, PD patients showed a more atherogenic lipid profile than HD patients, so statin therapy could have had a more evident effect on reducing sd-LDL. There is another important effect to be considered: peritoneal dialysis patients have a mean dialytic age shorter than hemodialysis patients, in general. This is due to the shorter duration of the technique compared to hemodialysis. Thus, it might be that the use of statins can provide a better outcome in patients on PD because they are closer to the status of an incident patient rather than that of a long-lasting prevalent patient. If this is the case, a study comparing the effects on incident patients versus prevalent patients in hemodialysis should be performed. Our sample size is too small to make such a comparison in the present study, however a prospective analysis in this line would be strongly recommended. In this light, the use of statins in CKD, could find a more appropriate use in the earlier phases of the disease when an advanced atherosclerotic damage has not occurred yet.

Limitations of the Study

Our study had some limitations. First, we did not investigate other factors that are known to affect the production of LDL subfractions, such as C-reactive protein, plasma fibrinogen, HOMA-IR, body mass index and hepatic lipase activity. Second, statin and control groups differed in terms of number of patients and of percentages of patients with hypertension and diabetes mellitus. This was a retrospective study, so we could not divide the population into equal numbers. Third, we did not compare the effect of each statin on sd-LDL subfraction. Actually, when we divided subjects in accordance with the type of statin, some groups were too small to analyze. However, we believe that further studies are needed to obtain more exact results.

Conclusion

Our study suggests that statin therapy may be effective in reducing both the absolute amount and the proportion of sd-LDL in patients with a more overtly abnormal lipid profile, such as patients undergoing peritoneal dialysis. Statins do not seem to be effective in altering sd-LDL levels in patients undergoing hemodialysis with other factors that can influence LDL subfractions generation, such as hypertension and diabetes mellitus. If and when our results prove to be reproducible in large-scale studies, such studies should provide new insights into sd-LDL and its actual role in atherogenesis in patients undergoing hemodialysis or peritoneal dialysis.

References

1 Shoji T, Nishizawa Y, Nishitani H, et al: Roles of hypoalbuminemia and lipoprotein lipase on hyperlipoproteinemia in continuous ambulatory peritoneal dialysis. Metabolism 1991;40:1002–1008.

2 Hörkkö S, Huttunen K, Läärä E, et al: Effects of three treatment modes on plasma lipids and lipoproteins in uraemic patients. Ann Med 1994;26:271–282.

3 Baigent C, Landray MJ, Reith C, et al: The effects of lowering LDL cholesterol with simvastatin plus ezetimibe in patients with chronic kidney disease (Study of Heart and Renal Protection): a randomised placebo-controlled trial. Lancet 2011;377:2181–2192.

4 Franceschini G, Cassinotti M, Vecchio G, et al: Pravastatin effectively lowers LDL cholesterol in familial combined hyperlipidemia without changing LDL subclass pattern. Arterioscler Thromb 1994;14:1569–1575.

5 Kronenberg F, Lingenhel A, Neyer U, et al: Prevalence of dyslipidemic risk factors in hemodialysis and CAPD patients. Kidney Int Suppl 2003;84:S113–S116.

6 Bredie SJ, Bosch FH, Demacker PN, et al: Effects of peritoneal dialysis with an overnight icodextrin dwell on parameters of glucose and lipid metabolism. Perit Dial Int 2001;21:275–281.

7 van den Akker JM, Bredie SJ, Diepenveen SH, et al: Atorvastatin and simvastatin in patients on hemodialysis: effects on lipoproteins, C-reactive protein and in vivo oxidized LDL. J Nephrol 2003;16:238–244.

8 Lins RL, Matthys KE, Billiouw JM, et al: Lipid and apoprotein changes during atorvastatin up-titration in hemodialysis patients with hypercholesterolemia: a placebo-controlled study. Clin Nephrol 2004;62:287–294.

9 Rizzo M, Berneis K, Spinas GA, et al: Quantitative and qualitative effects of rosuvastatin on LDL-cholesterol: what is the clinical significance? Int J Clin Pract 2009;63:478–485.

10 Choi CU, Seo HS, Lee EM, et al: Statins do not decrease small, dense low-density lipoprotein.Tex Heart Inst J 2010;37:421–428.

Prof. Claudio Ronco
Department of Nephrology, Dialysis and Transplantation, San Bortolo Hospital
Viale Rodolfi 37
IT–36100 Vicenza (Italy)
Tel. +39 0 444 753650, E-Mail cronco@goldnet.it

Ronco C, Rosner MH, Crepaldi C (eds): Peritoneal Dialysis – State-of-the-Art 2012.
Contrib Nephrol. Basel, Karger, 2012, vol 178, pp 116–123

Phosphate Control in Peritoneal Dialysis

Mario Cozzolino[a] · Andrea Stucchi[a] · Maria Antonietta Rizzo[a] · Irene Brenna[a] · Francesca Elli[a] · Paola Ciceri[a] · Jordi Bover[b] · Daniele Cusi[a] · Maurizio Gallieni[a]

[a]Renal Division and Laboratory of Experimental Nephrology, Dipartimento di Medicina e Chirurgia, Facoltà di Medicina e Chirurgia, Università di Milano, Milan, Italy, [b]Fundació Puigvert, IB Sant Pau, Barcelona, Spain

Abstract

Chronic kidney disease (CKD) is characterized by phosphorus retention and, in more advanced stages, by high serum phosphorus (P) levels. During the last decade, it has been elucidated the central role of P in the pathogenesis of CKD mineral bone disorder (CKD-MBD), determining both renal osteodystrophy and cardiovascular disease. Unfortunately, at least one third of patients on chronic dialysis have high serum P levels, with a consequent higher serum PTH levels, commonly associated with vitamin D deficiency, increased vascular calcification and the highest ratios of morbidity and mortality. In patients with CKD stage 5 on dialysis, therapeutic approaches to reduce serum P levels should include restriction of dietary phosphate intake, optimal dialysis treatment, and use of P binders. In this context, the use of P binders appears to be an essential treatment to control P overload in CKD patients. In this review, we analyzed the use of calcium-based and calcium-free P binders in peritoneal dialysis patients.

The risk of hyperphosphatemia has been clearly reported for population treated with both hemodialysis (HD) and peritoneal dialysis (PD) [1]. During the last 10 years, the role of hyperphosphatemia as a principle actor in the development and progression of vascular calcification has been well documented in patients affected by chronic kidney disease. This evidence is not only related to a passive deposition of calcium and phosphate in vessels, but it is also due to the capacity of inorganic phosphate to directly induce a kind of 'ossification' of the tunica media. In fact, in vitro evidences showed that vascular smooth muscle cells calcify or transform into osteoblast-like cells in a high phosphate medium [2–4]. In addition, lack of inhibitory proteins, such as fetuin-A and matrix Gla protein (MGP), plays an important role on calcium-phosphate deposition in extra-skeletal tissues.

The presence of strong associations between phosphate accumulation and diseases of the bone-vascular axis defined a new clinical syndrome: chronic kidney disease – mineral bone disorder (CKD-MBD). This definition has been coined in 2006 and introduced in a position statement by the Kidney Disease: Improving Global Outcomes (KDIGO) organization [5]. Vascular calcification is considered into the concept of CKD-MBD and since vascular calcifications are predictive of higher morbidity and mortality, the control

Table 1. Factors involved in calcium transfer in PD patients

Regulation by diffusion and convection
Regulation by serum calcium levels
Regulation by calcium concentration in dialysate
Regulation by dialysis dextrose concentration

of serum phosphorus in CKD patients becomes crucial in management of both secondary hyperparathyroidism and probably in the prevention of cardiovascular disease [6].

Serum phosphate levels in uremic patients can be controlled by the reduction of oral phosphate intake, an adequate dialysis schedule and the use of intestinal phosphate binders. Nowadays, several effective phosphate binders are available [7]: aluminum salts, calcium salts, and calcium and aluminum-free phosphate-binders, such as Sevelamer and lanthanum carbonate (LC). Since numerous alternative phosphate binders have become available and there is no ability to predict a safe aluminum dose, the KDIGO initiative unanimously voted that the long-term use of aluminum phosphate binders should be avoided [5].

In PD patients, many abnormalities of calcium and phosphate metabolism are described [8]. Compared to hemodialysis (HD), patients undergoing PD appear to have an increased prevalence of low turnover bone disease defined as adinamic bone disease (ABD). One of the many reasons able to explain this phenomenon is the frequent presence of a positive calcium balance, which may result in an oversuppression of PTH [9]. Moreover, without phosphate binding therapy, all PD patients show a positive phosphorus balance. So that management of hyperphosphatemia seems to be essential to reduce its clinical impact on bone metabolism and cardiovascular system.

Phosphate Balance in Peritoneal Dialysis

Elevated serum phosphate levels induce secondary hyperparathyroidism (SHPT) through indirect and direct mechanisms [10]. Hyperphosphatemia is able to directly stimulate PTH gene expression by mitogenic effects, but it also indirectly inhibits calcitriol production, with subsequent hypocalcemia, which represents a major stimulating factor on parathyroids hyperplasia. In fact, dietary phosphorus restriction appears to prevent parathyroid cell replication and the increase in parathyroid gland size [11].

Interestingly, several studies have described the picture of renal osteodystrophy in PD patients. In one of them, Moe [12] pointed out that patients undergoing PD seem to have an increase prevalence of low turnover bone disease, defined as ABD, as mentioned before. The same data have been previously summarized by Kurz et al. [13]. The most important risk factors for ABD are age, oversuppression of PTH with vitamin D, diabetes, circulating antagonist PTH fragments, and possibly calcium overload from calcium salts or high calcium dialysate. Moreover, the frequent presence of a positive calcium balance results in oversuppression of PTH and in a loss of the normal oscillatory secretion pattern of PTH [9].

In PD, calcium transfer across the peritoneum is regulated by two different mechanisms known like diffusion and convection. These processes depend on serum calcium levels, calcium concentration in the dialysate, and dialysis dextrose concentration (table 1). Sanchez et al. [14] compared the effects on bone metabolism of low calcium PD fluid (1.25 mmol/l) with the effects of a standard calcium dialysate (1.75 mmol/l). They found a significant increase in serum PTH levels and a higher intake of calcium salts in the low calcium group. Nevertheless, patients with a negative dialysate calcium balance may show an overall positive calcium balance, if they are concomitantly treated with calcium-containing phosphate binders, especially when coupled with vitamin D. It is important to emphasize that the KDIGO 2009 guidelines [5] recommend a 1.25–1.50 calcium dialysate for both HD and PD, and this is an additional consideration that should be taken into account when choosing the phosphate binder.

In a multicenter study, 490 Italian PD patients [15] were analyzed for the main parameters of mineral metabolism like serum phosphorus, albumin corrected total serum calcium, and PTH levels. Clearly, a significant number of patients were persistently outside of the guidelines' recommendations. Moreover, in a cohort study from the Netherlands [16], it was found that the presence of plasma phosphorus and Ca-P product concentrations greater than K/DOQI targets increased all-cause mortality risk in both HD and PD patients.

Without phosphate-binding therapy, all patients undergoing PD are in a positive phosphorus balance, unless they are severely malnourished. As mentioned before, the reduction of oral phosphate intake, an adequate dialysis schedule and the use of intestinal phosphate binders are three strategies used to manage hyperphosphatemia in dialysis patients [17]. Inevitably, in the long term, patients rarely observe rigid dietary phosphate restriction [18], especially in the context of PD where a higher number of patients are prescribed a less restrictive diet with a higher content of dietary protein. Thus, in addition to the optimization of dialysis regimens, phosphate binders seem to be essential to control phosphate overload and to improve outcomes in dialysis patients.

Regarding PD therapy, a study with 43 prevalent adult PD patients was conducted to evaluate peritoneal phosphate clearances and its relationship with standard small solute and ultrafiltration adequacy target, and with automated PD (APD) regimen. Results showed that phosphate transfer across the peritoneal membrane is almost exclusively diffusive and can be improved by increasing the number of APD cycles and cycle dwell time [19]. Importantly enough, this study confirmed also that phosphate control showed a major impact on morbidity and mortality than KT/V urea, within the ranges usually achieved.

Phosphate Binders in Peritoneal Dialysis

In the past, in addition to dietary phosphate restriction and dialysis treatment efficiency, the standard treatment for the hyperphosphatemia in CKD patients consisted of administration of phosphate-binders like aluminum and calcium salts. Unfortunately, this 'old generation' therapy is not free of complications. New calcium- and aluminum-free phosphate binders, such as Sevelamer and LC, may open new perspectives in preventing vascular and extravascular calcifications [20] (table 2).

Table 2. Phosphate management in PD patients

Diet
Dialysis
Phosphate binders
Calcium salts
Sevelamer
Lanthanum

Calcium-Containing Phosphate Binders

Calcium salts are effective and well-tolerated intestinal phosphate binders; they are available in two formulations: calcium carbonate and calcium acetate. They were introduced in the 1980s and largely administered also at high dosage, especially for the concept that high calcium level was helpful for a better management of PTH secretion.

Instead, nowadays calcium salts are considered not free of side effects. In fact, they may give a positive calcium balance, especially when used in association with vitamin D or high calcium dialyzing solutions. High calcium balance may oversuppress PTH, exiting in a state of ABD, which is as dangerous as a high bone turnover state. Moreover, it is becoming more crucial that the excess of calcium may lead to tissue and vascular calcifications, increasing cardiovascular mortality. Finally, the minimal requirement of daily calcium intake for an adequate bone turnover remains not well defined because a normal serum calcium level is not really representative of exposure to calcium overload [21].

Regarding PD patients, poor data about administration of calcium phosphate binders are available. Studies comparing Sevelamer and calcium salts in HD patients showed similar efficacy in controlling hyperphosphatemia [6].

Nevertheless, some of these trials, like the Treat to Goal Study, in HD patients treated with calcium salts compared to the Sevelamer group, found more episodes of hypercalcemia (5% in the Sevelamer group vs. 16% in calcium carbonate group, p = 0.004), progression of coronary calcification (6% Sevelamer group vs. calcium carbonate group 25%, p = 0.002) and progression of aortic calcification (5% Sevelamer group 28% vs. calcium salts, p = 0.002) [6]. In contrast, the Care-2 study did not show a significant difference in progression of coronary and aortic calcification in a study comparing calcium acetate and Sevelamer in HD patients (35% in the calcium acetate group vs. 39% in the Sevelamer group) [22].

Regarding all-cause mortality, results by recent studies are discordant. In the RIND study, the authors found that all-cause mortality after 4 years was higher in calcium acetate-treated patients than in the Sevelamer-treated group (p = 0.005) [23]. In the DCOR study instead, the authors did not find a difference between the calcium salt- and Sevelamer-treated groups regarding both all-cause and specific-cause mortality rates (p = 0.4) [24]. An improvement in survival was seen in >65-year-olds in secondary analysis, although St. Peter et al. [25] did not confirm these findings but observed a beneficial effect on multiple all-cause hospitalizations and hospital days (secondary outcomes) in patients treated with Sevelamer. Finally, in a very recent multicenter, prospective, randomized, nonblinded study by Di Iorio et al. [26], 212 patients with CKD 3–4 stages were randomized to either Sevelamer (n = 107) or calcium carbonate (n = 105). Results showed that the all-cause mortality rate was significantly higher among patients receiving calcium carbonate (p = 0.05). Nevertheless, the authors did not observe differences in the inception of dialysis for the two groups. Unfortunately, the main limitation of this study is the sample size, so larger studies are needed to confirm these results.

These discordant data do not permit a 'more correct' strategy for management of hyperphosphatemia to be defined, but they certainly confirm at the same time the efficacy of calcium salts and the potential role of them in developing calcifications. Even if they remain a good choice of treatment, they have to be administered carefully, considering the clinical status of each patient. Current international guidelines suggest that it is reasonable to use information on vascular calcification to guide the management of CKD-MBD [5], and it is suggested that restricting the dose of calcium-based phosphate binders should be considered in the presence of arterial calcification and/or adynamic bone disease and/or if serum PTH levels are persistently low.

Calcium-Free Phosphate Binders

Sevelamer hydrochloride (HCl) was the first calcium- and aluminum-free phosphate binder developed for hyperphosphatemia management in dialysis patients [27]. Sevelamer HCL is an anion-exchange resin containing several amines separated by one carbon from the polymer backbone. Being a nonabsorbable hydrogel, these amines bind phosphorus and bile acids in the intestinal tract [28].

Few data about Sevelamer administration in PD patients are available. A multicenter, open-label study, randomizing 143 adult patients on PD with serum phosphorus >5.5 mg/dl to 12 weeks of administration of Sevelamer HCl or calcium acetate showed the same efficacy of both treatments in management of serum phosphorus and PTH levels. In contrast, serum calcium levels increased in calcium acetate treated patients compared to those receiving Sevelamer HCl (18 vs. 2%, respectively, p = 0.001). Finally, both treatments were well tolerated as previously showed in HD patients [29].

More recently, in a cohort of 317 Canadian PD patients, it has been shown that Sevelamer was able to ameliorate CKD-MBD parameters within suggested target ranges, reducing dosages of elemental calcium [30].

Since data on adverse reactions of Sevelamer in PD patients are poor, the most commonly side effects in dialysis patients treated with Sevelamer HCl are related to the gastrointestinal tract including dyspepsia, diarrhea, nausea, and constipation, and metabolic acidosis. A study of 89 PD patients, 12 of whom were taking Sevelamer HCl, was performed to evaluate the acid-base status. No evidence of acidosis in both groups was found. It has been speculated that persistent exposure to PD solutions containing high lactate or bicarbonate concentration might prevent any effect on the acid-base status [31].

It has been hypothesized that a higher rate of diarrhea and constipation might increase the risk of peritonitis caused by Gram-negative micro-organisms due to trans-mural migration of bacteria [32, 33]. Thus, Evenepoel et al. [29] also evaluated the association between Sevelamer administration and risk of peritonitis in PD patients: although peritonitis occurred in 11% of the patients in the Sevelamer group and in 4% of the patients on calcium-containing phosphate binders, no significant increase in the risk of peritonitis was found.

Moreover, in a recent retrospective analysis conducted in 48 patients treated with Sevelamer, both Sevelamer use and its mean daily intake were not significantly associated with a higher risk for peritonitis (mean peritonitis incidence rate 0.5/patient year) [34].

Regarding nonclassical or so-called pleiotropic effects, Sevelamer was found to decrease serum levels of low density lipoprotein and increase high density lipoproteins in HD patients [35]. These data were also confirmed in an uncontrolled cross-sectional studies conducted in PD patients [36].

Sevelamer carbonate (SC) is a new formulation derived by Sevelamer HCl, where carbonate replaces chloride as the anion. SC has been found to have the same safety and efficacy profile as Sevelamer HCl in HD patients [37]. SC showed a better control of metabolic acidosis and optimal tolerance as described in a study by Ketteler et al. [38] in CKD patients not on dialysis. Its availability as powder formulation, and not only as tablet, may be beneficial especially for the elderly and pediatric populations, and preferable in patients treated with a large number of pills. A review compared characteristics of Sevelamer HCl and SC to evaluate the roles of these two drugs in the management of the hyperphosphatemia in CKD patients receiving HD or PD: results showed that both agents appeared to have the same action in lowering serum phosphate levels, while only SC did not show a decrease in serum bicarbonate in contrast with Sevelamer HCl. Therefore, SC may be more appropriate for patients at risk for metabolic acidosis [39].

Lanthanum Carbonate

LC is a new nonaluminum- and noncalcium-containing phosphate binder that has more recently become available for the management of hyperphosphatemia in patients with end-stage renal disease in 2004. It is a rare earth element whose atomic number is 57 and its binding capacity is very high, similar to that of aluminum hydroxide [40]. It is administered orally and it acts inducing formation and then excretion of highly insoluble complexes with dietary phosphate in the gastrointestinal tract [41].

Data by Lacour et al. [42] in 5/6 nephrectomized rats showed that oral administration of LC may cause lanthanum accumulation in liver, lung and kidneys suggesting that uremia might increase the intestinal absorption of lanthanum. To evaluate the liver toxicity, the effects of intravenous administration of LC at 20,000 times higher concentrations than those used in dialysis patients, was investigated in dogs. Clearly, only a mild liver inflammation was found with no liver toxicity, but only with liver 'handling' [43].

LC efficacy has been reported in some clinical trials in CKD patients [41, 44]. In particular, LC significantly reduced serum phosphorus levels when administered at doses between 2,250 and 3,000 mg/day over 4–6 weeks.

In a recent, multicenter study, 2,763 dialysis patients were converted to LC monotherapy after the washout period for other phosphate binders.

Results demonstrated the same efficacy compared to the other phosphate binders, but with a reduced daily dose and tablet burden, improving patient satisfaction [45].

Effects of LC on bone were specifically evaluated in 98 CKD patients randomized to receive LC or calcium carbonate for 1 year. In the LC group, the number of patients with adynamic bone, osteomalacia or high turnover decreased from 36% at baseline to 18%, while in the calcium carbonate group, bone alterations increased from 43 to 53% [46]. Finally, no histological evidence of osteomalacia was observed in CKD patients treated with LC for up to 5 years [47].

Unfortunately, less evidence and studies are available for patients undergoing PD. An open, noncomparative dose-escalation study in subjects with hyperphosphatemia undergoing continuous ambulatory PD (CAPD) evaluated safety and efficacy of LC to reduce serum phosphate levels [48]. These results demonstrated that LC was generally well tolerated. Moreover, 75% of the patients reached the therapeutic target level in 2 months at doses between 750 and 2,250 mg taken after meals, suggesting that the efficacy dose was lower than that for HD patients. This evidence is probably related to a slow and continuous transfer of phosphate between plasma and dialysate during the 24-hour period of CAPD.

Conclusions

It has been well documented that abnormalities in mineral and bone metabolism in CKD patients associate with increased morbidity and mortality. Elevated serum P levels play an important role in the pathogenesis of vascular calcification in dialysis patients and also appear to be associated with increased cardiovascular mortality. Therefore, control of P retention is now an even more crucial target of treatment in patients affected by CKD. The 'classical' treatment of hyperphosphatemia in CKD patients consisted of calcium based P binders that are not free of complications. New calcium free P binders, such as Sevelamer and lanthanum, can be used to treat hyperphosphatemia in PD patients, not only to control secondary hyperparathyroidism but also to potentially reduce the atherosclerotic process and prevent vascular calcification.

References

1 Melamed ML, Eustace JA, Plantinga L, Jaar BG, Fink NE, Coresh J, Klag MJ, Powe NR: Changes in serum calcium, phosphate, and PTH and the risk of death in incident dialysis patients: a longitudinal study. Kidney Int 2006;70:351–357.

2 Cozzolino M, Brancaccio D, Gallieni M, Slatoposlky E: Pathogenesis of vascular calcification in chronic kidney disease. Kidney Int 2005;68:429–436.

3 Jono S, McKee MD, Murry CE, Shioi A, Nishizawa Y, Mori K, Morii H, Giachelli CM: Phosphate regulation of vascular smooth muscle cell calcification. Circ Res 2000;87: E10–17.

4 Ciceri P, Volpi E, Brenna I, Arnaboldi L, Neri L, Brancaccio D, Cozzolino M: Combined effects of ascorbic acid and phosphate on rat VSMC osteoblastic differentiation. Nephrol Dial Transplant 2012;27:122–127.

5 Kidney Disease: Improving Global Outcomes (KDIGO) CKD-MBD Work Group. Kidney Int Suppl 2009;113:S1–S130.

6 Chertow GM, Burke SK, Raggi P, Treat to Goal Working Group: Sevelamer attenuates the progression of coronary and aortic calcification in hemodialysis patients. Kidney Int 2002;62:245–252.

7 Tonelli M, Pannu N, Manns B: Oral phosphate binders in patients with kidney failure. N Engl J Med 2010;362:1312–1324.

8 Cozzolino M, Gallieni M, Chiarelli G, Brancaccio D: Calcium and phosphate handling in peritoneal dialysis. Contrib Nephrol. Basel, Karger, 2006, vol 150, pp 214–225.

9 Schmitt CP, Schaefer F, Huber D, et al: 1,25(OH)2-vitamin D_3 reduces spontaneous and hypocalcemia-stimulated pulsatile component of parathyroid hormone secretion. J Am Soc Nephrol 1998;9:54–62.

10 Cozzolino M, Brancaccio D, Gallieni M, et al: Pathogenesis of parathyroid hyperplasia in renal failure. J Nephrol 2005;18:5–8.

11 Denda M, Finch J, Slatopolsky E: Phosphorus accelerated the development of parathyroid hyperplasia and secondary hyperparathyroidism in rats with renal failure. Am J Kidney Dis 1996;28:596–602.

12 Moe SM: Management of renal osteodystrophy in peritoneal dialysis patients. Perit Dial Int 2004;24:209–216.

13 Kurz P, Tsobanelis T, Roth P, et al: Differences in calcium kinetic pattern between CAPD and HD patients. Clin Nephrol 1995;44:255–261.
14 Sanchez C, Lopez-Barea F, Sanchez-Cabezudo J, Bajo A, Mate A, Martinez E, Selgas R, Collaborators of the Multicentre Study Group: Low vs. standard calcium dialysate in peritoneal dialysis: differences in treatment, biochemistry and bone histomorphometry. A randomized multicentre study. Nephrol Dial Transplant 2004;19:1587–1593.
15 Gallieni M, Borgatti P, Bottalico D, et al: Mineral metabolism in 490 peritoneal dialysis patients: The ROCK-PD (Renal Osteodystrophy and Calcifications: Key Factors in Peritoneal Dialysis) Multicenter Study. J Am Soc Nephrol 2005;16:456A.
16 Noordzij M, Korevaar JC, Boeschoten EW, Dekker FW, Bos WJ, Krediet RT, Netherlands Cooperative Study on the Adequacy of Dialysis (NECOSAD) Study Group: The kidney disease outcomes quality initiative (K/DOQI) guideline for bone metabolism and disease in CKD: association with mortality in dialysis patients. Am J Kidney Dis 2005;46:925–932.
17 Ketteler M: The control of hyperphosphatemia in chronic kidney disease: which phosphate binders? Int J Artif Organs 2009;32:95–100.
18 Kalantar-Zadeh K, Gutekunst L, Mehrotra R, et al: Understanding sources of dietary phosphorus in the treatment of patients with chronic kidney disease. Clin J Am Soc Nephrol 2010;5:519–530.
19 Botelho C, Rodrigues A, Santos O: Phosphate removal in peritoneal dialysis regimens: an underestimated adequacy parameter. NDT Plus 2010;33(suppl 3):477–478.
20 Cozzolino M, Galassi A, Gallieni M, Brancaccio D: Preventive measures and new pharmacological approaches of calcium and phosphate disorders. Contrib Nephrol. Basel, Karger, 2008, vol 161, pp 234–239.
21 Cozzolino M, Mazzaferro S, Brandenburg V: The treatment of hyperphosphataemia in CKD: calcium-based or calcium-free phosphate binders? Nephrol Dial Transplant 2011;26:402–407.
22 Qunibi W, Moustafa M, Muenz LR, He DY, Kessler PD, Diaz-Buxo JA, CARE-2 Investigators: A 1-year randomized trial of calcium acetate versus Sevelamer on progression of coronary artery calcification in hemodialysis patients with comparable lipid control: the Calcium Acetate Renagel Evaluation-2 (CARE-2) study. Am J Kidney Dis 2008;51:952–965.
23 Block GA, Raggi P, Bellasi A, Kooienga L, Spiegel DM: Mortality effect of coronary calcification and phosphate binder choice in incident hemodialysis patients. Kidney Int. 2007;71:438–441.
24 Suki WN, Zabaneh R, Cangiano JL, et al: Effects of Sevelamer and calcium-based phosphate binders on mortality in hemodialysis patients. Kidney Int 2007;72:1130–1137.
25 St. Peter WL, Liu J, Weinhandl E, Fan Q: A comparison of Sevelamer and calcium-based phosphate binders on mortality, hospitalization, and morbidity in hemodialysis: a secondary analysis of the Dialysis Clinical Outcomes Revisited (DCOR) randomized trial using claims data. Am J Kidney Dis 2008;51:445–454.
26 Di Iorio B, Bellasi A, Russo D, on behalf of the INDEPENDENT Study Investigators: Mortality in kidney disease patients treated with phosphate binders: a randomized study. Clin J Am Soc Nephrol 2012;7:487–493.
27 Raggi P, Vukicevic S, Moyse's R M, Wesseling K, Spiegel DM: Ten-year experience with Sevelamer and calcium salts as phosphate binders. Clin J Am Soc Nephrol 2010;5(suppl 1): S31–S40.
28 Slatopolsky EA, Burke SK, Dillon MA: RenaGel, a nonabsorbed calcium-and aluminium-free phosphate binder, lowers serum phosphorus and parathyroid hormone. The RenaGel Study Group. Kidney Int 1999;55:299–307.
29 Evenepoel P, Selgas R, Caputo F, et al: Efficacy and safety of Sevelamer hydrochloride and calcium acetate in patients on peritoneal dialysis. Nephrol Dial Transplant 2009;24:278–285.
30 Soroka SD, Beard KM, Mendelssohn DC, Cournoyer SH, Da Roza GA, Geary DF: Mineral metabolism management in Canadian peritoneal dialysis patients. Clin Nephrol 2011;75:410–415.
31 Pagé D, Knoll G: Peritoneal dialysis patients using Sevelamer do not present the acidosis problems that hemodialysis patients do. Adv Periton Dial 2005;21:185–187.
32 Singharetnam W, Holley JL: Acute treatment of constipation may lead to transmural migration of bacteria resulting in Gram-negative, polymicrobial, or fungal peritonitis. Perit Dial Int 1996;16:423–425.
33 Bender FH, Bernardini J, Piraino B: Prevention of infectious complications in peritoneal dialysis: best demonstrated practices. Kidney Int 2006;103:S44–54.
34 Kerschbaum J, Konig P, Hausdorfer J, Mayer G, Rudnicki M: Sevelamer use and incidence of peritonitis in peritoneal dialysis. Wien Klin Wochenschr 2011;123:204–208.
35 Chertow GM, Burke SK, Dillon MA, Slatopolsky E: Long-term effects of Sevelamer hydrochloride on the calcium × phosphate product and lipid profile of haemodialysis patients. Nephrol Dial Transplant 1999;14:2907–2914.
36 Ramos R, Moreso F, Borras M, et al: Sevelamer hydrochloride in peritoneal dialysis patients: results of a multicenter cross-sectional study. Perit Dial Int 2007;27:697–701.
37 Delmez J, Block G, Robertson J, et al: A randomized, double-blind, crossover design study of Sevelamer hydrochloride and Sevelamer carbonate in patients on hemodialysis. Clin Nephrol 2007;68:386–391.
38 Ketteler M, Rix M, Fan S, et al: Efficacy and tolerability of Sevelamer carbonate in hyperphosphatemic patients who have chronic kidney disease and are not on dialysis. Clin J Am Soc Nephrol 2008;3:1125–1130.
39 Pai AB, Shepler BM: Comparison of Sevelamer hydrochloride and Sevelamer carbonate: risk of metabolic acidosis and clinical implications. Pharmacotherapy 2009;29: 554–561.
40 Pennick M, Damment SJP, Gill M: The pharmacokinetics and tissue distribution of lanthanum carbonate (Fosrenol®) a novel non-aluminium, non-calcium phosphate binder. Poster 36th Ann Meet Am Soc Nephrology, San Diego, 2003.

41 Albaaj F, Hutchison AJ: Lanthanum carbonate for the treatment of hyperphosphataemia in renal failure and dialysis patients. Expert Opin Pharmacother 2005;6:319–28.
42 Lacour B, Lucas A, Auchèere D, Ruellan N, de Serre Patey NM, Drüeke TB: Chronic renal failure is associated with increased tissue deposition of lanthanum after 28-day oral administration. Kidney Int 2005;67:1062–1069.
43 Hutchison A: Analysis of liver function and hepatobiliary adverse event data from 2000 dialysis patients participating in clinical trials on the new phosphate binder, lanthanum carbonate. Nephrol Dial Transplant 2005;20(suppl 5):V93.
44 Finn WF, Joy MS, LAM-308 Study Group: A long-term, open-label extension study on the safety of treatment with lanthanum carbonate, a new phosphate binder, in patients receiving hemodialysis. Curr Med Res Opin 2005;21:657–664.
45 Vemuri N, Michelis MF, Matalon A: Conversion to lanthanum carbonate monotherapy effectively controls serum phosphorus with a reduced tablet burden: a multicenter open-label study. BMC Nephrol 2011;12:49.
46 D'Haese, PC, Spasovski GB, Sikole A, et al: A multicenter study on the effects of lanthanum carbonate (Fosrenol™) and calcium carbonate on renal bone disease in dialysis patients. Kidney Int 2003;63:S73–S78.
47 Malluche HH, Faugere M-C, Wang G, et al: No evidence of osteomalacia in dialysis patients treated with lanthanum carbonate up to 5 years. J Am Soc Nephrol 2004;15:270A.
48 Kawanishi H, Ishida M, Ishizaki M, Takuma Y, Tamura H, Kobayashi S, Tamura T, Ohashi H, Hiramatsu M, Minakuchi J, Hirakata H, Shigematsu T: Lanthanum Carbonate treatment of patients with hyperphosphatemia undergoing CAPD. Perit Dial Int 2008;28:673–682.

Mario Cozzolino, MD, PhD
DMCO, University of Milan, Renal Division, Azienda Ospedale San Paolo
Via A. di Rudinì, 8
IT–20142 Milano (Italy)
Tel. +39 02 81844381, E-Mail mario.cozzolino@unimi.it

Ronco C, Rosner MH, Crepaldi C (eds): Peritoneal Dialysis – State-of-the-Art 2012.
Contrib Nephrol. Basel, Karger, 2012, vol 178, pp 124–142

Role of Vitamin D Receptor Activators in Peritoneal Dialysis

J. Bover[a] · M.J. Lloret[a] · I. DaSilva[a] · M. Furlano[a] · M. Díaz[a] · A. Herreros[a] · M. Cozzolino[b] · J. Ballarín[a]

[a]Fundació Puigvert, IB Sant Pau, Barcelona, Spain; [b]Renal Division and Laboratory of Experimental Nephrology, Dipartimento di Medicina e Chirurgia, Facoltà di Medicina e Chirurgia, Università di Milano, Milan, Italy

Abstract

Chronic kidney disease (CKD), including patients on peritoneal dialysis (PD), is linked to an important increase in mortality risk. Within the new systemic term CKD-MBD, alterations in vitamin D metabolism are also included. Many adverse events have been associated with vitamin D deficiency or lack of vitamin D receptor (VDR) activation both in the general population and CKD patients, and these associations seem to be maintained in PD patients. Particularities of PD in vitamin D metabolism, calcium balance, low PTH levels and the high prevalence of adynamic bone disease are discussed. We also review the associations of clinical or survival benefits with vitamin D supplementation, VDR or selective VDR activation, although they are low-graded and most of them obtained from HD databases. Nevertheless, we think that the combined approach to secondary hyperparathyroidism seems also to be appropriate in PD patients, and vitamin D (native plus VDR or selective VDR activation) seem an important part of the required integral approach. The later may provide additional benefits but definitive prove is still lacking.

Chronic kidney disease (CKD), and particularly end-stage renal disease (ESRD), is linked to accelerated atherosclerosis with an important increase in mortality risk, mostly of cardiovascular (CV) origin [1–3]. As with hemodialysis (HD), half of the mortality in peritoneal dialysis (PD) patients is due to cardiovascular CV causes [4, 5]. The unexpected and disproportionate mortality in ESRD appears to be due not only to classical but also to other nonclassical (CV) risk factors, including several disturbances related to mineral metabolism [6–10]. Thus, in observational studies in dialysis patients laboratory parameters such as serum calcium, phosphorus, alkaline phosphatase, calcidiol, calcitriol (CTR), fibroblast growth factor-23 (FGF-23), klotho and parathyroid hormone (PTH) levels have been repeatedly associated with bone disease, vascular and/or valvular calcification (VC), arterial dysfunction, and most importantly, with an increased morbidity and mortality, including sudden death [7, 8, 11–13]. It has also been reported that a sustained control of some of these parameters within published targets (i.e. time within target) is also a strong predictor of survival in HD patients [14].

All these studies have prompted these parameters to be considered as non-classical CV risk factors, and the new term chronic kidney disease-mineral and bone disorder (CKD-MBD) has been adopted to acknowledge the systemic consequences of mineral metabolism derangements and their relationship with damage to organs beyond bone, including the cardiorenal syndrome type IV [15, 16]. This term is now universally accepted [10] and alterations in vitamin D metabolism are included in CKD-MBD definition [10, 17, 18]. The circulating levels of calcitriol (1,25-OH-vitamin D) significantly decrease across the stages of CKD, related or not with increasing levels of FGF-23, as a response to chronic phosphate loading or to the direct effect of phosphorus retention on the renal 1α-hydroxylase, contributing to the development of secondary hyperparathyroidism [19–22]. However, as will be discussed later, many pleiotropic effects have also been attributed to vitamin D and thus vitamin D receptor (VDR) activation is considered an important step for both the management of secondary hyperparathyroidism and the beneficial systemic effects of this 'hormone' [23, 24].

Vitamin D Deficiency and Disease

Nomenclature for vitamin D and VDR activators (VDRAs) has become increasingly complex and inconsistent. We shall essentially use the nomenclature of table 1, adapted from previous publications [10, 25, 26].

Beyond CKD, a very high and unexpected prevalence of vitamin D deficiency, as measured by calcidiol (25-OH-vitamin D; classically considered the storage form of vitamin D) levels is being increasingly recognized in the general population and those with chronic inflammatory disorders. Moreover, the importance of vitamin D deficiency as a health issue is increasing because it has been shown that around 3% of the human genome is regulated by the vitamin D endocrine system and that the VDR is almost ubiquitously expressed [20, 27–29]. Thus, it may not be surprising that vitamin D deficiency has been linked to disturbances of immunity, inflammation, cell proliferation and differentiation, VC, neoplasms (e.g. colon, breast, prostate), infection (including the relationship between tuberculosis and sun exposure), and diabetes, as well as in patients with ESRD to atherosclerosis, arterial dysfunction and/or survival [20, 27, 30–32]. Specifically, in PD patients it has been reported that treatment with active vitamin D (calcitriol) is associated with a lower risk of peritonitis [33]. In experimental studies, it had previously been shown that calcium and calcitriol enhanced the antimicrobial function of macrophages isolated from PD patients [34], and that treatment of peritoneal macrophages with calcitriol increased superoxide generation and bactericidal activity [35]. The importance of measuring calcidiol levels is supported not only by these previously described associations but also by the awareness that in addition to VDR, an extrarenal 1α-hydroxylase is expressed at many sites outside the kidney [36]. The extrarenal pool of 1α-hydroxylase may remain intact in kidney disease. This locally produced calcitriol seems to have 'autocrine' or 'paracrine' effects, potentially explaining the additional roles for vitamin D beyond its classical functions in respect of mineral metabolism [37].

Vitamin D Deficiency in Dialysis Patients

Vitamin D deficiency is also very common in patients with CKD [38–40]. Many publications from several different geographical areas now confirm that as many as 80% of patients with nondialysis CKD show calcidiol plasma levels below 30 ng/ml (75 nmol/l). Classically, vitamin D insufficiency has been defined by levels between 16 and 30 ng/ml (40–75 nmol/l), deficiency by levels between 5 and 15 ng/ml (12–37 nmol/l) and severe deficiency by levels below 5 ng/ml (12 nmol/l) [41]. There is, however, no general consensus on these values. The aforementioned 80% value is even higher in dialysis patients and it is only lower, but still present, in some countries with a high-intensity UVB radiation [42]. Wang et al. [43] found that up to 87% of PD patients have insufficient or deficient vitamin D levels, while Taskapan et al. [44] reported the prevalence of vitamin D deficiency in PD to be 92% (43.6% of patients had severe vitamin D deficiency, 48.4% had vitamin D deficiency), with

Table 1. Nomenclature

KDIGO 2011	Description	Name	Molecule	Standardized nomenclature
Vitamin D	Native vitamin D (also known as 'nutritional' or 'natural' vitamin D)	cholecalciferol	vitamin D_3	native vitamin D
		ergocalciferol	vitamin D_2	
	Product of the first liver 25-hydroxylation of vitamin D *	calcidiol (also known as ercalcidiol or calcifediol)	25-hydroxy-vitamin D	calcidiol
Active vitamin D	Product of the second renal 1α-hydroxylation of vitamin D; binds the VDR directly with high affinity	calcitriol	1,25-dihydroxy-vitamin D_3	calcitriol (CTR)
	A synthetic analog of calcitriol, converted to calcitriol in the liver before binding the VDR	alfacalcidol	1α-hydroxyvitamin D_3	1α-calcidol
Selective VDR activator	Act as synthetic agonists to the VDR, but are not converted to calcitriol before binding. Selectively activate downstream pathways (i.e. less effects on Ca and P absorption in the gut, vascular calcification, etc.)	paricalcitol	19-NOR-1α-dihydroxy-vitamin D_2	selective VDR activator (sVDRA)
		maxacalcitol	22-oxa-1,25 dihydroxy-vitamin D_3	selective VDR activator

For the purposes of common nomenclature, we use the terms on the right column along the paper, a combination of nomenclature used in KDIGO 2009 guidelines, Spanish 2011 guidelines and others [10, 94, 130].
*Calcidiol actually binds the vitamin D receptor (VDR), although to a much lower affinity compared to calcitriol. However, calcidiol plasma levels are much higher [24].

a further 4.4% having vitamin D insufficiency and only 3.6% having adequate vitamin D stores. Thus, it seems that PD patients have an increased risk for vitamin D deficiency as compared to HD patients [45]. The former tend to lose vitamin D-binding protein (VDBP) and bound metabolites in the dialysate fluid [45–48]. The calcidiol level in the dialysate fluid has been found to be higher than that in serum in PD patients [45]. These observations may explain not only why calcidiol levels are lower in PD patients but also why higher doses are required to normalize stores [49]. Moreover, during episodes of peritonitis the loss of proteins may also be augmented [50]. Recently, it has been disputed whether, in PD pediatric patients, losses of VDBP contribute to vitamin D deficiency; however, Prytula et al. [51] have observed that peritoneal VDBP losses mirror both dialysate and urinary losses, and are associated with a longer dialysis vintage. Among PD patients, several authors have described a greater prevalence of vitamin D deficiency in women, those with diabetes and somewhat surprisingly, in those without residual renal function [44, 52].

Vitamin D production is influenced by age, diet (limited food intake, dietary restrictions or malnutrition), and sunlight exposure [53]. In CKD patients it is also associated with urinary protein loss (especially nephrotic syndrome), chronic inflammation, corticosteroid treatment, diabetes, obesity, black race, postmenopausal status and dialysis vintage [51, 54, 55]. It has also been recently suggested that uremia by itself may induce an impaired dermal vitamin D synthesis by decreasing photoconversion of provitamin D to cholecalciferol. Furthermore, it has been shown in uremic rats that hepatic synthesis of calcidiol is decreased secondary to a PTH-mediated reduction in liver CYP450 isoforms [27, 56]. As a final consequence, patients with CKD suffering from calcidiol deficiency may also display circulating calcitriol deficiency. In parallel with the deterioration in kidney function, there is a decrease in renal 1α-hydroxylase activity also driven by the early and marked elevation of FGF-23 in response to derangements in phosphate metabolism [22]. FGF-23 also increases the activity of 24,25-vitamin D-hydroxylase, an enzyme involved in the degradation of calcitriol [57]. Actually, new drugs blocking this enzyme with CYP24A1 inhibitors are being developed for CKD patients [58].

Other Pleiotropic Effects of Vitamin D

As mentioned above, vitamin D has been associated with antiproliferative effects and also with regulatory actions on extracellular matrix production (the balance between synthesis and degradation). Thus, vitamin D deficiency has been associated with vascular and myocardial dysfunction, chronic heart failure and acute pulmonary edema, stroke, peripheral artery disease, myocardial infarction, and sudden death in the general population [59, 60]. Consequently, decreased VDR activation has also been associated with the observed increase in CV morbidity and mortality in CKD patients. The role of vitamin D on CV protection has recently been reviewed [61, 62], and several plausible mechanistic hypotheses have been formulated.

Several experimental studies suggest that CV benefits of vitamin D and VDR activation are due to inhibition of the renin-angiotensin system (RAS) [63]. Vitamin D deficiency has also been linked to inflammation, atherosclerosis, left ventricular hypertrophy (LVH) and VC in animal studies [20, 61, 62, 64–66]. Importantly, it has recently been shown in a double-blind, placebo-controlled intervention that vitamin D supplementation had great benefits as an anti-inflammatory agent in infants with chronic heart failure [67]. It helped to accelerate the clinical improvement and cytokine profile balance, causing significant improvements in the heart failure score, left-ventricular (LV) end-diastolic diameter, LV end-systolic diameter, LV ejection fraction %, and myocardial performance index together with markedly increased serum calcidiol and interleukin (IL)-10 and decreased PTH, IL-6, and TNF-α levels compared with the placebo group [67].

In experimental animals, it has been shown that in addition to inhibition of RAS by vitamin D, some VDRAs and selective VDRA (sVDRA) may even significantly decrease the expression of cardiac renin in hypertensive rats and improve certain anatomical, functional, biochemical and molecular cardiac disturbances, including left ventricular dysfunction parameters [68]. Diastolic dysfunction seems to be an strong predictor of death in CKD patients [69], and pilot studies even suggested that vitamin D, and specifically the sVDRA paricalcitol, could protect against LVH and/or improve diastolic dysfunction in HD patients [68, 70]. As will be reviewed later, clinical data in HD patients have suggested that vitamin D administration is associated with reduction in LVH and CV mortality [70–74]. In a prospective study with native vitamin D (cholecalciferol), Matias et al. [72] recently reported an improvement in LVH, as measured by echocardiography, and inflammation markers (PCR) in a cohort of 158 HD patients after 1 year of follow-up. Eighty percent of the patients were insufficient for vitamin and 44% were receiving paricalcitol. These results were observed despite the demonstration that experimental animals null for 1α-hydroxylase develop LVH in the setting of elevated levels of calcidiol and almost absent levels of calcitriol [75]. In this model, LVH is attenuated following calcitriol administration, suggesting that the active hormone has the greatest effect on modification of this end point, and it has been considered unlikely that native vitamin D supplementation (ergocalciferol or cholecalciferol) of similar duration modifies LVH [76]. Despite all these preliminary data, the results of the recently published prospective, randomized, controlled study PRIMO (Paricalcitol Benefits in Renal Disease Induced Cardiac MOrbidity Study) are somewhat disappointing ($p = 0.06$ in a trend not clinically meaningful but favoring placebo) [76]. This study was performed in CKD stage III-IV non-dialysis patients with mild-to-moderate LVH, and the primary end-point of the study evaluating the progression of LVH became clearly negative. Some consider that the cohort had only mild LVH and that a positive effect of paricalcitol, on top of RAS inhibitors in most patients, would have been difficult to demonstrate. Some potentially positive effects were also observed [76]. We shall discuss additional results of this study later in the review.

Through similar mechanisms of RAS inhibition, vitamin D has been also associated with reduction of proteinuria both in experimental and clinical studies [77–80]; these studies have included a prospective clinical trial with the sVDRA paricalcitol in diabetic patients not on dialysis, administered on top of RAS inhibitors, which suggested a potentially additive renoprotective effect [81]. This antiproteinuric action of paricalcitol has also been shown in a small cohort of PD patients with residual renal function [82]. Paricalcitol was started at an initial dose of 1–2 μg daily depending on the level of PTH. Patients whose doses of paricalcitol were maintained at 3 months showed a reduction in proteinuria from 3.1 ± 2.7 to 2.1 ± 2.1 g/l ($p = 0.04$) and from 5.0 ± 6.1 to 2.3 ± 2.1 g/day ($p = 0.012$) [82].

In addition to its direct effects on the CV system or RAS, vitamin D may influence upon other classical and nonclassical CV risk factors such as hypertension [61, 83], dyslipidemia, and improvement of insulin resistance [29, 84, 85]. Inflammation through different pathways (Wnt/β-catenin, NFκB, RAS) has been recognized as an important mediator in many systemic diseases, and anti-inflammatory properties have been attributed to vitamin D [20, 86]. Protection against VC has also been associated with vitamin D (although high doses of vitamin D together with a high phosphorus diet is a known and easy model of VC in uremic rats) [20, 87]. A dose-dependent effect (high pharmacological versus more physiological doses) and the influence of phosphate loading are definitely present. London et al. [13] have found an association between low calcidiol and calcitriol levels with arteriosclerosis and endothelial dysfunction in HD patients. In 50 prevalent nondiabetic PD patients, dialysate glucose exposure was recently shown in a preliminary study to be an independent predictor of coronary artery calcification score, in addition to serum calcium and Kt/V (urea) in multivariate analysis [88]. Also in PD patients with vitamin D deficiency, the effect of vitamin D replacement was evaluated on physical performance tests, static and dynamic balance tests and isometric strength tests [89]. Vitamin D supplementation improved muscle strength, functional ability and balance in these patients. As a final point, it is necessary to consider that vitamin D and reduction of renal 1α-hydroxylase activity are very well-known stimulators of PTH synthesis and secretion, and proliferation of the parathyroid cells [19]. The effect of PTH has also been associated to many deleterious systemic effects which could be potentially controlled by VDRAs [19, 90]. In table 2, we summarize some of the many pleiotropic effects attributed to vitamin D.

Peritoneal Dialysis and Low PTH Levels

It is important to remember that both high and low PTH levels are associated with increased mortality in CKD patients, although the PTH levels identified as entailing risk are quite variable and depend on the considered geographical area as well [10, 26, 91–94]. Recently, Floege et al. [91] have shown that HD patients with intact PTH, calcium and phosphate levels within the KDOQI 2003 target ranges have a lower risk of mortality than patients outside those target ranges [41, 91]. For this and other reasons, the 2011 Spanish Guidelines on CKD-MBD [94] suggested that the intact PTH target range should still be maintained at 150–300 pg/ml as targets (and that levels <100 or >500 pg/ml 'corrected' for the PTH assay should in particular be avoided as they represent extremes of risk; a concept similar to that used in the KDIGO 2009 guidelines). The importance of taking into account 'trends' is also recognized, and it is acknowledged that PTH levels should not be considered an 'emergency' leading to rapid changes in drug doses [10, 94]. These goals are different than the intact PTH levels associated with a high specificity for the diagnosis of either high or low bone turnover according to the KDIGO 2009 guidelines (2–9 times the upper limit of normal for the PTH assay) [10].

Adynamic bone disease (ABD) is characterized by a low bone formation rate (without the increase in osteoid volume diagnostic of osteomalacia). Potential causative factors include specially the presence of relatively low PTH levels [18, 95–97]. It seems that ABD is related to several complications including an impairment of the bone calcium-buffering ability of bone in handling any extra calcium load [98]. Consequently, ABD has also been associated with VC since calcium may be deposited in vessels instead of bone [18]. It is known that PD patients suffer from a higher prevalence of ABD than their HD counterparts (biopsy-confirmed ABD has been observed in 60% and 36% of patients, respectively) [96, 97, 99, 100]. Furthermore, some studies in PD patients have established an independent correlation between a femoral low bone mineral density and increased VC, arterial stiffness and peripheral artery disease [101–103]. The higher frequency of relatively low PTH levels in PD patients or skeletal resistance to the action of PTH in CKD is not completely understood. Several factors may explain these observations such as a greater prevalence of diabetic patients in PD programs and a positive calcium balance [104]. This positive calcium balance is linked not only to the use of calcium-based phosphate binders in patients with low PTH but also to a potentially positive balance from the high concentration of the peritoneal fluid for long periods [103]. Calcium flux during PD is an important determinant of overall calcium balance. The calcium concentration of the dialysate therefore should be adjusted to optimize the total body calcium load [10]. Theoretically, this strategy should help to improve bone health by reducing calcium flux during PD in patients with ABD and extraskeletal calcification, and by inducing a positive calcium flux if needed. However, the strategy has not been adequately investigated prospectively neither in either HD or PD patients. Calcium balance in PD is especially complex since these patients have a protein loss in the dialysate fluid and thus calcium levels should be calculated as a function of albumin levels or directly assessed by ionized calcium.

It is also worth emphasizing that in some European countries a dialysate calcium concentration of 1.75 mmol/l (3.5 mEq/l) is still used (e.g. 75% of PD patients in Spain are receiving it), though this concentration has been widely abandoned in HD except after parathyroidectomy or symptomatic hypocalcemia. The KDIGO 2009 guidelines (and indirectly the 2011 Spanish Society ones) suggest that a PD calcium concentration as high as 1.75 mmol/l should be avoided to prevent calcium overload and the induction of ABD [10, 94]. Therefore, similar calcium concentrations are now recommended for both HD and PD [10]. In addition, in these patients and those with suspicion of ABD, calcium-based phosphate binders and/or nonselective VDRAs, both of which have a lower therapeutic window, have shown an association with hypercalcemia and, at least in experimental animals and some studies, a faster progression of VC [103, 105, 106]. VC

Table 2. Experimental effects of vitamin D receptor activators beyond bone

Cardiovascular effects
Reduction of myocyte hypertrophy and proliferation
(improvement of anatomical profile; attenuation of progression of LVH not proven in CKD patients)
Inhibition of arterial calcification (low doses)
Paricalcitol is less pro-calcifying than others at equipotent doses and independently of calcium and phosphate
Increased arterial calcification (at pharmacological doses, especially in the presence of a phosphate load and/or kidney disease)
Improvement of systolic and diastolic myocardial dysfunction
Improvement of functional profile; not proven in humans
Improvement of left atrial volume
Modulation of calcium flux and contractility
Modulation of extracellular matrix turnover: ↑ degradation, ↓ synthesis
Anti-atherogenic
Improvement of endothelial dysfunction
Reduction of vascular cell proliferation
Antihypertensive effects
PTH suppression (effects beyond bone)
Decreases natriuretic peptides (BNP)
Downregulates endothelin receptors
Downregulates EGFR
Kidney effects
Renin-angiotensin-aldosterone system inhibition
Increases nephrin expression in podocytes
Antifibrotic glomerular and tubular effects: modulation of extracellular matrix turnover including epithelial-mesenchymal transition
Decreases glomerular cell growth
Antiproteinuric action (experimental and human)
Anti-inflammatory effects
(mediate many of the effects mentioned above)
Reduction of C-reactive protein
Decreases MCP-1
Decreases TNF-α, IL-1, IL-6
Decreases the expression of NF-κB
Increases IL-10, IL-4
Reduces TACE activity (TNF-angiotensin-converting enzyme)
Competitive antagonism with endothelial nitric oxide synthase
Other
(mediate many of the effects mentioned above)
Antithrombotic
Decreases oxidative stress
Modulation of the immune system
Bactericidal
Upregulation of VDR and calcium-sensing receptor
Upregulation of osteopontin, MGP, calbindin, megalin
Upregulation of p21, p27
Upregulation of insulin receptor and influence on pancreatic β-cell function
Improves EPO resistance

will be further analyzed below. Despite the aforementioned considerations, the choice of dialysate calcium (and CKD-MBD treatments) should be individualized whenever possible in order to meet specific patient requirements (for instance, taking into account age for a growing patient, PTH levels, PTH plus alkaline phosphatase serum levels, concomitant use of VDRAs or calcimimetics, etc.). It is our belief that calcium-based phosphate binders or antiparathyroid agents (VDRAs or calcimimetics) should be carefully monitored in PD patients dialyzed with high calcium fluids [103]. Nevertheless, there have not been significant differences when the proportion of patients taking VDRAs were compared between PD patients with or without VC [107–109]. A closer follow-up in this particular population is probably needed.

Vitamin D and Association with Survival

As a consequence of the above-mentioned associations, low plasma calcidiol levels have been uniformly linked to decreased survival in the general population and in CKD and dialysis patients [30, 43, 59, 110]. In an American study, Wolf et al. [110] performed a cross-sectional analysis of 825 consecutive patients from within a prospective cohort of incident HD patients; they found, in an elegant nested case-control analysis, that low calcidiol and calcitriol serum levels were significantly associated with 90-day all-cause and CV mortality [110]. Similarly, the NECOSAD Dutch study [111] described an increased total and CV-mortality risk in vitamin-D deficient (≤10 ng/ml) dialysis patients, including 36% on PD. Analysis of a longer follow-up showed that the association between vitamin D levels and survival was stronger after 6 months than after 3 years. No relationship was found between vitamin D status and non-CV mortality, but the number of patients and events likely lacked sufficient statistical power. This study also revealed that the impact of calcidiol levels on clinical events was modified by PTH status, with low calcidiol levels meaningfully affecting outcomes only in patients with PTH levels above the median of 123 pmol/l [111].

Wang et al. performed the first observational study in 230 prevalent PD patients and then they followed these patients prospectively for 3 years or until death [43]. They confirmed in this cohort the association between serum vitamin D status and increase in CV events. Adjusting for clinical and demographic factors, every 1-unit increase (nmol/l) in log-transformed serum calcidiol was associated with a 44% reduction in the risk of fatal or nonfatal cardiovascular events (95% CI 0.35–0.91). Furthermore, serum calcidiol status appeared to show a differential influence on CV outcomes of PD patients depending on the degree of left ventricular hypertrophy and systolic dysfunction. Kaplan-Meier estimates revealed a significantly greater fatal or non-fatal CV event-free survival probability among patients with serum calcidiol above the median (>45.7 nmol/l) than among patients with concentrations ≤45.7 nmol/l. In addition, patients with calcidiol >45.7 nmol/l had a significantly higher CV event-free survival probability than did patients with calcidiol ≤45.7 nmol/l in the stratified analysis for patients with left ventricular mass index less than the median ($p = 0.013$) or normal systolic function ($p = 0.005$). Interestingly enough, the association between calcidiol levels and outcomes was lost when residual renal function and echocardiographic parameters were considered, potentially suggesting that vitamin D may link the loss of residual renal function and CV mortality in these patients. Thus, the serum calcidiol status appeared to exert a differential influence on the CV outcomes of PD patients depending on the degree of LVH and systolic dysfunction. As a result, in patients with an ejection fraction ≤50% or a ventricular mass index ≥206 g/m^2, the vitamin D status had no influence on CV survival. This may suggest that vitamin D plays an important role in less severe forms of cardiac disease, that it may influence diastolic function more than systolic function, that different models of cardiac disease (e.g. with or without renal failure, phosphate loading, etc.) may lead to distinct pathway mechanisms, or that vitamin D affects cardiac anatomical structure less predictably than cardiac function [68, 75, 112–115].

Although observational and experimental studies establish a quite unidirectional and uniform relationship between vitamin D and mortality, vitamin D is also a surrogate marker of nutritional and overall health status, creating some potential biases in the absence of prospective randomized controlled studies. In this context, the results of the recently published prospective, randomized and controlled PRIMO study were unexpected [76]. PRIMO showed that 48 weeks of therapy with high doses of paricalcitol (2 μg/day, doses sufficient to suppress serum intact PTH) did not alter left ventricular mass index, as measured by cardiovascular magnetic resonance imaging, or improve certain Doppler measures of diastolic dysfunction in patients with stage 3–4 CKD. Eligibility criteria included mild-to-moderate LVH (septal wall thickness of 1.1–1.7 cm in women and 1.2–1.8 cm in men), left-ventricular ejection fraction greater than 50%, and estimated glomerular filtration rate of 15–60 ml/min/1.73 m^2. Individuals taking RAS inhibitors followed the same regimen for at least 1 month prior to screening and throughout the study. Nevertheless, paricalcitol did reduce CV hospitalizations, primarily for congestive heart failure and, in post hoc analysis, it also reduced left atrial volume, a measure linked to adverse CV events, particularly congestive heart failure, and attenuated the increase in blood levels of brain natriuretic peptide (BNP), particularly in those with prominent LVH at baseline [76]. BNP and the N-terminal fragment of B-type natriuretic peptide (NT-proBNP) are highly correlated with calcidiol levels in PD patients [116]. At least the N-terminal fragment of B-type natriuretic peptide (NT-proBNP) has been shown to be a reliable predictor of death risk independently of the effect of dialysis modality on fluid volume control in a prospective multicenter cohort of 753 prevalent adult patients on PD (continuous ambulatory PD or automated PD) and HD [117]. Accordingly, future outcome studies with paricalcitol should target patients with CKD and a history of congestive heart failure with preserved systolic function [76]. Although it does not directly affect PD patients, the focus of our article, we think that it is important to consider that more frequent episodes of hypercalcemia at this high dose of paricalcitol were linked to a higher number of patients reaching ESRD [76], since hypercalcemia can decrease residual renal function if not properly monitored.

Treatment with Vitamin D and Survival

Native Vitamin D Replacement and Survival in CKD Patients

In a recent meta-analysis, supplementation of native vitamin D in deficient patients appeared to reduce mortality as compared to placebo in the general population [118]. A nutritional trial focusing on the role of vitamin D in the primary prevention of CV disease started in January 2010, this being one more than 200 vitamin D trials ongoing in the general population. Since the KDOQI 2003 recommendations were published [41], an increasing number of reports devoted to vitamin D supplementation in CKD patients with either cholecalciferol (mostly in Europe) or ergocalciferol (mostly in the United States) have been published. In some countries, calcidiol itself is used as a 'native' vitamin D supplement for the sake of convenience, but strictly speaking calcidiol may act directly upon VDR [24] and the conversion 1:1 in international units (IU) leads to overdosage, especially if plasma levels are not being monitored. Nonetheless, the use of any of these forms of vitamin D has been shown to correct most vitamin D deficiencies even in HD and PD patients, and supplementation is considered in most current guidelines when low levels of vitamin D are present [10, 94]. The best cut-off (i.e. >20 to >30 ng/ml) is still under dispute [27, 41, 94, 119–122], even within the same country [94, 122]. However, nonuniform effects on mineral metabolism parameters have been reported in CKD patients [123]. It has even been suggested that calcidiol levels should be evaluated and replaced in CKD patients regardless of PTH and independently of whether they are receiving a VDRA [94, 124].

Whether native vitamin D supplementation in CKD and dialysis patients reduces mortality and CV events is still a burning question. As mentioned before, current knowledge on this topic is based on only in a few observational studies [27]. However, almost none have evaluated hard endpoints or outcomes with native vitamin D, and only some epidemiological descriptions have been reported [123]. The ideal vitamin D therapy for CKD patients should be the one that improves survival irrespective of suggested or imposed target ranges for arbitrary or opinion-based surrogate endpoints [123]. Although we think that randomized controlled trials are needed to verify which agents offer superior survival advantages, we still give some priority to sVDRAs, which at least have been associated with improved survival (see below). Additionally, a recent meta-analysis showed that higher calcidiol levels are associated with significantly improved survival in patients with CKD and dialysis patients [62, 111, 125]. Nevertheless, to our knowledge, not even an association between treatment with native vitamin D and survival has yet been described. Finally, it has been shown that the relationship between calcidiol levels and mortality disappeared when patients were treated with active forms of vitamin D (mostly paricalcitol) [110]. This observation may be explained, at least partially, by the fact that an active vitamin D (i.e. calcitriol) seems to be necessary to improve the in-vitro cellular uptake of calcidiol (i.e. by 1α-containing cells such as macrophages) and the relative importance of active versus native vitamin D [24, 36, 76, 126, 127].

Beyond its role in decreasing PTH levels, observed in some but not all studies in CKD patients [123], supplementation with native vitamin D may be strictly necessary in some other circumstances; one such case involved a growing adolescent on HD who had osteomalacia, previously treated with paricalcitol [128]. Most importantly, Matias et al. [72] observed a significant increase in serum albumin and a decrease in PCR as well as in erythropoietin needs in cholecalciferol-treated HD patients. Furthermore, BNP plasma levels and LVH as measured by echocardiography were significantly reduced at the end of the 1-year treatment.

It may be concluded that randomized controlled trials are needed to elucidate whether vitamin D supplementation in dialysis patients indeed reduces CV risk or mortality. Although most of the current recommendations are opinion based, it is our belief that strong and uniform associations of mineral metabolism disorders with poor outcomes in CKD patients have been repeatedly documented. Consequently, the Spanish guidelines do suggest the use and monitoring of calcidiol in all CKD patients (including PD and HD patients) until and unless there is a clear-cut proof that vitamin D supplementation is not of value.

Although it would appear that supplementation should be simple, safe, and cost-effective (it may even decrease the need for more expensive forms of active vitamin D), the requirements are still a matter of debate. High doses are probably undesirable [129] and calcidiol treatment may also increase 24,25-vitamin D-hydroxylase [24, 126]. Thus, the direct use of calcidiol on a monthly basis should not be considered equivalent to daily doses of native vitamin D from the academic point of view, and consequently split doses could be preferred [24, 122]. Recently released guidelines for the general population suggest a daily dose of 600 IU till 70 years of age and 800 IU thereafter, and the maximum daily dose was been increased from 2,000 to 4,000 IU/day for the American general population [119]. On the other hand, an upper limit of normality has not been clearly established, either for the general population or for CKD patients, and some labs still report 300 ng/ml as the upper limit of normality. Actually, calcidiol levels higher than 200 ng/ml would be needed to maintain normal levels of calcitriol through the action of extrarenal 1α-hydroxylase in anephric patients [24]. In HD patients, levels higher than 100 ng/ml [50] have been related to toxicity [24, 130]. Levels above or below the target range seem to confer a significantly increased in risk for CV disease, and thus a U-shaped curve or a reverse J curve may describe quite well the relationship between adverse systemic or vascular effects and the vitamin D status [18, 131]. sVDRAs may increase this therapeutic window [18, 131].

Activation of VDR and Survival in CKD Patients

Survival benefits have been associated with the use of different VDRAs (not considering calcidiol) in both nondialysis and dialysis patients and paricalcitol in dialysis patients [71, 73, 74, 110, 132–134], independently of calcium, phosphate and PTH control to a certain extent [20, 135, 136]. These results are statistically powerful since very large numbers of patients have been analyzed and an important consistency in the results has been observed. Nevertheless, there is still the possibility that unrecognized confounding variables may account for the described benefits, and the lack of a prospective intervention somehow diminishes the strength of these results to some extent.

Following the initial description by Marco et al. [74] in Spain calcitriol was found to be independently associated with improved survival among HD patients in all multivariant models they used in a study devoted to the analysis of VDR polymorphisms. The study by Shoji et al. [71] that showed that 1α-calcidol too was associated with an improvement in CV mortality in a small Japanese cohort. Many observational and retrospective studies also demonstrated treatment with VDRAs to be linked to decreased mortality in patients on HD. Several years later these results were confirmed when examining much larger HD databases. Thus, Teng et al. [136] observed an approximate 20% reduction in global and CV mortality in 51,037 American patients, with a better outcome in those receiving an intravenous (i.v.) VDRA (paricalcitol or calcitriol) than in those not receiving vitamin D. Later, Naves-Díaz et al. [134] reported a similar observation in the CORES Latino-American HD cohort where a VDRA (96.7% oral calcitriol) was also independently associated with improved survival. In the latter study, not only global but also CV, infectious and neoplastic mortality rates were improved by the use of VDRAs [134]. Similarly, Kalantar-Zadeh et al. [137] analyzed 58,058 HD US patients from a different database (DaVita) and found that the use of paricalcitol was associated with an improved survival compared to those patients not receiving it, even after correcting for inflammation. Interestingly, it has been reported that these beneficial effects on survival were progressively attenuated with increasing doses of calcitriol [134] or paricalcitol [137]. In these studies, the benefit of calcitriol was lost at doses >1 μg/day [134] and the benefit of paricalcitol at doses >15 μg/week [137]. In both cases, higher doses of VDRAs are obviously associated with the need for higher PTH levels. Thus, the attenuation of the improvement in survival may also represent a more severe form of secondary hyperparathyroidism and other comorbidities (such as inflammation in a similar mirror image of EPO hyporesponsiveness). Interestingly, Shinaberger et al. [138] showed in a retrospective analysis that higher weekly paricalcitol dosage per each unit of serum PTH seems to have an incremental association with greater survival in maintenance HD patients. However, the observed dosage-response phenomenon needs to be confirmed in clinical trials and we think that a combination treatment with calcimimetics (such as the usual approach for hypertension or immunosuppression in kidney transplantation) is more reasonable [9, 26, 94, 139–142] since it cannot be completely ruled out that high doses of vitamin D may directly overcome the beneficial effects [18, 130, 131]. In addition, we would emphasize that to our knowledge no increased mortality has been shown in any adult study using VDRAs.

It is also worth mentioning that VDRA survival benefit was observed regardless of mineral metabolism parameters, suggesting that VDRAs could exert benefits beyond the classical effects. Even in the subgroup of patients with PTH ≤150 pg/ml, a PTH value at which VDRAs are not usually indicated, VDRAs were associated with improved survival [73, 134, 136]. These results have recently been confirmed in the Italian FARO study [92, 93]. Thus, although most guidelines recommend minimization or withdrawal of VDRAs when PTH is persistently low or when the combination of PTH and alkaline phosphatase values is suggestive of ABD, some authors believe that a minimal weekly dose should be given to any dialysis patient to ensure activation of the VDR, especially if calcidiol levels are not being monitored [18, 94, 124, 137]. Increased mortality in patients with ABD or low PTH levels could potentially also be due to the common withdrawal of VDRAs in these patients [18, 20, 92].

Although these points may probably apply to the PD population as well, there are few studies in PD. Melamed et al. [143] analyzed 1,007 incident dialysis patients (only 26% of whom were on PD) and accidentally found a lower global mortality in patients treated with calcitriol.

Differences among Different VDRAs in Respect of Effects and Survival

Although it is clear that a prospective randomized controlled clinical trial to prove that vitamin D or VDRAs affect hard clinical outcomes in dialysis patients is still needed and can be ethically conducted (especially considering the rather surprising results of the PRIMO study) [144, 145], the consistency of previous retrospective studies on outcomes is obvious and cannot be underestimated [146]. On the other hand, the issue of whether there are differences in hard outcomes when administering different vitamin D compounds is still the subject of much controversy [73, 136, 144, 145].

Calcitriol, pro-hormones 1α-calcidol and doxercalciferol, and sVDRAs (e.g. paricalcitol and maxacalcitol) quite clearly seem to have different effects on serum calcium, phosphorus and PTH [147]. The development of various compounds was driven by the need to treat secondary hyperparathyroidism through VDR activation without the induction of hypercalcemia and/or hyperphosphatemia. Thus, sVDRAs appear to have a greater selectivity for the parathyroid gland than for intestinal receptors. This may explain the less frequent episodes of hypercalcemia and hyperphosphatemia attributed to these sVDRAs, providing a seemingly wider therapeutic window [148]. Accordingly, a tenfold dose of paricalcitol, compared with calcitriol, was needed in experimental animals to produce the same increases in serum calcium levels [149, 150]. In a randomized study including PD and HD patients, paricalcitol reduced PTH with minimal effects on calcium levels [151]. The aforementioned and other experimental differences could be due to differential interaction with the ubiquitous VDR in diverse tissues (intestinal, vascular, bone, metabolic or inflammatory pathways, etc.), coactivator recruitment and cell/tissue selectivity, or activating or inhibiting genes with a vitamin D receptor element (VDRE) in the promotor DNA region [24]. Beyond serum mineral metabolism parameters, experimental and small animal studies have also suggested that paricalcitol may exert different effects on bone compared with calcitriol, but no human bone biopsy data are as yet available to verify these observations [95, 152, 153].

Few randomized clinical trials have compared the efficacy of different VDRAs in PD patients. When oral calcitriol and doxercalciferol were compared, no significant differences were observed in 60 pediatric PD patients [154]. Likewise, in a recent preliminary study no differences were found between oral calcitriol and paricalcitol in 66 PD patients over 24 weeks of treatment [155]. In another retrospective study including as many as 1,372 PD patients, differences were not found in bone mineral parameters when oral forms of calcitriol, doxercalciferol and paricalcitol were compared (Data on file with DaVita Clinical Research, October 2010 in ref. [156]).

Another important finding indicating a differential effect, shown consistently but only in experimental rat studies, is that when equipotent doses of the sVDRAs paricalcitol and calcitriol are administered, the former induces less VC than calcitriol [64, 157, 158]. Thus, paricalcitol appears to have fewer experimental procalcifying effects than other forms of VDRA, this being attributable not only to a lower serum calcium, phosphate or calcium x phosphate product but also to the fact that paricalcitol does not induce the expression of Cbf-α1 (Runx-2), a nuclear transcription factor which triggers the transformation of vascular smooth muscle cells [158]. Recent research developments and newly available treatments have contributed in shifting the focus of nephrologists from the control of laboratory parameters, mainly PTH values or bone health, to a more integral management, as supported by the CKD-MBD concept, where the main goal is global outcomes. In the KDIGO guidelines, it is suggested that in CKD stages 3–5D, a lateral abdominal radiograph (the Spanish 2011 guidelines do not specify the view of choice and it is stated 'by any means'), can be used to detect the presence or absence of VC, and an echocardiogram can be used to detect the presence or absence of valvular calcification, as reasonable alternatives to computed tomography-based imaging [10]. It is suggested that patients with CKD stages 3–5D and known vascular/valvular calcification be considered at highest cardiovascular risk (evidence 2A) [10]. Thus, it is reasonable to use this information to guide management of CKD-MBD (not graded) [10]. In the Spanish guidelines, it is considered that this information should be considered in any patient whenever the presence or absence of VC is going to influence the medical decision of the nephrologist in care. However, it is recognized that this approach has not really been tested, or proven a hard-outcome benefit [10, 94].

Very few data are available in PD patients but the current evidence suggests that vascular and valvular calcifications are equally highly prevalent complications in the PD population [159]. In two small surveys, at least 60–80% of the PD patients had the complication of coronary artery calcification [160]. The prevalence of cardiac valvular calcification ranges from 32 to 47% in PD patients, in contrast to 19 to 84% in hemodialysis patients [161, 162]. The reasons behind these discrepancies are not clear.

Finally, some nonrandomized studies show survival advantages with sVDRAs in HD patients [18]. In a huge retrospective study evaluating 63,399 patients, i.v. paricalcitol appeared to provide an additional survival benefit (16% lower all-cause mortality) as compared to i.v. calcitriol [73]. Importantly, the analysis found out that patients who switched from calcitriol to paricalcitol showed improved survival as compared to those who switched from paricalcitol to calcitriol. As in other studies, these results were also seen in most of the subgroup analyses including those relating to calcium, phosphate or PTH level. This observation suggests that the beneficial effects of sVDRAs (paricalcitol) may be independent of mineral metabolism parameters and/or distinct pleiotropic effects (such as effects on VC) among different vitamin D compounds. However, it is our understanding that control of other mineral metabolism parameters is also important. For instance in this study, it appeared that the advantage of paricalcitol over calcitriol was lost at higher levels of serum phosphate [73].

Nevertheless, differences between different VDRA are still under dispute [144]. In the recent retrospective analysis in PD patients mentioned above, although it included a much smaller number of patients (data on file with DaVita Clinical Research, October 2010 in ref. [156]), those receiving oral calcitriol showed a bit lower mortality (9.33 deaths per 100 patient-years) than those receiving either doxercalciferol (12.20 deaths per 100 patient-years) or paricalcitol (12.27 deaths per 100 patient-years). However, any statistics or p values are reported. Other studies have not shown differences among different VDRAs [144, 163]. Thus, while vitamin D therapy has been shown to be associated with lower mortality in adjusted time-varying standard regression models and time-varying marginal structural models, no significant differences in mortality were observed using an 'instrumental' variable model [144]. Tentori et al. [144] stated that a randomized controlled trial of vitamin D and clinical outcomes is still needed and can be ethically conducted. A prospective study was previously initiated in 2003 but terminated in 2006 because the enrollment target had not been reached, likely because of investigator and ethics committee biases against enrolling patients [164]. Although some authors have drawn attention to the inconveniences of using paricalcitol after publication of the PRIMO trial [146], we still use it as the vitamin D of choice in our practice, at least in dialysis patients. We also believe that any VDRA is probably better than none. However, it is obvious that use of paricalcitol cannot just be justified by the presence of LVH in a CKD patient. When comparing sVDRAs to calcimimetics in dialysis patients, the preliminary results of the IMPACT trial seemed to show some differences between sVDRA-based vs. calcimimetic-based therapy, including cost considerations [165]. However, superiority of oral paricalcitol over cinacalcet could not be demonstrated.

Administration of VDRAs in PD Patients

Different routes of administration are possible in PD patients. In contrast to the situation in HD patients, i.v. administration is typically not feasible because PD is essentially a home dialysis technique; instead the oral route in the most widely used [166]. The oral preparation became available in 2006 in the United States and in the following years in several European countries. It is used basically for the prevention and treatment of secondary hyperparathyroidism in patients with CKD stages 3–5D, including PD patients [166]. As with the use of insulin in diabetic PD patients, some studies have evaluated the intraperitoneal (i.p.) route as an alternative, especially in patients with resistant secondary hyperparathyroidism. In pediatric PD patients the i.p. route was shown to be safe and effective [167]. Other old studies did not show differences [168]. One of the main concerns regarding the i.p. route is that higher doses of vitamin D are needed since it seems that part of the vitamin D adsorbs to the dialysis bags [167]. Salusky et al. [169] evaluated adherence of the sterol to dialysate bags and found that the percentage of ^{3}H-calcitriol recovered from the dialysate outflow reached 62 ± 6% of the amount initially added to vials. To minimize surface contact between the hormone and the plastic components of the dialysate delivery system, they injected the hormone directly into the peritoneal cavity through the adapter of the catheter instead of adding the sterol dose to the whole bag of PD solution [169]. Overall, the best route remains to be defined, since all options offer advantages and drawbacks in relation to bioavailability and secondary effects [170].

Conclusions

Most of the studies in the literature on vitamin D treatment in CKD patients have been done in patients other than those on PD. The same holds true for dialysis patients, since most studies have been performed in HD. Thus, the best available evidence is not only generally low-graded because of the lack of prospective studies with hard outcomes, but such evidence as exists has also been described in HD rather than PD. In general, we believe that beyond some small considerations, the approach in PD patients should probably be similar to HD patients. Nevertheless, knowledge on the potentially positive calcium balance in patients treated with calcium concentrations beyond the KDIGO guidelines should be expanded, and some caution is appropriate given the high incidence of ABD in PD, probably beyond the presence of diabetic patients. The combined approach to secondary hyperparathyroidism seems to be also appropriate in these patients, and vitamin D (both native plus VDRAs or native plus sVDRAs) seems an important part of the required integral approach, since PD patients probably need vitamin D or activation of the VDR at least as much as HD patients. sVDRAs may provide additional benefits but a definitive prove is lacking.

Acknowledgements

The research group belongs to a Consolidated Research Catalan Group (AGAUR 2009/SGR-1116), Catalonia, Spain. The research group is also integrated in the Spanish Renal Network for Research (16/06, RETICS), Instituto de Investigación Carlos III. M. Díaz is sponsored by FRIAT (Fundación Renal Iñigo Alvarez de Toledo).

Disclosure Statement

Dr. J. Bover has given lectures sponsored by Abbott, Amgen, Genzyme and Shire. Dr. J. Bover has also participated in national and international advisory boards for Abbott, Amgen, and Genzyme. Dr. M. Cozzolino has given lectures and participated in advisory boards for Abbott.

References

1 Lindner A, Charra B, Sherrard DJ, Scribner BH: Accelerated atherosclerosis in prolonged maintenance hemodialysis. N Engl J Med 1974;290:697–701.
2 Go AS, Chertow GM, Fan D, et al: Chronic kidney disease and the risks of death, cardiovascular events, and hospitalization. N Engl J Med 2004;351:1296–1305.
3 Fernandez-Llama P, Bover J: Is albuminuria a marker of arterial remodeling? J Hypertens 2008;26:633–635.
4 Gotch FA: The CANUSA study. Canada-USA. Perit Dial Int 1997;17(suppl 2):S111–S114.
5 Burkart J: The future of peritoneal dialysis in the United States: optimizing its use. Clin J Am Soc Nephrol 2009;4(suppl 1):S125–S131.
6 Zoccali C: Traditional and emerging cardiovascular and renal risk factors: an epidemiologic perspective. Kidney Int 2006;70:26–33.
7 Block GA, Klassen PS, Lazarus JM, et al: Mineral metabolism, mortality, and morbidity in maintenance hemodialysis. J Am Soc Nephrol 2004;15:2208–2218
8 Bover J, Canal C, Marco H, et al: Diagnostic procedures and rationale for specific therapies in chronic kidney disease-mineral and bone disorder. Contrib Nephrol. Basel, Karger, 2008, vol 161, pp 222–233.
9 Bover J, Andres E, Lloret MJ, et al: Dietary and pharmacological control of calcium and phosphate metabolism in dialysis patients. Blood Purif 2009;27:369–386.
10 KDIGO Clinical Practice Guideline for the Diagnosis, Evaluation, Prevention, and Treatment of Chronic Kidney Disease-Mineral and Bone Disorder (CKD-MBD). Kidney Int 2009;76:S1–S130.
11 Tentori F, Blayney MJ, Albert JM, et al: Mortality risk for dialysis patients with different levels of serum calcium, phosphorus, and PTH: the Dialysis Outcomes and Practice Patterns Study (DOPPS). Am J Kidney Dis 2008;52:519–530.
12 Isakova T, Xie H, Yang W, et al: Fibroblast growth factor 23 and risks of mortality and end-stage renal disease in patients with chronic kidney disease. JAMA 2011;305:2432–2439.
13 London GM, Guerin AP, Verbeke FH, et al: Mineral metabolism and arterial functions in end-stage renal disease: potential role of 25-hydroxyvitamin D deficiency. J Am Soc Nephrol 2007;18:613–620.
14 Danese MD, Belozeroff V, Smirnakis K, Rothman KJ: Consistent control of mineral and bone disorder in incident hemodialysis patients. Clin J Am Soc Nephrol 2008;3:1423–1429.
15 Ronco C, Haapio M, House AA, et al: Cardiorenal syndrome. J Am Coll Cardiol 2008;52:1527–1539.
16 Ronco C, Cozzolino M: Mineral metabolism abnormalities and vitamin D receptor activation in cardiorenal syndromes. Heart Fail Rev 2011, Feb 13, [Epub ahead of print].
17 Cozzolino M: KDIGO on CKD-MBD: a new classification for an old problem? G Ital Nefrol 2009;26:645.
18 Bover J, Cozzolino M: Mineral and bone disorders in chronic kidney disease and end-stage renal disease patients: new insights into vitamin D receptor activation. Kidney Int 2011;1(suppl):122–129.
19 Llach F, Bover J: Renal osteodystrophies; in Brenner BM (ed.): The Kidney, ed 6. Philadelphia, Saunders, 2000, pp 2103–2186.
20 Andress DL: Vitamin D in chronic kidney disease: a systemic role for selective vitamin D receptor activation. Kidney Int 2006;69:33–43.
21 Cozzolino M, Mazzaferro S: The fibroblast growth factor 23: a new player in the field of cardiovascular, bone and renal disease. Curr Vasc Pharmacol 2010;8:404–411.
22 Vervloet MG, Larsson TE: Fibroblast growth factor 23 and klotho in chronic kidney disease. Kidney Int 2011;(suppl 1):130–135.
23 Valdivielso JM, Cannata-Andia J, Coll B, Fernandez E: A new role for vitamin D receptor activation in chronic kidney disease. Am J Physiol Renal Physiol 2009;297:F1502–F1509.
24 Dusso AS: Kidney disease and vitamin D levels: 25-hydroxyvitamin D, 1,25-dihydroxyvitamin D and VDR activation. Kidney Int 2011;(suppl 1):107–110.
25 Cozzolino M, Bover J, Vervloet M, Brandenbrug VM: A multidisciplinary review of the science of vitamin D receptor activation. Kidney Int 2011;(suppl 1):111–115.
26 Torregrosa JV, Bover J, Cannata AJ: Spanish Society of Nephrology recommendations for controlling mineral and bone disorder in chronic kidney disease patients (SEN-MBD). Introduction. Nefrologia 2011;31(suppl 1):1–2.
27 Rojas-Rivera J, De La PC, Ramos A, et al: The expanding spectrum of biological actions of vitamin D. Nephrol Dial Transplant 2010;25:2850–2865.
28 Holick MF: Vitamin D deficiency. N Engl J Med 2007;357:266–281.
29 Bouillon R, Carmeliet G, Verlinden L, et al: Vitamin D and human health: lessons from vitamin D receptor null mice. Endocr Rev 2008;29:726–776.
30 Melamed ML, Michos ED, Post W, Astor B: 25-hydroxyvitamin D levels and the risk of mortality in the general population. Arch Intern Med 2008;168:1629–1637.
31 Liu PT, Stenger S, Li H, et al: Toll-like receptor triggering of a vitamin D-mediated human antimicrobial response. Science 2006;311:1770–1773.
32 Byers SW, Rowlands T, Beildeck M, Bong YS: Mechanism of action of vitamin D and the vitamin D receptor in colorectal cancer prevention and treatment. Rev Endocr Metab Disord 2012;13:31–38.
33 Rudnicki M, Kerschbaum J, Hausdorfer J, et al: Risk factors for peritoneal dialysis-associated peritonitis: the role of oral active vitamin D. Perit Dial Int 2010;30:541–548.
34 Carozzi S, Nasini MG, Schelotto C, et al: Ca^{++} and $1,25(OH)_2D_3$ enhance peritoneal macrophage (PMPhi) antimicrobial functions in CAPD. Adv Perit Dial 1989;5:103–110.
35 Levy R, Klein J, Rubinek T, et al: Diversity in peritoneal macrophage response of CAPD patients to 1,25-dihydroxyvitamin D_3. Kidney Int 1990;37:1310–1315.
36 Dusso A, Lopez-Hilker S, Rapp N, Slatopolsky E: Extra-renal production of calcitriol in chronic renal failure. Kidney Int 1988;34:368–375.
37 Morris HA, Anderson PH: Autocrine and paracrine actions of vitamin D. Clin Biochem Rev 2010;31:129–138.

38 Craver L, Marco MP, Martinez I, et al: Mineral metabolism parameters throughout chronic kidney disease stages 1–5–achievement of K/DOQI target ranges. Nephrol Dial Transplant 2007;22:1171–1176.
39 Levin A, Bakris GL, Molitch M, et al: Prevalence of abnormal serum vitamin D, PTH, calcium, and phosphorus in patients with chronic kidney disease: results of the study to evaluate early kidney disease. Kidney Int 2007;71:31–38.
40 Bover J, Gorriz JL, Martin de Francisco AL, et al: Unawareness of the K/DOQI guidelines for bone and mineral metabolism in predialysis chronic kidney disease: results of the OSERCE Spanish multicenter-study survey. Nefrologia 2008;28:637–643.
41 K/DOQI clinical practice guidelines for bone metabolism and disease in chronic kidney disease. Am J Kidney Dis 2003;42:S1–S201.
42 Foucan L, Ducros J, Merault H: Vitamin D status in dark-skinned patients undergoing hemodialysis in a continually sunny country. J Nephrol 2012 Jan 17:0. doi: 10.5301/jn.5000079, [Epub ahead of print].
43 Wang AY, Lam CW, Sanderson JE, et al: Serum 25-hydroxyvitamin D status and cardiovascular outcomes in chronic peritoneal dialysis patients: a 3-y prospective cohort study. Am J Clin Nutr 2008;87:1631–1638.
44 Taskapan H, Ersoy FF, Passadakis PS, et al: Severe vitamin D deficiency in chronic renal failure patients on peritoneal dialysis. Clin Nephrol 2006;66:247–255.
45 Sahin G, Kirli I, Sirmagul B, et al: Loss via peritoneal fluid as a factor for low 25(OH)D3 level in peritoneal dialysis patients. Int Urol Nephrol 2009;41:989–996.
46 Morton AR: 25-hydroxyvitamin D in peritoneal dialysis patients: a substrate for investigation. Perit Dial Int 2005;25:343–347.
47 Aloni Y, Shany S, Chaimovitz C: Losses of 25-hydroxyvitamin D in peritoneal fluid: possible mechanism for bone disease in uremic patients treated with chronic ambulatory peritoneal dialysis. Miner Electrolyte Metab 1983;9:82–86.
48 Joffe P, Heaf JG: Vitamin D and vitamin-D-binding protein kinetics in patients treated with continuous ambulatory peritoneal dialysis (CAPD). Perit Dial Int 1989;9:281–284.
49 Shany S, Rapoport J, Goligorsky M, et al: Losses of 1,25- and 24,25-dihydroxycholecalciferol in the peritoneal fluid of patients treated with continuous ambulatory peritoneal dialysis. Nephron 1984;36:111–113.
50 Lin CY, Huang TP: Enhancement of ionized calcium and 1,25-dihydroxycholecalciferol loss from peritoneal fluid during peritonitis in patients treated with continuous ambulatory peritoneal dialysis. Nephron 1991;59:90–95.
51 Prytula A, Wells D, McLean T, et al: Urinary and dialysate losses of vitamin D-binding protein in children on chronic peritoneal dialysis. Pediatr Nephrol 2012;27:643–649.
52 Elder GJ, Mackun K: 25-Hydroxyvitamin D deficiency and diabetes predict reduced BMD in patients with chronic kidney disease. J Bone Miner Res 2006;21:1778–1784.
53 Calvo MS, Whiting SJ, Barton CN: Vitamin D intake: a global perspective of current status. J Nutr 2005;135:310–316.
54 Bindal ME, Taskapan H: Hypovitaminosis D and insulin resistance in peritoneal dialysis patients. Int Urol Nephrol 2011;43:527–534.
55 Barreto DV, Barreto FC, Liabeuf S, et al: Vitamin D affects survival independently of vascular calcification in chronic kidney disease. Clin J Am Soc Nephrol 2009;4:1128–1135.
56 Michaud J, Naud J, Ouimet D, et al: Reduced hepatic synthesis of calcidiol in uremia. J Am Soc Nephrol 2010;21:1488–1497.
57 Prosser DE, Jones G: Enzymes involved in the activation and inactivation of vitamin D. Trends Biochem Sci 2004;29:664–673.
58 Petkovich M, Jones G: CYP24A1 and kidney disease. Curr Opin Nephrol Hypertens 2011;20:337–344.
59 Wang TJ, Pencina MJ, Booth SL, et al: Vitamin D deficiency and risk of cardiovascular disease. Circulation 2008;117:503–511.
60 Zittermann A, Schleithoff SS, Tenderich G, et al: Low vitamin D status: a contributing factor in the pathogenesis of congestive heart failure? J Am Coll Cardiol 2003;41:105–112.
61 Pilz S, Tomaschitz A, Dreschsler C, de Boer RA: Vitamin D deficiency and heart disease. Kidney Int 2011;(suppl 1):111–115.
62 Pilz S, Tomaschitz A, Marz W, et al: Vitamin D, cardiovascular disease and mortality. Clin Endocrinol (Oxf) 2011;75:575–584.
63 Li YC, Kong J, Wei M, et al: 1,25-Dihydroxyvitamin D(3) is a negative endocrine regulator of the renin-angiotensin system. J Clin Invest 2002;110:229–238.
64 Cardus A, Panizo S, Parisi E, et al: Differential effects of vitamin D analogs on vascular calcification. J Bone Miner Res 2007;22:860–866.
65 Noonan W, Koch K, Nakane M, et al: Differential effects of vitamin D receptor activators on aortic calcification and pulse wave velocity in uraemic rats. Nephrol Dial Transplant 2008;23:3824–3830.
66 Becker M, et al: Vascular Calcification. American Society of Nephrology-Renal Week. J Am Soc Nephrol 2008 (abstr).
67 Shedeed SA: Vitamin D supplementation in infants with chronic congestive heart failure. Pediatr Cardiol 2012 Feb 18, [Epub ahead of print].
68 Bodyak N, Ayus JC, Achinger S, et al: Activated vitamin D attenuates left ventricular abnormalities induced by dietary sodium in Dahl salt-sensitive animals. Proc Natl Acad Sci USA 2007;104:16810–16815.
69 Pecoits-Filho R, Bucharles S, Barberato SH: Diastolic heart failure in dialysis patients: mechanisms, diagnostic approach, and treatment. Semin Dial 2012;25:35–41.
70 Yakupoglu U, Cigerli O, Ozdemir N: Advantages of selective VDR analogs in CV dysfunctions of HD patients (abstract). World Congress of Nephrology, 2009, M550.
71 Shoji T, Shinohara K, Kimoto E, et al: Lower risk for cardiovascular mortality in oral 1alpha-hydroxy vitamin D3 users in a haemodialysis population. Nephrol Dial Transplant 2004;19:179–184.

72 Matias PJ, Jorge C, Ferreira C, et al: Cholecalciferol supplementation in hemodialysis patients: effects on mineral metabolism, inflammation, and cardiac dimension parameters. Clin J Am Soc Nephrol 2010;5:905–911.
73 Teng M, Wolf M, Lowrie E, et al: Survival of patients undergoing hemodialysis with paricalcitol or calcitriol therapy. N Engl J Med 2003;349:446–456.
74 Marco MP, Craver L, Betriu A, et al: Influence of vitamin D receptor gene polymorphisms on mortality risk in hemodialysis patients. Am J Kidney Dis 2001;38:965–974.
75 Chen S, Law CS, Grigsby CL, et al: Cardiomyocyte-specific deletion of the vitamin D receptor gene results in cardiac hypertrophy. Circulation 2011;124:1838–1847.
76 Thadhani R, Appelbaum E, Pritchett Y, et al: Vitamin D therapy and cardiac structure and function in patients with chronic kidney disease: the PRIMO randomized controlled trial. JAMA 2012;307:674–684.
77 Agarwal R, Acharya M, Tian J, et al: Antiproteinuric effect of oral paricalcitol in chronic kidney disease. Kidney Int 2005;68:2823–2828.
78 Alborzi P, Patel NA, Peterson C, et al: Paricalcitol reduces albuminuria and inflammation in chronic kidney disease: a randomized double-blind pilot trial. Hypertension 2008;52:249–255.
79 Fishbane S, Chittineni H, Packman M, et al: Oral paricalcitol in the treatment of patients with CKD and proteinuria: a randomized trial. Am J Kidney Dis 2009;54:647–652.
80 Szeto CC, Chow KM, Kwan BC, et al: Oral calcitriol for the treatment of persistent proteinuria in immunoglobulin A nephropathy: an uncontrolled trial. Am J Kidney Dis 2008;51:724–731.
81 De ZD, Agarwal R, Amdahl M, et al: Selective vitamin D receptor activation with paricalcitol for reduction of albuminuria in patients with type 2 diabetes (VITAL study): a randomised controlled trial. Lancet 2010;376:1543–1551.
82 Coronel F, Rodriguez-Cubillo B, Cigarran S, Gomis A: Effects of oral paricalcitol on hyperparathyroidism and proteinuria in peritoneal dialysis patients. Adv Perit Dial 2011;27:130–133.
83 Lind L, Hanni A, Lithell H, et al: Vitamin D is related to blood pressure and other cardiovascular risk factors in middle-aged men. Am J Hypertens 1995;8:894–901.
84 Pittas AG, Chung M, Trikalinos T, et al: Systematic review: vitamin D and cardiometabolic outcomes. Ann Intern Med 2010;152:307–314.
85 Takiishi T, Gysemans C, Bouillon R, Mathieu C: Vitamin D and diabetes. Endocrinol Metab Clin North Am 2010;39:419–46.
86 Li YC: Vitamin D: roles in renal and cardiovascular protection. Curr Opin Nephrol Hypertens 2012;21:72–79.
87 Mathew S, Lund RJ, Chaudhary LR, et al: Vitamin D receptor activators can protect against vascular calcification. J Am Soc Nephrol 2008;19:1509–1519.
88 Sevinc: Int Urol Nephrol, 2012.
89 Taskapan H, Baysal O, Karahan D, et al: Vitamin D and muscle strength, functional ability and balance in peritoneal dialysis patients with vitamin D deficiency. Clin Nephrol 2011;76:110–116.
90 Massry SG: Parathyroid hormone: a uremic toxin. Adv Exp Med Biol 1987;223:1–17.
91 Floege J, Kim J, Ireland E, et al: Serum iPTH, calcium and phosphate, and the risk of mortality in a European haemodialysis population. Nephrol Dial Transplant 2011;26:1948–1955.
92 Cozzolino M: Italian FARO study. NDT Plus 2011:4.
93 Brancaccio D, Cozzolino M, Cannella G, et al: Secondary hyperparathyroidism in chronic dialysis patients: results of the Italian FARO survey on treatment and mortality. Blood Purif 2011;32:124–132.
94 Torregrosa JV, Bover J, Cannata AJ, et al: Spanish Society of Nephrology recommendations for controlling mineral and bone disorder in chronic kidney disease patients (SEN-MBD). Nefrologia 2011;31(suppl 1):3–32.
95 Andress DL: Adynamic bone in patients with chronic kidney disease. Kidney Int 2008;73:1345–1354.
96 Frazao JM, Martins P: Adynamic bone disease: clinical and therapeutic implications. Curr Opin Nephrol Hypertens 2009;18:303–307.
97 Brandenburg V, Floege J: Adynamic bone disease-bone and beyond. NDT Plus 2008;3:135–147.
98 Kurz P, Monier-Faugere MC, Bognar B, et al: Evidence for abnormal calcium homeostasis in patients with adynamic bone disease. Kidney Int 1994;46:855–861.
99 Sherrard DJ, Hercz G, Pei Y, et al: The spectrum of bone disease in end-stage renal failure–an evolving disorder. Kidney Int 1993;43:436–442.
100 Carmen SM, Auxiliadora BM, Selgas R, et al: Parathormone secretion in peritoneal dialysis patients with adynamic bone disease. Am J Kidney Dis 2000;36:953–961.
101 Adragao T, Herberth J, Monier-Faugere MC, et al: Low bone volume – a risk factor for coronary calcifications in hemodialysis patients. Clin J Am Soc Nephrol 2009;4:450–455.
102 Adragao T, Branco P, Birne R, et al: Bone mineral density, vascular calcifications, and arterial stiffness in peritoneal dialysis patients. Perit Dial Int 2008;28:668–672.
103 Demirci MS, Ozkahya M, Asci G, et al: The influence of dialysate calcium on progression of arterial stiffness in peritoneal dialysis patients. Perit Dial Int 2009;29(suppl 2):S15–S17,
104 Cotovio P, Rocha A, Rodrigues A: Peritoneal dialysis in diabetics: there is room for more. Int J Nephrol 2011:914849.
105 Goodman WG, Goldin J, Kuizon BD, et al: Coronary-artery calcification in young adults with end-stage renal disease who are undergoing dialysis. N Engl J Med 2000;342:1478–1483.
106 Chertow GM, Burke SK, Raggi P: Sevelamer attenuates the progression of coronary and aortic calcification in hemodialysis patients. Kidney Int 2002;62:245–252.
107 Al HH, Al-Hilali N, Ahmad AA, et al: Vascular calcification in dialysis patients. Transplant Proc 2005;37:4183–4186.
108 Moe SM: Vascular calcification: the three-hit model. J Am Soc Nephrol 2009;20:1162–1164.
109 Moe SM: Management of renal osteodystrophy in peritoneal dialysis patients. Perit Dial Int 2004;24:209–216.
110 Wolf M, Shah A, Gutierrez O, et al: Vitamin D levels and early mortality among incident hemodialysis patients. Kidney Int 2007;72:1004–1013.

111 Drechsler C, Verduijn M, Pilz S, et al: Vitamin D status and clinical outcomes in incident dialysis patients: results from the NECOSAD study. Nephrol Dial Transplant 2011;26:1024–1032.
112 Bae S, Yalamarti B, Ke Q, et al: Preventing progression of cardiac hypertrophy and development of heart failure by paricalcitol therapy in rats. Cardiovasc Res 2011;91:632–639.
113 Przybylski R, McCune S, Hollis B, Simpson RU: Vitamin D deficiency in the spontaneously hypertensive heart failure (SHHF) prone rat. Nutr Metab Cardiovasc Dis 2010;20:641–646.
114 Simpson RU, Hershey SH, Nibbelink KA: Characterization of heart size and blood pressure in the vitamin D receptor knockout mouse. J Steroid Biochem Mol Biol 2007;103:521–524.
115 Repo JM, Rantala IS, Honkanen TT, et al: Paricalcitol aggravates perivascular fibrosis in rats with renal insufficiency and low calcitriol. Kidney Int 2007;72:977–984.
116 Obineche EN, Saadi H, Benedict S, et al: Interrelationships between B-type natriuretic peptides and vitamin D in patients on maintenance peritoneal dialysis. Perit Dial Int 2008;28:617–621.
117 Paniagua R, Ventura MD, vila-Diaz M, et al: NT-proBNP, fluid volume overload and dialysis modality are independent predictors of mortality in ESRD patients. Nephrol Dial Transplant 2010;25:551–557.
118 Autier P, Gandini S: Vitamin D supplementation and total mortality: a meta-analysis of randomized controlled trials. Arch Intern Med 2007;167:1730–1737.
119 Institute of Medicine of the National Academies: Dietary reference intakes for calcium and vitamin D. Released November 30, 2010. http://www.iom.edu/Reports/2010/Dietary-Reference-Intakes-for-Calcium-and-Vitamin-D.aspx (last visited 2/29/2012).
120 Sattar N, Welsh P, Panarelli M, Forouhi NG: Increasing requests for vitamin D measurement: costly, confusing, and without credibility. Lancet 2012;379:95–96.
121 Torregrosa JV, Cannata AJ, Bover J, et al: SEN Guidelines. Recommendations of the Spanish Society of Nephrology for managing bone-mineral metabolic alterations in chronic renal disease patients. Nefrologia 2008;28(suppl 1):1–22.
122 Prados-Garrido MD, Bover J, González-Alvarez MT, Hervás JG, Ocharan-Corcuera J, Foraster A, Llopis A, Fernández E, Dusso A, Cannata-Andía JB: 2010-Guías de práctica clínica de la Sociedad Española de Diálisis y Trasplante (SEDYT) de las alteraciones del metabolismo mineral y óseo de la enfermedad renal crónica (CKD-MBD). Dial Transplant 2011;32:108–118.
123 Kalantar-Zadeh K, Kovesdy CP: Clinical outcomes with active versus nutritional vitamin D compounds in chronic kidney disease. Clin J Am Soc Nephrol 2009;4:1529–1539.
124 Wolf M: Should activated vitamin D be used in patients with end-stage renal disease and low levels of parathyroid hormone? Semin Dial 2011;24:428–430.
125 Pilz S, Iodice S, Zittermann A, et al: Vitamin D status and mortality risk in CKD: a meta-analysis of prospective studies. Am J Kidney Dis 2011;58:374–382.
126 Gallieni M, Kamimura S, Ahmed A, et al: Kinetics of monocyte 1 alpha-hydroxylase in renal failure. Am J Physiol 1995;268:F746–F753.
127 Dusso A, Lopez-Hilker S, Lewis-Finch J, et al: Metabolic clearance rate and production rate of calcitriol in uremia. Kidney Int 1989;35:860–864.
128 Hernandez JD, Wesseling K, Boechat MI, et al: Osteomalacia in a hemodialysis patient receiving an active vitamin D sterol. Nat Clin Pract Nephrol 2007;3:227–232.
129 Sanders KM, Stuart AL, Williamson EJ, et al: Annual high-dose oral vitamin D and falls and fractures in older women: a randomized controlled trial. JAMA 2010;303:1815–1822.
130 Cozzolino M, Bover J, Vervloet M, Brandenburg VM: A multidisciplinary review of the science of vitamin D recptor activation. Kidney Int 2011;(suppl 1):107–110.
131 Cozzolino M, Brandenburg V: Paricalcitol and outcome: a manual on how a vitamin D receptor activator (VDRA) can help us to get down the 'U'. Clin Nephrol 2009;71:593–601.
132 Shoben AB, Rudser KD, de BI, et al: Association of oral calcitriol with improved survival in non-dialyzed CKD. J Am Soc Nephrol 2008;19:1613–1619.
133 Kovesdy CP, Kalantar-Zadeh K: Vitamin D receptor activation and survival in chronic kidney disease. Kidney Int 2008;73:1355–1363.
134 Naves-Diaz M, varez-Hernandez D, Passlick-Deetjen J, et al: Oral active vitamin D is associated with improved survival in hemodialysis patients. Kidney Int 2008;74:1070–1078.
135 Teng M, Wolf M, Lowrie E, et al: Survival of patients undergoing hemodialysis with paricalcitol or calcitriol therapy. N Engl J Med 2003;349:446–456.
136 Teng M, Wolf M, Ofsthun MN, et al: Activated injectable vitamin D and hemodialysis survival: a historical cohort study. J Am Soc Nephrol 2005;16:1115–1125.
137 Kalantar-Zadeh K, Kuwae N, Regidor DL, et al: Survival predictability of time-varying indicators of bone disease in maintenance hemodialysis patients. Kidney Int 2006;70:771–780.
138 Shinaberger CS, Kopple JD, Kovesdy CP, et al: Ratio of paricalcitol dosage to serum parathyroid hormone level and survival in maintenance hemodialysis patients. Clin J Am Soc Nephrol 2008;3:1769–1776.
139 Bover J, Ortiz-Herbener F, Ballarin J, et al: New therapy strategies in secondary hyperparathyroidism on dialysis. I. New concepts, new treatments. Nefrologia 2005;25(suppl 2):100–108.
140 Bover J, Farre N, Andres E, et al: Update on the treatment of chronic kidney disease-mineral and bone disorder. J Ren Care 2009; 35(suppl 1):19–27.
141 Rodriguez ME, Almaden Y, Canadillas S, et al: The calcimimetic R-568 increases vitamin D receptor expression in rat parathyroid glands. Am J Physiol Renal Physiol 2007;292:F1390–F1395.
142 Carrillo-Lopez N, varez-Hernandez D, Gonzalez-Suarez I, et al: Simultaneous changes in the calcium-sensing receptor and the vitamin D receptor under the influence of calcium and calcitriol. Nephrol Dial Transplant 2008;23:3479–3484.
143 Melamed ML, Eustace JA, Plantinga L, et al: Changes in serum calcium, phosphate, and PTH and the risk of death in incident dialysis patients: a longitudinal study. Kidney Int 2006;70:351–357.

144 Tentori F, Albert JM, Young EW, et al: The survival advantage for haemodialysis patients taking vitamin D is questioned: findings from the Dialysis Outcomes and Practice Patterns Study. Nephrol Dial Transplant 2009;24:963–972.
145 Tentori F, Hunt WC, Stidley CA, et al: Mortality risk among hemodialysis patients receiving different vitamin D analogs. Kidney Int 2006;70:1858–1865.
146 Anker SD, von HS: Vitamin D in chronic kidney disease: more questions than answers. JAMA 2012;307:722–723.
147 Bover J, Ballarin J, Andres E, et al: New therapeutic strategies in secondary hyperparathyroidism on dialysis. II. Vitamin D analogues and calcium-mimetics. Nefrologia 2005; 25(suppl 2):109–116.
148 Slatopolsky E, Cozzolino M, Finch JL: Differential effects of 19-nor-1,25-(OH)(2)D(2) and 1alpha-hydroxyvitamin D(2) on calcium and phosphorus in normal and uremic rats. Kidney Int 2002;62:1277–1284.
149 Slatopolsky E, Cozzolino M, Finch JL: Differential effects of 19-nor-1,25-(OH)(2)D(2) and 1alpha-hydroxyvitamin D(2) on calcium and phosphorus in normal and uremic rats. Kidney Int 2002;62:1277–1284
150 Slatopolsky E, Finch J, Ritter C, Takahashi F: Effects of 19-nor-1,25(OH)$_2$D$_2$, a new analogue of calcitriol, on secondary hyperparathyroidism in uremic rats. Am J Kidney Dis 1998;32:S40–S47.
151 Ross EA, Tian J, Abboud H, et al: Oral paricalcitol for the treatment of secondary hyperparathyroidism in patients on hemodialysis or peritoneal dialysis. Am J Nephrol 2008;28:97–106.
152 Balint E, Marshall CF, Sprague SM Effect of the vitamin D analogues paricalcitol and calcitriol on bone mineral in vitro. Am J Kidney Dis 2000;36:789–796.
153 Monier-Faugere MC, Mawad H, Malluche HH: Opposite effects of calcitriol and paricalcitol on the parathyroid hormone-(1–84)/large carboxy-terminal-parathyroid hormone fragments ratio in patients with stage 5 chronic kidney disease. Clin J Am Soc Nephrol 2007;2:1255–1260.
154 Wesseling-Perry K, Pereira RC, Sahney S, et al: Calcitriol and doxercalciferol are equivalent in controlling bone turnover, suppressing parathyroid hormone, and increasing fibroblast growth factor-23 in secondary hyperparathyroidism. Kidney Int 2011;79:112–119.
155 Ong LM, Punitha N, Goh HK, et al: A randomized controlled trial to compare the safety and efficacy of oral paricalcitol with calcitriol in dialysis patiets with secondary hyperparathyroidism. J Am Soc Nephrol-Renal Week 2010 (abstr).
156 Krishnan M, McCarley P: Comparative effectiveness of active oral vitamin D agents in patients on peritoneal dialysis. Nephrol News Issues 2011;25:27–30.
157 Lopez I, Mendoza FJ, guilera-Tejero E, et al: The effect of calcitriol, paricalcitol, and a calcimimetic on extraosseous calcifications in uremic rats. Kidney Int 2008;73:300–307.
158 Mizobuchi M, Finch JL, Martin DR, Slatopolsky E: Differential effects of vitamin D receptor activators on vascular calcification in uremic rats. Kidney Int 2007;72:709–715.
159 Wang AY: Vascular and valvular calcification in chronic peritoneal dialysis patients. Int J Nephrol 2011:198045.
160 Ammirati AL, Dalboni MA, Cendoroglo M, et al: The progression and impact of vascular calcification in peritoneal dialysis patients. Perit Dial Int 2007;27:340–346.
161 Huting J: Mitral valve calcification as an index of left ventricular dysfunction in patients with end-stage renal disease on peritoneal dialysis. Chest 1994;105:383–388.
162 Wang AY, Woo J, Wang M, et al: Association of inflammation and malnutrition with cardiac valve calcification in continuous ambulatory peritoneal dialysis patients. J Am Soc Nephrol 2001;12:1927–1936.
163 Tentori F, Hunt WC, Stidley CA, et al: Mortality risk among hemodialysis patients receiving different vitamin D analogs. Kidney Int 2006;70:1858–1865.
164 Fishbane S, et al: Prospective trial comparing mortality between paricalcitol and calcitriol in hemodialysis patients (abstract). World Congress of Nephrology, M642, 2009.
165 Ketteler M: Improved management of iPTH with paricalcitol-centered therapy vs. cinacalcet therapy with low-dose vitamin D in hemodialysis patients with secondary hyperparathyroidism. Results of the IMPACT SHPT study (abstract). Nephrol Dial Transplant, EDTA Congress, Prague, 2011.
166 Brancaccio D, Cozzolino M, Pasho S, et al: New acquisitions in therapy of secondary hyperparathyroidism in chronic kidney disease and peritoneal dialysis patients: role of vitamin D receptor activators. Contrib Nephrol. Basel, Karger, 2009, vol 163, pp 219–226.
167 Cano FJ, Azocar MA, Guerrero JL, et al: Intraperitoneal calcitriol in infants on peritoneal dialysis. Perit Dial Int 2007;27:681–686.
168 Jones CL, Vieth R, Spino M, et al: Comparisons between oral and intraperitoneal 1,25-dihydroxyvitamin D$_3$ therapy in children treated with peritoneal dialysis. Clin Nephrol 1994;42:44–49.
169 Salusky IB, Kuizon BD, Belin TR, et al: Intermittent calcitriol therapy in secondary hyperparathyroidism: a comparison between oral and intraperitoneal administration. Kidney Int 1998;54:907–914.
170 Wesseling K, Salusky IB: Vitamin D therapy in children on dialysis. Perit Dial Int 2007;27:651–653.

Dr. Jordi Bover
Nephrology Department, Fundació Puigvert
C. Cartagena 340
ES–08025 Barcelona (Spain)
E-Mail jbover@fundacio-puigvert.es

Ronco C, Rosner MH, Crepaldi C (eds): Peritoneal Dialysis – State-of-the-Art 2012.
Contrib Nephrol. Basel, Karger, 2012, vol 178, pp 143–149

Calcimimetics in Peritoneal Dialysis Patients

Piergiorgio Messa · Claudia Castelnovo · Antonio Scalamogna

Nephrology, Dialysis and Renal Transplant, Fondazione IRCCS Ca' Granda OMP, Milan, Italy

Abstract

Though the prevalence of secondary hyperparathyroidism (SHP) and the related mineral metabolism (MM) changes have been reported at almost the same rate in peritoneal dialysis (PD) as in hemodialysis (HD) patients, PD patients have a higher prevalence of adynamic bone disease (ABD), suggesting that their bone is less sensitive for a given level of PTH. Furthermore, the phosphorus control seems to be better and vitamin D deficiency is more common in PD patients than in HD patients. So, the therapeutic approach to SHP and MM changes in PD patients might be different from the one applied to HD patients. Vitamin D metabolites and phosphate binders, though effective in controlling SHP of CKD patients, are not equally effective in controlling at the same extent calcium and/or phosphorus levels. Recently, a new drug (Cinacalcet) has been introduced in the clinical practice which significantly increased the chance of obtaining a simultaneous control of both PTH and MM parameters. However, only scanty data are present in the literature regarding the use of Cinacalcet in PD patients. The few studies produced in PD retraced the results obtained in hemodialysis patients, confirming that both in the short- and long-term Cinacalcet induced a more pronounced reduction of PTH in a larger percentage of patients as compared with standard therapy (ST), and this effect was associated with a decrease in both calcium and phosphorus concentrations, though the extent of the percentage decrease of phosphorus was lower than in HD patients. The safety/tolerability profile was again the same as in HD patients, with gastrointestinal symptoms representing the more frequently reported side effects. In our experience, given that a severe form of SHP is less frequent, the control of phosphate is usually better and vitamin D deficiency is more frequent in PD than in HD patients, making the former patients more prone to hypo- rather than hypercalcemia, the need for the use of the most recent and potent drugs for the control of SHP, including Cinacalcet, is usually lower in PD than in HD patients.

Background

Secondary hyperparathyroidism (SHP) and mineral metabolism (MM) changes are among the most frequent complications in patients with chronic kidney disease (CKD) and they have long been considered to be uniquely related to the CKD-associated bone disease [1].

In the last decades, many observational studies have strongly suggested that increased blood levels of phosphorus, calcium and PTH might contribute to a certain extent to the increased prevalence of the vascular calcification process, cardiovascular (CV) morbidity/mortality and to the general mortality rate which are all observed with an exceedingly high rate in CKD patients [2, 3].

These were the reasons why the nephrology community was prompted to coin the newly named syndrome defined as chronic kidney disease-mineral bone disorder (CKD-BMD) [4].

It is for these reasons that both K/DOQI and K-DIGO guidelines underlined that the goals of the therapy of SHP and the related MM disorders in CKD patients should not be directed only to prevent and/or cure the SHP-related bone disease, but also to avoid or possibly reduce the negative impact on the CV system [5, 6].

For quite some time, vitamin D metabolites and phosphate binders were the basic drugs for controlling SHP of CKD patients. However, it has been well acknowledged that this therapy is not equally effective in controlling at the same time PTH, calcium and phosphorus levels. Recently, a new drug (Cinacalcet) started out in this therapeutic field which significantly increased the chance of obtaining a simultaneous control of both PTH and MM parameters [7, 8].

However, it is worth underlining that most of the literature on these topics derives from studies carried out mainly in hemodialysis (HD) patients. So, most of the recommendations for peritoneal dialysis (PD) patients are simply transferred from the HD experiences.

For these reasons, before specifically addressing the main topic of our paper, we will briefly deal with some aspects of SHP characteristics of PD patients.

Specific Aspects of CKD-MBD in Peritoneal Dialysis

Prevalence of CKD-MBD in PD

There are only scanty data reporting on the prevalence of CKD-MBD in PD patients, as compared to those referring to HD patients.

In a single-center experience, the percentage of patients with values of PTH, calcium and phosphorus above, within or under the K/DOQI targets was not different between HD and PD patients [9]. In the cohorts of our local HD (n = 112) and PD (n = 63) patients (fig. 1), the prevalence of Ca levels above or under the K/DOQI targets was almost the same in the two cohorts; on the other hand, the percentage of PD patients with a PTH or a phosphorus level within the target was significantly higher than the one observed in the HD cohort (i-PTH 76.2 vs. 35.7, $p < 0.01$; phosphorus 80 vs. 54%, $p < 0.01$), the latter result suggesting a better control of phosphate balance by peritoneal dialysis. However, it is also well acknowledged that this better control of phosphorus levels might be mostly dependent on a higher likelihood of maintaining a residual renal function in PD patients [10], which can consistently contribute to phosphorus excretion [11].

At variance with these almost overlapping biochemical conditions, PD patients have a quite different prevalence of the various types of bone disease as compared to HD patients. In fact, the few studies where a bone biopsy was performed show that the prevalence of adynamic bone disease (ABD) is consistently higher in PD than in HD patients, while the rate of high turnover bone disease (HTBD) in PD has been reported to be either lower or equal to that observed in HD patients [12]. Though there is no definitive explanation for these findings, it seems likely to suppose that a more positive calcium balance, due to a more frequent utilization of a relatively high dialysate calcium concentration (1.75 mmol/l) in PD than in HD, might in part explain the lower bone turnover rate in PD patients [12, 13]. Other potential causal factors which might contribute to the lower bone turnover rate in PD patients could be the suggested reduced sensitivity of bone to PTH, the higher glucose supply by peritoneal dialysis fluid, infectious episodes, etc.

Furthermore, though most CKD patients have some degree of vitamin D deficit, assessed by the serum levels of 25-OH-vitamin D, it has also been widely reported that PD patients have lower vitamin D levels as compared with the HD patients [14]. Among the multiple causes which might explain the higher prevalence of vitamin D deficiency in PD patients (discussed in other parts of this book), the peritoneal loss of vitamin D binding protein probably plays an overwhelming role.

Though the impact of all these changes on bone health is well established, it is still a matter of intense debate whether they might be in some way related also to the general clinical outcomes of these patients [15–17].

Summarizing, though the prevalence of SHP in PD patients has been reported to be almost the same as in HD patients, the higher prevalence of ABD in the former patients suggests that the bone of PD patients is less sensitive for a given level of PTH. Furthermore, the phosphorus control

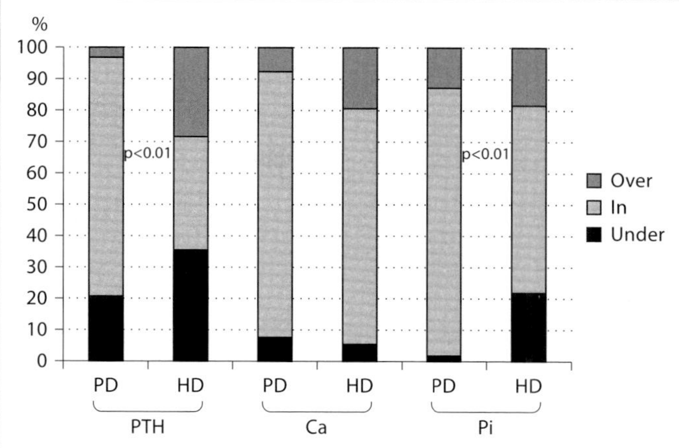

Fig. 1. Percent prevalence of HD and PD patients within, under, or over the K/DOQI target for the mean annual values of PTH, calcium and phosphorus levels, in our prevalent local population on dialysis treatment from the 1st of January 2011 to the 31st December 2011 (HD = 112; PD = 63).

seems to be better in PD, at least until when the residual renal function is maintained. Finally, PD patients are more prone to suffer from vitamin D deficiency than HD patients.

Taking into account all these considerations, the therapeutic approach to CKD-MBD in PD patients might be slightly but consistently different from the one applied to HD patients.

Cinacalcet: Some General Aspects

After a calcium-sensing receptor (CaSR), expressed on the cellular membrane of parathyroid cells and responsible for the calcium controlled PTH release and synthesis, was cloned and characterized [18], a great number of compounds able to modulate CaSR activity have been discovered and studied. However, to this day, only the drug Cinacalcet has been introduced in clinical practice due to its favorable pharmacokinetic and pharmachodynamic characteristics. Cinacalcet, formerly approved by the Regulatory Authorities (FDA, EMA) for the treatment of SHP in patients on dialysis treatment and in patients with parathyroid carcinoma, received more recently the indication also for the treatment of those patients with hypercalcemic primary hyperparathyroidism who cannot be candidates for surgical treatment.

Cinacalcet HCl, the R-enantiomer of AMG 073, has been proven to induce a dose dependent inhibition of PTH secretion and a consequent reduction of Ca^{2+} concentration. It has a good bioavailability after oral administration (>70–75%), which increases proportionally to the increase in an administered oral dose of up to a dose of 200 mg. Cinacalcet bioavailability is also consistently increased (about 70%) if administered after a meal as compared with the fasting condition.

This drug is mainly metabolized in the liver (cytochrome 2D6, 1A2, 3A4), and in the presence of liver impairment an increased bioavailability (increased efficacy and potentially toxicity) might be expected. On the other hand, no significant impact of the degree of renal function or of different dialysis treatment types on Cinacalcet metabolism and/or clearance have been reported.

A more comprehensive coverage of this topic has been given in a previous review [19].

Cinacalcet: Its Use in PD Patients

As already mentioned, most of the published clinical studies regarding the use of Cinacalcet for the treatment of SHP in ESRD patients have been performed in the setting of HD [7, 8]. In the biggest randomized, double-blind, placebo-controlled multicenter study [7], 741 HD patients, with SHP not controlled by the standard therapy (ST) (phosphate binders and vitamin D metabolites), were treated with Cinacalcet or placebo in addition to the ST for 26 weeks. The main result of this study was that the percentage of patients achieving the established target levels for intact PTH (150–250 pg/ml) was about eightfold higher in Cinacalcet plus ST treated patients as compared with placebo and ST treated patients (43 vs. 5%). Furthermore, in Cinacalcet-treated patients a 6.8 and 8.4% reduction of calcium and phosphate, respectively, was observed, at variance with no change or a trend toward an increase in the placebo group. The most frequently reported side effects were related to an excess of efficacy, often associated with hypocalcemia, and to the appearance of gastrointestinal symptoms (nausea, vomiting, diarrhea, stomach discomfort). Though these side effects were usually of moderate intensity, in some cases they were the cause for the withdrawal of the drug.

Though this study gave an unequivocally important basis for the treatment of SHP of ESRD patients, it suffers some important limitations. First, since it was designed before the K/DOQI were published, the target of PTH was too narrow and probably too low. Second, the use of standard therapy was left to the local habits in each participating center, which implied an uncontrolled large variability. Third, the treatment period was relatively short. Finally, no peritoneal dialysis patient was included in the study.

To partially overcome at least the first two limitations, a subsequent study explored the efficacy and safety of Cinacalcet plus ST versus ST alone, used according to an algorithm shared by all participating centers, with the aim of achieving the K/DOQI targets for the three main MM parameters: PTH, calcium, and phosphorus [8]. The main results of this study were that patients on Cinacalcet plus ST treatment had a significantly higher chance of achieving the K/DOQI targets for all the three MM parameters contemporarily than patients on the ST alone (59 vs. 16%). As an additional finding, a 22% reduction in the vitamin D dose in the Cinacalcet group was reported, at variance with no change or a slight increase in the control group.

Further studies looked at the other two limitations: the proof of efficacy also in PD patients and the efficacy and safety in the long term.

In the study of Lindberg et al. [20], a total of 395 patients on dialysis (349 on HD and 46 on PD) were enrolled. Two-hundred and ninety-four patients (260 HD, 34 PD) were treated with once-daily oral Cinacalcet (titrated from 30 to 180 mg/day), while the remaining 101 patients (89 HD, 12 PD) were on placebo in addition to the ongoing ST. This study almost exactly retraces the characteristics of the study of Block et al. [7], as far as the associated ST and PTH targets to be achieved were concerned, therefore maintaining the same related limitations. Also, this study confirmed that Cinacalcet induced a more pronounced reduction of PTH in a larger percentage of patients as compared with ST, with no major difference in the percentage of patients on HD and on PD treatment achieving a PTH level lower than 250 pg/ml (39 and 38%, respectively). Again, Cinacalcet treatment was associated with a slight, but significant, decrease in both calcium and phosphorus concentrations as compared with patients treated with the ST only. However, though the percentage reduction of calcium was almost the same in HD and PD patients (–6.3 and –7.4%, respectively), the extent of the percentage decrease of phosphorus was consistently different: –8.0% in HD vs. –1.5% in PD patients. This relevant finding might probably be secondary to the lower levels of phosphorus which also characterized this cohort of PD patients as compared with HD patients: 5.0 ± 0.2 vs. 5.5 ± 0.1 mg/dl, respectively (mean ± SE). The safety/tolerability profile traced the results of the previous studies, with gastrointestinal symptoms representing the more frequently reported side effects. However, no difference was observed between HD and PD patients in the incidence or type of the reported adverse events.

For addressing the question of the maintenance of the efficacy/safety profile, Sprague et al. [21] carried out an extension study on 589 of 1,184 patients who completed one or more of lead-in double-blind RCTs. Both patients treated with the experimental drug and patients on placebo during the original studies were treated with Cinacalcet for an overall study period lasting 164 weeks. The study included a small number of PD patients, all sourced from the previously mentioned study [20]; however, the results concerning this limited cohort are not reported separately by the AA. Also, this study reinforced the established results of a simultaneous control of all the three main MM parameters in over 30% of the patients treated with the calcimimetic, whether they belonged to the originally Cinacalcet-treated or the placebo group. Most importantly, these effects were maintained over the whole treatment period, without any relevant variation in the efficacy and safety profile.

Summarizing, Cinacalcet is effective in reducing PTH levels, with a concomitant better control of both calcium and phosphorus levels in ESRD patients on either HD or PD dialysis treatment. The safety profiles derived from the published studies and from the every-day clinical experience confirms that the most disturbing side effects are related to the gastrointestinal tract, in addition to some hypocalcemic episodes. Most of these side effects are usually mild; however, in some limited cases they may lead to the physician discontinuing the use of the drug.

It is worth underlining that the number of patients on PD treatment included in the available studies is very small and much of the information needs to be arbitrarily drawn from the experience in HD patients.

Table 1. Types of therapy and drug doses used for the control of SHP in our local cohort of patients (n = 63) treated with PD from the 1st of January 2011 to the 31st December 2011

	Number (%) of patients on treatment	Median (range) of the drug dose per day
Calcitriol	18 (28.6)	0.18 µg/day (0.10–0.50)
Paricalcitol	2 (3.2)	1 µg (1–1)
Cinacalcet	2 (3.2)	22.5 mg/day (15–30)
Calcifediol/ cholecalciferol	29 (46)	950 IU/day (800–1,200)
Calcium carbonate	29 (46)	1 g/day (0.5–3)
Sevelamer	27 (43)	2.4 g/day (0.8–4.8)
Lanthanum carbonate	4 (6.4)	1.875 g/day (1.5–3.0)

Conclusions and Opinions

SHP prevalence has not been reported to be different in PD patients as compared to HD patients. However, in our experience a severe form of SHP is an unusual finding in PD patients. Furthermore, the control of phosphate is usually better in PD than in HD patients, at least until the residual diuresis is maintained. Another specific characteristic of patients treated with PD is the higher tendency to status of Vitamin D deficiency which might make these patients more prone to hypo rather than hypercalcemia. For all these reasons, it is possible to predict that the need for the use of the most recent and potent drugs which are nowadays available for the control of SHP, including Cinacalcet, might be lower in PD than in HD patients.

However, when necessary, the use of Cinacalcet can be adopted with the same indications and limitations as in the HD patients, with expected overlapping side effects.

In clinical practice, our therapeutic approach to SHP in PD patients starts with the optimization of dialysis schedule and adjustment of phosphate binder use, for maximizing phosphorus control, then correcting vitamin D deficiency, using low doses of either cholecalciferol or calcifediol (800–100 UI/day), adding calcitriol or paricalcitol only when, after the first two described steps, the PTH levels are stable at 450–500 pg/ml or show a clear increasing trend in the absence of relatively high calcium (>10.0 mg/dl) and/or phosphorus (>5.5 mg/dl) levels. In these latter cases, we use Cinacalcet starting with low doses (30 mg/day or on alternate days), increasing the dose only if a failed response is observed over at least 2 months, and associating calcitriol when calcium and phosphorus levels return under the above-described limits. The expensive association of cinacalcet and paricalcitol is reserved for the most severe cases of SHP. With this policy, in our experience most of our PD patients have a well-controlled SHP status (63.5% with all the 3 MM parameters within the K/DOQI targets simultaneously) with a very limited use of the most expensive drugs (table 1).

Finally, it is well worth considering that the newly available therapeutic tools have greatly improved the chance of controlling biochemical parameters related to SHP in dialysis patients. However, how much of this better biochemical control might translate into an improvement on bone health or possibly on the general clinical outcomes is still far from being demonstrated.

Acknowledgements

This study was supported by the grant: 'Project Glomerulonephritis' in memory of Pippo Neglia.

References

1 Levin A, Bakris GL, Molitsh M, et al: Prevalence of abnormal serum vitamin D, PTH, calcium, and phosphorus in patients with chronic kidney disease: results of the study to evaluate early kidney disease. Kidney Int 2007;71:31–38.

2 Block G, Port FK: Calcium phosphate metabolism and cardiovascular disease in patients with chronic kidney disease. Semin Dial 2003;16:140–147.

3 Young EW, Albert JM, Satayathum S, et al: Predictors and consequences of altered mineral metabolism: the Dialysis Outcomes and Practice Patterns Study. Kidney Int 2005;67:1179–1187.

4 Moe SM, Drüeke T, Lameire N, Eknoyan G: Chronic kidney disease-mineral-bone disorder: a new paradigm. Adv Chronic Kidney Dis 2007;14:3–12.

5 National Kidney Foundation: K/DOQI clinical practice guidelines on bone metabolism and disease. Am J Kidney Dis 2003;42(S3):1–201.

6 Kidney Disease: Improving Global Outcomes (KDIGO) CKD-MBD Work Group. KDIGO clinical practice guideline for the diagnosis, evaluation, prevention, and treatment of Chronic Kidney Disease-Mineral and Bone Disorder (CKD-MBD). Kidney Int Suppl 2009;113:S1–S130.

7 Block GA, Martin KJ, de Francisco AL, Turner SA, Avram MM, Suranyi MG, Hercz G, Cunningham J, Abu-Alfa AK, Messa P, Coyne DW, Locatelli F, Cohen RM, Evenepoel P, Moe SM, Fournier A, Braun J, McCary LC, Zani VJ, Olson KA, Drüeke TB, Goodman WG: Cinacalcet for secondary hyperparathyroidism in patients receiving hemodialysis. N Engl J Med 2004;350:1516–1525.

8 Messa P, Macario F, Yagoob M, et al: The optima study: assessing a new cinacalcet (Sensipar/Mimpara) treatment algorithm for secondary hyperparathyroidism. Clin J Am Soc Nephrol 2008;3:36–45.

9 Noordzij M, Korevaar JC, Bos WJ, Boeschoten EW, Dekker FW, Bossuyt PM, Krediet RT: Mineral metabolism and cardiovascular morbidity and mortality risk: peritoneal dialysis patients compared with haemodialysis patients. Nephrol Dial Transplant 2006;21:2513–2520.

10 Bernardo AP, Contesse SA, Bajo MA, Rodrigues A, Del Peso G, Ossorio M, Cabrita A, Selgas R: Peritoneal membrane phosphate transport status: a cornerstone in phosphate handling in peritoneal dialysis. Clin J Am Soc Nephrol 2011;6:591–597.

11 Messa P, Gropuzzo M, Cleva M, Boscutti G, Mioni G, Cruciatti A, Mazzolini S, Malisan MR: Behaviour of phosphate removal with different dialysis schedules. Nephrol Dial Transplant 1998;13(suppl 6):43–48.

12 Moe SM: Management of renal osteodystrophy in peritoneal dialysis patients. Perit Dial Int 2004;24:209–216.

13 Yamamoto H, Kasai K, Hamada C, Hasegawa H, Higuchi C, Hiramatsu M, Hosoya T, Itami N, Kawanishi H, Kubota M, Masakane I, Minakuchi J, Mitarai T, Nakao T, Suzuki H, Tomo T, Kawaguchi Y, Japan Peritoneal Dialysis-Mineral Bone Disorders (PD-MBD) Research Group: Differences in corrective mode for divalent ions and parathyroid hormone between standard- and low-calcium dialysate in patients on continuous ambulatory peritoneal dialysis – result of a nationwide survey in Japan. Perit Dial Int 2008;28(suppl 3):S128–S130.

14 Gracia-Iguacel C, Gallar P, Qureshi AR, Ortega O, Mon C, Ortiz M, Villarreal I, Garcia-Lacalle C, Olieta A, Sánchez M, Herrero JC, Vigil A, Lindholm B, Carrero JJ: Vitamin D deficiency in dialysis patients: effect of dialysis modality and implications on outcome. J Ren Nutr 2010;20:359–367.

15 Avram MM, Mittman N, Myint MM, Fein P: Importance of low serum intact parathyroid hormone as a predictor of mortality in hemodialysis and peritoneal dialysis patients: 14 years of prospective observation. Am J Kidney Dis 2001;38:1351–1357.

16 Wang AY, Lam CW, Sanderson JE, Wang M, Chan IH, Lui SF, Sea MM, Woo J: Serum 25-hydroxyvitamin D status and cardiovascular outcomes in chronic peritoneal dialysis patients: a 3-y prospective cohort study. Am J Clin Nutr 2008;87:1631–1638.

17 Palmer SC, Hayen A, Macaskill P, Pellegrini F, Craig JC, Elder GJ, Strippoli GF: Serum levels of phosphorus, parathyroid hormone, and calcium and risks of death and cardiovascular disease in individuals with chronic kidney disease: a systematic review and meta-analysis. JAMA 2011;305:1119–1127.
18 Brown EM, Gamba G, Riccardi D, et al: Cloning and characterization of an extracellular $Ca^{(2+)}$-sensing receptor from bovine parathyroid. Nature 1993;366:575–580.
19 Messa P, Alfieri C, Brezzi B: Cinacalcet: pharmacological and clinical aspects. Expert Opin Drug Metab Toxicol 2008;4:1551–1560.
20 Lindberg JS, Culleton B, Wong G, Borah MF, Clark RV, Shapiro WB, Roger SD, Husserl FE, Klassen PS, Guo MD, Albizem MB, Coburn JW: Cinacalcet HCl, an oral calcimimetic agent for the treatment of secondary hyperparathyroidism in hemodialysis and peritoneal dialysis: a randomized, double-blind, multicenter study. J Am Soc Nephrol 2005;16:800–807.
21 Sprague SM, Evenepoel P, Curzi MP, González MT, Husserl FE, Kopyt N, Sterling LR, Mix C, Wong G: Simultaneous control of PTH and CaxP Is sustained over three years of treatment with cinacalcet HCl. Clin J Am Soc Nephrol 2009;4:1465–1476.

Piergiorgio Messa, MD
Nephrology, Dialysis and Renal Transplant Unit, Fondazione IRCCS Ca' Granda OMP
Via Commenda 15
IT–20122 Milano (Italy)
Tel. +39 0255034551/2, E-Mail pmessa@policlinico.mi.it

Ronco C, Rosner MH, Crepaldi C (eds): Peritoneal Dialysis – State-of-the-Art 2012.
Contrib Nephrol. Basel, Karger, 2012, vol 178, pp 150–156

Factors Affecting Loss of Residual Renal Function(s) in Dialysis

Jochen G. Raimann[a,b] · Thomas M. Kitzler[c] · Nathan W. Levin[a,b]

[a]Renal Research Institute and [b]Beth Israel Medical Center, New York, N.Y., USA; [c]McGill University, Montreal, Que., Canada

Abstract

Many physiological processes relate to two aspects of kidney function: (1) excretory and secretory (excretion of electrolytes and water, elimination of metabolic end products and uremic toxins, regulation of the acid-base status), and (2) endocrine functions (regulating bone and mineral metabolism and red blood cell production). Decreases in renal functions are known to be associated with shortened survival. The exact mechanisms for this are still to be elucidated but evidence in the literature suggests mechanisms such as adverse effects of accumulation of uremic toxins, fluid overload, inflammation and possibly loss of antioxidant functions. Knowledge of factors affecting decrease of residual renal function is currently based on observational data only. Possible strategies to preserve residual renal function have been suggested but require confirmation in adequately powered prospective trials to test their effectiveness.

Residual renal function (RRF) represents the ability of a failing kidney to maintain its functions to the point which is life threatening without additional clearance of uremic toxins by dialysis and iatrogenic substitution of endogenous hormones. Declining RRF is associated with increased mortality [1–3] and hospitalization [4] in both hemodialysis (HD) and peritoneal dialysis (PD) patients.

Excretory Functions

The kidney regulates excretion and reabsorption of salt and water by expressing aquaporins in the tubuli (stimulated by vasopressin), but also by the functions of the enzyme renin which, via the renin-angiotensin-aldosterone system, induces vasoconstriction and secretion of aldosterone, which leads to increased reabsorption of sodium and subsequently water in the kidney. Failure of these functions leads to accumulation of salt and water, elevated blood pressure, potassium overload and hyperaldosteronism. With cardiovascular disease being the major cause of death in PD and HD patients, the implications of fluid overload are most relevant and with strong associations to left-ventricular mass (LVM). In HD patients, reduction of LVM improved survival in an interventional prospective trial, where normotension was achieved by progressive post-HD weight reduction and the use of antihypertensive drugs [5]. A recently concluded randomized trial showed an improved composite of mortality and LVM reduction achieved by more frequent hemodialysis [6]. In a Turkish study, similar effects were achieved by salt restriction and strict volume control [7].

Endocrine Functions

The two main hormones of the kidney, calcitriol and erythropoietin, regulate bone and mineral metabolism and red blood cell production, respectively.

Calcitriol (Vitamin D)

To a lesser extent, vitamin D is absorbed with food in the intestines, but the major part of circulating vitamin D is endogenously produced. Its metabolic precursor cholecalciferol, which is available following ultraviolet light-mediated breakdown of cholesterol in the skin or by gastrointestinal absorption, is hydroxylated in the liver to 25-hydroxycholecalciferol. This major circulating vitamin D metabolite, which is almost entirely bound to vitamin D binding protein (DBP), is hydroxylated by proximal tubular epithelial cells (PTEC) to its active form calcitriol (1,25-dihydroxycholecalciferol). Approximately 90% of this takes place after the complex (consisting of DBP and 25-hydroxycholecalciferol) has been freely filtered by the glomerulus. After filtration, the complex enters the PTEC through receptor dependent endocytosis, where DBP is degraded and the released 25-hydroxycholecalciferol serves as a source for calcitriol production through the enzyme 1α-hydroxylase [8]. Alternative pathways exist, but animal models suggest that 80–90% of calcitriol is generated through this mechanism [8, 9].

This suggests that calcitriol levels may be directly related to the declining levels of glomerular filtration rate (GFR). GFR reduction has also been associated with increased levels of inflammatory markers [10]. In this context vitamin D may be a key modulator of the immune response and of the antimicrobial peptide pathway [11]. Human cathelicidin antimicrobial protein (hCAP18) belongs to a class of widely conserved antimicrobial peptides produced by mammalian species as part of the innate immune system and has broad activity against Gram-positive and Gram-negative bacteria [11, 12]. The cathelicidin gene is reported to be a direct target of the vitamin D receptor and its expression appears regulated by active vitamin D [13], the production of which in turn relates to GFR. Hence, sufficient expression of cathelicidin depends on calcitriol plasma levels, which in turn are a direct function of the GFR and the filtered 25-hydroxycholecalciferol/DBP complex. Wolf et al. [14] demonstrated that long-term survival in HD patients is directly correlated to 25-hydroxycholecalciferol levels. Moreover, a study in healthy subjects revealed a clear correlation between 25-hydroxycholecalciferol levels and cathelicidin [15]. A recent study by Gombart et al. [16] showed low baseline plasma levels of cathelicidin to be predictive of infectious disease 1-year mortality in 81 incident HD patients.

Erythropoietin

Lack of erythropoietin (produced by peritubular interstitial cells) and subsequent renal anemia is a well-known consequence of progressive CKD. Anemia affects between 60 and 80% of patients with CKD, reduces quality of life and has also been identified as an independent risk factor for early death in CKD patients [17].

The exact mechanisms by which preserved RRF leads to improvement of survival in CKD patients are only partially understood. The highly complex functions of the kidney (e.g. regulation of hydration status, cardiac afterload, mineral metabolism, inflammatory status, and tissue oxygenation) render approaches focusing solely on any one of those aspects likely to be ineffective. Moreover, the methodological separation of exocrine and endocrine function seems to be impractical in a clinical setting, as both systems appear to be highly interwoven. The observation that filtration of 25-hydroxycholecalciferol is needed for sufficient calcitriol production, which then further regulates bone mineral metabolism and the immune status, perfectly illustrates this point of view. Considering the architecture of the kidney it seems reasonable to conclude that calcitriol production is more reliant on GFR than erythropoietin. The hypothetical functional dissociation between erythropoietin levels and calcitriol, where the latter more rapidly declines paralleling the declining GFR, whilst erythropoietin levels diminish over a longer period of time, as the kidney fails due to atrophy, may be considered a research question of interest.

Factors Affecting Residual Renal Function

Blood Pressure

A difference between residual renal function (RRF) in PD and HD, respectively, is well established [18–21]. The reasons for this are not entirely understood, but fluid overload and volume management have been hypothesized to be responsible. A recent study showed no significant difference in degree of overhydration between HD (prior to treatment) and PD patients, but showed a significantly lower degree after HD, where overhydration was surprisingly absent [22]. Along these lines data published by Jansen et al. [23] suggest intradialytic hypotension to cause a steeper decline of RRF. Data in PD patients published by Davenport et al. [24] suggest a close relation between fluid status and RRF based on univariate analyses relating 24-hour urine output to the ratio of extracellular volume over total body water (ECV/TBW, $r = -0.25$, $p < 0.0001$). Stratification of all 550 PD patients into 3 groups of residual urine volume correlated significantly with ECV/TBW. A relationship between the ratio of ECV over height and GFR ($r = -0.4$, $p < 0.016$) has been reported in a cross-sectional study of 37 PD patients [25]. Although a PD treatment (particularly during fluid instillation) induces substantial hemodynamic changes, HD patients are subject to mechanical ultrafiltration during a shorter period so that relative blood volume reduction is much greater, which may be considered relatively less physiological as compared to reaching an osmotic equilibrium between fluid in the peritoneal cavity and the blood, which is the physicochemical mechanism, used for ultrafiltration in PD patients. Rapid fluid removal during HD depletes the intravascular compartment, particularly pronounced in the presence of high ultrafiltration rates, potentially leading to hypotension and hypoperfusion of organs. During hypoperfusion, functional reduction of aquaporins and renal vasoconstriction, but also structural changes in the tubular system may occur. Along these lines a negative correlation between dialysis vintage and the ratio of kidney weight to body weight in 58 pediatric HD patients ($r = -0.42$, $p < 0.01$) was reported, which may be considered due to structural changes following longstanding hemodynamic challenges during HD [26]. The relative roles of overhydration and changes in fluid status are not yet clear and remain to be studied.

The actual impact of blood pressure on RRF is at this point only based on observational data. Misra et al. [19] showed no significant effect of hypertension on starting GFR or on the rate of decline, whereas Moist et al. [20] reported a significant effect of post-HD mean arterial pressure on decline of RRF with higher post-HD values associated with increased preservation of RRF in HD patients. In CKD patients prior to dialysis initiation, a history of hypertension and higher mean arterial pressure was associated with an increased slope of GFR reduction [27], and Jansen et al. [23] reported in HD and PD patients a worsening effect on RRF by higher diastolic blood pressure and confirms earlier work by Brazy et al. [28], who also showed an aggravated decline of RRF by higher diastolic but not systolic blood pressure.

Age

Hung et al. [29] reported a significant effect of age on decline of RRF in 174 chronic HD patients. Contrary effects of age on RRF decline have been reported [19, 20]. Jansen et al. did report age to not be a significant influence on residual GFR in 522 incident HD and PD patients [23]. Hunsicker et al. [27] reported age to not be a significant predictor of GFR decline in CKD patients prior to dialysis initiation. In summary, age appears not to be a consistent predictor of decline in RRF. A possible explanation for the influence of age on decline of RRF given by Hung et al. could be that the rate of progression of different diseases might potentially differ between age groups [29].

Underlying Diseases and Comorbidities
Without a doubt underlying diseases do significantly affect progression of decline of RRF. Hunsicker et al. [27] identified presence of polycystic kidney disease and glomerular disease as being associated with decline of GFR in CKD patients. Jansen et al. [23] reported significant influences of comorbidities, quantified per the Davies' score on decline of RRF, Lysaght et al. [18] identified diabetes as a significant predictor in PD patients, which was confirmed in the studied cohort by Moist et al. [20] in PD patients only.

Gender
Contrary results on effect of gender have been reported by several authors. Hung et al. reported no significant influence on the decline of RRF [29], whereas Moist et al. [20] report a borderline significant relation between female gender and decline of GFR compared to males. Results from Hunsicker et al. [27] and Tangri et al. [30] also reported female gender to be associated with a lower risk of decline of GFR. In summary decline of RRF appears less pronounced in women as compared to men.

Race
The data on the impact of race on RRF and decline of GFR are controversial. Hung et al. [29] reported no significant influence on the decline of RRF. Hunsicker et al. [27] showed a faster GFR decline in black CKD patients and similar findings were shown by Moist et al. [20] in multivariable analysis in PD patients only.

Drugs
The nephroprotective effects of angiotensin-converting enzyme (ACE) inhibitors and angiotensin receptor blockers (ARB) has been reported in CKD patients prior to dialysis initiation. Moist et al. [20] found a significant influence of ACE inhibitors (adjusted odds ratio AOR: 0.7, $p < 0.02$) and calcium channel blockers (AOR: 0.71, $p < 0.02$) on preservation of RRF in PD patients only (in HD patients ACE inhibitors were borderline significant) and statins (AOR: 0.56, $p < 0.03$) in HD patients only. Suzuki et al. [40] reported ARBs as being associated with reduced loss of RRF in a randomized study in 34 incident PD patients over 2 years. There was a significant increase of urine volume and creatinine clearance after the start of valsartan in the study population. However, prospective research in a larger population studying the effectiveness of these drugs in HD and PD patients is needed to evaluate the potential to alter the progress of RRF decline.

All nephrotoxic agents should be avoided in patients with impaired renal function and those on dialysis. This includes nephrotoxic radiocontrast agents, nonsteroidal anti-inflammatory drugs, antibiotics (aminoglycosides, cephalosporines, etc.), chemotherapeutic agents (cisplatin, etc.) and many other drugs used in clinical medicine.

Bone and Mineral Metabolism
Hung et al. [29] and Penne et al. [32] reported better calcium and phosphate control in patients with higher RRF patients than in those with lower RRF. Moist et al. [20] found a protective effect on RRF by higher calcium levels and worsening effect of higher phosphate in univariate analysis. An association between fibroblast growth factor-23 and decline in RRF, which remained significant in multivariable analysis [β –0.19 ($p < 0.002$)], has also been reported. The relation of this finding to hard outcomes such as hospitalizations and mortality remains to be studied [33].

Lipid Metabolism
Moist et al. [20] report no significant effect of total cholesterol levels on the decline of RRF, however, parameters of the lipid panel may still be worth observing because Hunsicker et al. [27] reported a slower decline in GFR with higher HDL and Apolipoprotein A1 values.

Dialysis-Related Factors
Hung et al. [29] reported no significant influence of dialysis vintage on decline of RRF in HD patients. Cellulose membranes, in comparison

to more biocompatible membranes, were associated with accelerated RRF loss [34, 35], but this was not confirmed in all published observations [20]. Ultrapure water used for dialysate might be another factor preserving RRF [36]. For PD solutions pH neutrality and the concentration of glucose degradation products has shown better preservation of RRF when compared to a standard PD solution in a randomized cross-over trial [37].

Other Factors
Jansen et al. [23] reported the presence of proteinuria and lower serum albumin to be a significant predictor of decline in RRF and also identified serum albumin as a significant predictor. Hospitalizations, particularly those involving surgical interventions which may possibly lead to reduced organ perfusion could contribute to declines in RRF. Inflammation, reflected by an impaired activity in the glutathione antioxidant system that occurs early in the course of chronic uremia, may also be a factor associated with decrease of RRF [38]. Furthermore, modifiable lifestyle factors also appear to play a role in the decrease of RRF particularly the adverse effects of cigarette smoking [39] which also appears to be a predictor of GFR decline in CKD patients [27].

Strategies to Preserve Residual Renal Function

Data from prospective research to preserve residual renal function (RRF) are scarce and thus recommendations and suggestions are mainly based on observational data. Lifestyle modification such as smoking cessation and salt restriction which lowers interdialytic weight gain and consequently intradialytic hypotension caused by high ultrafiltration rates and blood volume reduction should be recommended to every patient. Furthermore, all exposure to nephrotoxic agents and or drugs which may potentially worsen the condition of an already damaged kidney should be avoided. On a dialysis treatment level, the lack of capability to launch an appropriate cardiovascular response to the intradialytic high filtration hemodynamic challenge has to be seen as important (potentially modifiable though by means of dialysate cooling, use of midodrine or other measures) factors potentially affecting RRF. PD solutions which are pH neutral and low on glucose degradation products may be considered alternatively to current solutions [37].

With regard to the considerably high hospitalization rates of dialysis patients close observation of hospitalized CKD patients at risk of hypotension of any cause is of importance to avoid any damage to the kidneys as discussed above.

The possibilities to support the preservation of RRF by means of a pharmaceutical regimen still need to be investigated in larger prospective studies, but some data suggest positive effects by angiotensin-converting enzyme inhibitors [20], angiotensin receptor blockers [40], N-acetlycysteine [41] and bardoxolone [42].

In conclusion, much more research is needed to give evidence-based recommendations on how to preserve RRF and thus improve outcomes. Studies in prospective settings, preferably in randomized controlled trials, are needed and should become a focus of the nephrology community in order to improve outcomes in dialysis patients. This research should focus on hard outcomes such as hospitalizations, cardiovascular events and mortality. More information needs to be gained on the variable relationships between filtration and other renal functions. While it is well recognized that even the lowest urea clearances still make a contribution to the total dialysis 'dose' it is quite possible that even the non-urine-producing kidney may have important metabolic and endocrine effects.

References

1 Shemin D, Bostom AG, Laliberty P, Dworkin LD: Residual renal function and mortality risk in hemodialysis patients. Am J Kidney Dis 2001;38:85–90.

2 Termorshuizen F, Korevaar JC, Dekker FW, van Manen JG, Boeschoten EW, Krediet RT: The relative importance of residual renal function compared with peritoneal clearance for patient survival and quality of life: an analysis of the Netherlands Cooperative Study on the Adequacy of Dialysis (NECOSAD)-2. Am J Kidney Dis 2003;41:1293–302.

3 Bargman JM, Thorpe KE, Churchill DN: Relative contribution of residual renal function and peritoneal clearance to adequacy of dialysis: a reanalysis of the CANUSA study. J Am Soc Nephrol 2001;12:2158–2162.

4 Brener ZZ, Thijssen S, Kotanko P, Kuhlmann MK, Bergman M, Winchester JF, Levin NW: The impact of residual renal function on hospitalization and mortality in incident hemodialysis patients. Blood Purif 2011;31:243–251.

5 London GM, Pannier B, Guerin AP, Blacher J, Marchais SJ, Darne B, Metivier F, Adda H, Safar ME: Alterations of left ventricular hypertrophy in and survival of patients receiving hemodialysis: follow-up of an interventional study. J Am Soc Nephrol 2001;12:2759–2767.

6 Chertow GM, Levin NW, Beck GJ, Depner TA, Eggers PW, Gassman JJ, Gorodetskaya I, Greene T, James S, Larive B, Lindsay RM, Mehta RL, Miller B, Ornt DB, Rajagopalan S, Rastogi A, Rocco MV, Schiller B, Sergeyeva O, Schulman G, Ting GO, Unruh ML, Star RA, Kliger AS: In-center hemodialysis six times per week versus three times per week. N Engl J Med 2010;363:2287–2300.

7 Ozkahya M, Ok E, Toz H, Asci G, Duman S, Basci A, Kose T, Dorhout Mees EJ: Long-term survival rates in haemodialysis patients treated with strict volume control. Nephrol Dial Transplant 2006;21:3506–3513.

8 Nykjaer A, Dragun D, Walther D, Vorum H, Jacobsen C, Herz J, Melsen F, Christensen EI, Willnow TE: An endocytic pathway essential for renal uptake and activation of the steroid 25-(OH) vitamin D_3. Cell 1999;96:507–515.

9 Berg JP: Vitamin D-binding protein prevents vitamin D deficiency and presents vitamin D for its renal activation. Eur J Endocrinol 1999;141:321–322.

10 Pecoits-Filho R, Heimburger O, Barany P, Suliman M, Fehrman-Ekholm I, Lindholm B, Stenvinkel P: Associations between circulating inflammatory markers and residual renal function in CRF patients. Am J Kidney Dis 2003;41:1212–1218.

11 Gombart AF: The vitamin D-antimicrobial peptide pathway and its role in protection against infection. Future Microbiol 2009;4:1151–1165.

12 Niyonsaba F, Iwabuchi K, Someya A, Hirata M, Matsuda H, Ogawa H, Nagaoka I: A cathelicidin family of human antibacterial peptide LL-37 induces mast cell chemotaxis. Immunology 2002;106:20–26.

13 White JH: Vitamin D as an inducer of cathelicidin antimicrobial peptide expression: past, present and future. J Steroid Biochem Mol Biol 2010;121:234–238.

14 Wolf M, Shah A, Gutierrez O, Ankers E, Monroy M, Tamez H, Steele D, Chang Y, Camargo CA Jr, Tonelli M, Thadhani R: Vitamin D levels and early mortality among incident hemodialysis patients. Kidney Int 2007;72:1004–1013.

15 Bhan I, Camargo CA Jr, Wenger J, Ricciardi C, Ye J, Borregaard N, Thadhani R: Circulating levels of 25-hydroxyvitamin D and human cathelicidin in healthy adults. J Allergy Clin Immunol 2011;127:1302–1304.

16 Gombart AF, Bhan I, Borregaard N, Tamez H, Camargo CA Jr, Koeffler HP, Thadhani R: Low plasma level of cathelicidin antimicrobial peptide (hCAP18) predicts increased infectious disease mortality in patients undergoing hemodialysis. Clin Infect Dis 2009;48:418–424.

17 Santos PR, Melo AD, Lima MM, Negreiros IM, Miranda JS, Pontes LS, Rabelo GM, Viana AC, Alexandrino MT, Barros FA, Neto BR, Brito AA, Da Silva Costa A: Mortality risk in hemodialysis patients according to anemia control and erythropoietin dosing. Hemodial Int 2011;15:493–500.

18 Lysaght MJ, Vonesh EF, Gotch F, Ibels L, Keen M, Lindholm B, Nolph KD, Pollock CA, Prowant B, Farrell PC: The influence of dialysis treatment modality on the decline of remaining renal function. ASAIO Trans 1991;37:598–604.

19 Misra M, Vonesh E, Van Stone JC, Moore HL, Prowant B, Nolph KD: Effect of cause and time of dropout on the residual GFR: a comparative analysis of the decline of GFR on dialysis. Kidney Int 2001;59:754–763.

20 Moist LM, Port FK, Orzol SM, Young EW, Ostbye T, Wolfe RA, Hulbert-Shearon T, Jones CA, Bloembergen WE: Predictors of loss of residual renal function among new dialysis patients. J Am Soc Nephrol 2000;11:556–564.

21 Rottembourg J, Issad B, Gallego JL, Degoulet P, Aime F, Gueffaf B, Legrain M: Evolution of residual renal function in patients undergoing maintenance haemodialysis or continuous ambulatory peritoneal dialysis. Proc Eur Dial Transplant Assoc 1983;19:397–403.

22 Devolder I, Verleysen A, Vijt D, Vanholder R, Van Biesen W: Body composition, hydration, and related parameters in hemodialysis versus peritoneal dialysis patients. Perit Dial Int 2010;30:208–214.

23 Jansen MA, Hart AA, Korevaar JC, Dekker FW, Boeschoten EW, Krediet RT: Predictors of the rate of decline of residual renal function in incident dialysis patients. Kidney Int 2002;62:1046–1053.

24 Davenport A, Sayed RH, Fan S: Is extracellular volume expansion of peritoneal dialysis patients associated with greater urine output? Blood Purif 2011;32:226–231.

25 Verbeke F, Van Biesen W, Pletinck A, Van Bortel LM, Vanholder R: Acute central hemodynamic effects of a volume exchange in peritoneal dialysis. Perit Dial Int 2008;28:142–148.

26 Ogata K: Clinicopathological study of kidneys from patients on chronic dialysis. Kidney Int 1990;37:1333–1340.

27 Hunsicker LG, Adler S, Caggiula A, England BK, Greene T, Kusek JW, Rogers NL, Teschan PE: Predictors of the progression of renal disease in the Modification of Diet in Renal Disease Study. Kidney Int 1997;51:1908–1919.

28 Brazy PC, Stead WW, Fitzwilliam JF: Progression of renal insufficiency: role of blood pressure. Kidney Int 1989;35:670–674.
29 Hung AM, Young BS, Chertow GM: The decline in residual renal function in hemodialysis is slow and age dependent. Hemodial Int 2003;7:17–22.
30 Tangri N, Stevens LA, Griffith J, Tighiouart H, Djurdjev O, Naimark D, Levin A, Levey AS: A predictive model for progression of chronic kidney disease to kidney failure. JAMA 2010;305:1553–1559.
31 Novak JE, Szczech LA: Triumph and tragedy: anemia management in chronic kidney disease. Curr Opin Nephrol Hypertens 2008;17:580–588.
32 Penne EL, van der Weerd NC, Grooteman MP, Mazairac AH, van den Dorpel MA, Nube MJ, Bots ML, Levesque R, ter Wee PM, Blankestijn PJ: Role of residual renal function in phosphate control and anemia management in chronic hemodialysis patients. Clin J Am Soc Nephrol 2010;6:281–289.
33 Viaene L, Bammens B, Meijers BK, Vanrenterghem Y, Vanderschueren D, Evenepoel P: Residual renal function is an independent determinant of serum FGF-23 levels in dialysis patients. Nephrol Dial Transplant 2011 Oct 24. [Epub ahead of print].
34 Van Stone JC: The effect of dialyzer membrane and etiology of kidney disease on the preservation of residual renal function in chronic hemodialysis patients. ASAIO J 1995;41:M713–M716.
35 McCarthy JT, Jenson BM, Squillace DP, Williams AW: Improved preservation of residual renal function in chronic hemodialysis patients using polysulfone dialyzers. Am J Kidney Dis 1997;29:576–583.
36 Schiffl H, Lang SM, Fischer R: Ultrapure dialysis fluid slows loss of residual renal function in new dialysis patients. Nephrol Dial Transplant 2002;17:1814–1818.
37 Williams JD, Topley N, Craig KJ, Mackenzie RK, Pischetsrieder M, Lage C, Passlick-Deetjen J: The Euro-Balance Trial: the effect of a new biocompatible peritoneal dialysis fluid (balance) on the peritoneal membrane. Kidney Int 2004;66:408–418.
38 Ceballos-Picot I, Witko-Sarsat V, Merad-Boudia M, Nguyen AT, Thevenin M, Jaudon MC, Zingraff J, Verger C, Jungers P, Descamps-Latscha B: Glutathione antioxidant system as a marker of oxidative stress in chronic renal failure. Free Radic Biol Med 1996;21:845–853.
39 Odoni G, Ogata H, Viedt C, Amann K, Ritz E, Orth SR: Cigarette smoke condensate aggravates renal injury in the renal ablation model. Kidney Int 2002;61:2090–2098.
40 Suzuki H, Kanno Y, Sugahara S, Okada H, Nakamoto H: Effects of an angiotensin II receptor blocker, valsartan, on residual renal function in patients on CAPD. Am J Kidney Dis 2004;43:1056–1064.
41 Feldman L, Shani M, Efrati S, Beberashvili I, Yakov-Hai I, Abramov E, Sinuani I, Rosenberg R, Weissgarten J: N-acetylcysteine improves residual renal function in peritoneal dialysis patients: a pilot study. Perit Dial Int 2011;31:545–550.
42 Pergola PE, Raskin P, Toto RD, Meyer CJ, Huff JW, Grossman EB, Krauth M, Ruiz S, Audhya P, Christ-Schmidt H, Wittes J, Warnock DG: Bardoxolone methyl and kidney function in CKD with type 2 diabetes. N Engl J Med 2011;365:327–336.

Jochen G. Raimann, MD
Renal Research Institute
207 East 94th Street, Suite 303
New York, NY 10128 (USA)
Tel. +1 212 360 4954, E-Mail j.raimann@gmx.net

Ronco C, Rosner MH, Crepaldi C (eds): Peritoneal Dialysis – State-of-the-Art 2012.
Contrib Nephrol. Basel, Karger, 2012, vol 178, pp 157–163

Prospective Safety Study of Bardoxolone Methyl in Patients with Type 2 Diabetes Mellitus, End-Stage Renal Disease and Peritoneal Dialysis

David G. Warnock[a] · Sudarshan Hebbar[b] · Joanne Bargman[c] · John Burkart[d] · Simon Davies[e] · Frederic O. Finkelstein[f] · Rajnish Mehrotra[g] · Claudio Ronco[h] · Isaac Teitelbaum[i] · Kingsley Urakpo[b] · Glenn M. Chertow[j]

[a]Division of Nephrology, Department of Medicine, and University of Alabama at Birmingham, Birmingham, Ala., [b]Reata Pharmaceuticals, Inc, Irving, Tex., [c]Division of Nephrology, Department of Medicine, University Health Network, Toronto General Hospital, Toronto, Ont., Canada, [d]Department of Nephrology, Wake Forest University Medical Center, Winston Salem, N.C., [e]Department of Nephrology, University Hospital of North Staffordshire, Hartshill, Stoke-on-Trent, UK, [f]Department of Medicine, Yale University, New Haven, Conn., [g]Department of Medicine, Harbor-UCLA Medical Center, Torrance, Calif., [h]Department of Nephrology Dialysis and Transplantation, International Renal Research Institute (IRRIV), San Bortolo Hospital, Vicenza, Italy, [i]University of Colorado at Denver Health Sciences Center, Division of Renal Diseases and Hypertension, Aurora, Colo., [j]Division of Nephrology, Department of Medicine, Stanford University School of Medicine, Palo Alto, Calif., USA

Abstract

Patients on peritoneal dialysis experience inflammation associated with advanced chronic kidney disease and the therapy itself. An important consequence of the inflammation may be acceleration of the rate of decline in residual renal function. The decline in residual renal function has been associated with an increased mortality for patients in this population. Bardoxolone methyl is a synthetic triterpenoid. To date, the effects of bardoxolone methyl on kidney function in humans have been studied in patients with type 2 diabetes mellitus. A large-scale event-driven study of bardoxolone methyl in patients with type 2 diabetes mellitus with stage 4 chronic kidney disease is underway. The safety of bardoxolone methyl has not been evaluated in patients with more advanced (stage 5) chronic kidney disease or patients on dialysis. This report describes a proposed double blind, prospective evaluation of bardoxolone methyl in patients with type 2 diabetes mellitus receiving peritoneal dialysis. In addition to assessing the safety of bardoxolone methyl in this population, the study will evaluate the effect of bardoxolone methyl on residual renal function over 6 months as compared to placebo.

Chronic kidney disease (CKD) is characterized by inflammation and oxidative stress that worsens as patients progress to end-stage renal disease (ESRD) [1]. Significantly higher levels of oxidative stress and impaired endothelial function, as compared to controls, are present in patients with ESRD being treated with peritoneal dialysis (PD) [2–4]. Hypertension, adiposity, insulin resistance, volume overload and infections are common in PD patients and all contribute to the inflammatory state. Glucose-based PD solutions exacerbate the inflammatory state by causing weight gain, hyperglycemia and dyslipidemia [5]. In addition, sterilization of the glucose-based PD solutions generates glucose degradation products that, when exposed to the peritoneal membrane, enhance the production of advanced glycation end products that activate RAGE receptors and downstream inflammatory cascades [6–8]. Sustained inflammation promotes angiogenesis and fibrosis, which can be associated with ultrafiltration failure, limiting the long-term effectiveness of PD [9].

Inflammation in Peritoneal Dialysis Patients and the Link to Residual Renal Function

The chronic inflammatory state in PD patients is associated with a decline in residual renal function (RRF). Singhal et al. [10], found a gradual decline in RRF in patients on PD, with 40% of patients developing anuria an average of 20 months after starting treatment. Risk factors associated with a more rapid decline in RRF include a larger body mass, diabetes mellitus, history of heart failure, use of diuretics, episodes of volume depletion, hypotension and peritonitis [11].

The decline in RRF is associated with poor patient outcomes. Maiorca et al. [12] first described the association between RRF and survival in patients on PD and hemodialysis. Since then, findings from multiple observational studies have strengthened the documentation of the association. Reanalysis of the Canada-United States (CANUSA) Study identified RRF as the most important factor associated with survival in PD patients [13]. The Adequacy of PD in Mexico (ADEMEX) study showed an 11% risk reduction in patient mortality associated with each 10 liters/week/1.73 m^2 increase in RRF [14]. The Netherlands Cooperative Study on the Adequacy of Dialysis (NECOSAD) also found for each increase in RRF of 1 ml/min/1.73 m^2, there was an associated 12% reduction in mortality rate [15]. Recognition of the importance of RRF to the success of PD treatment has led to KDOQI guidelines stressing the importance of monitoring and preserving RRF [16]. Recommendations for preserving RRF include careful attention to glycemic control, use of drugs inhibiting the renin-angiotensin-aldosterone system, avoiding nephrotoxic agents, reduction in glucose degradation products in peritoneal dialysate, and avoiding volume depletion [17]. Long-term prospective clinical trials will need to be performed to answer whether these approaches, alone or in combination, will attenuate the loss of RRF and enhance survival in patients on PD.

Bardoxolone Methyl: An Antioxidant and Inflammation Modulator

Bardoxolone methyl is a synthetic triterpenoid and an antioxidant and inflammation modulator. It is the most potent known inducer of the Keap1-Nrf2 pathway to enter clinical development [18]. Activation of Keap1-Nrf2 induces transcription of a large number of genes that increase cellular antioxidant content, suppress NF-κB activity, and restores redox homeostasis in areas of inflammation. The structure and activity profile resemble that of cyclopentenone prostaglandins, endogenous activators of Nrf2, which play an important role in the resolution of inflammation [19]. Activation of Nrf2 is suppressed in animal models of CKD; experiments conducted in mice with genetic deletion of Nrf2 demonstrate that Nrf2 plays an important role in maintaining the function and structure of the kidney [20–23].

Clinical Experience with Bardoxolone Methyl

Two recently published phase 2 trials have tested the effects of a crystalline formulation of bardoxolone methyl in patients with type 2 diabetes mellitus and CKD. The first trial was an open-label study that enrolled 20 patients with type 2 diabetes mellitus and stage 3b/4 CKD [24]. The study included a dose titrating regimen in which patients were administered 25 mg once daily for 4 weeks followed by 75 mg once daily for four additional weeks. Statistically significant increases in estimated glomerular filtration rate (eGFR) over the 8 weeks were observed in approximately 90% of patients and were corroborated by highly correlated reductions in blood urea nitrogen, phosphorus, uric acid, and magnesium, without a change in the 24-hour creatinine excretion rate. Circulating endothelial cells, markers of endothelial dysfunction and vascular injury were significantly decreased at the end of 8 weeks.

The second trial (Bardoxolone Methyl Treatment: Renal Function in CKD/Type 2 Diabetes, BEAM) was a multicenter, double-blind, placebo-controlled trial that evaluated bardoxolone methyl administered once daily for 52 weeks [25]. In this study, 227 adults with CKD (eGFR between 20 and 45 ml/min/1.73 m^2) and type 2 diabetes were randomized to receive either placebo or bardoxolone methyl at one of three titrated doses (25, 75 or 150 mg) of the crystalline formulation. The primary outcome was change in kidney function as assessed by eGFR following 24 weeks of treatment relative to placebo. Increases in eGFR, ranging from 8.3 ± 1.1 to 11.5 ± 1.1 ml/min/1.73 m^2, were observed in each bardoxolone methyl group, whereas a change of 0.1 ± 1.1 ml/min/1.73 m^2 was observed in the placebo group ($p < 0.001$ for each dose group relative to placebo). Improvement in eGFR from baseline plateaued with the 75 mg dose, and persisted through 52 weeks of treatment. The mean eGFR remained above baseline levels 4 weeks after discontinuation of bardoxolone methyl, suggesting the potential for a persisting effect off drug.

Muscle spasms were the most frequent adverse events in the bardoxolone methyl groups and were generally mild, self-limiting, and not associated with markers of muscle injury. Hypomagnesemia and mild increases in alanine aminotransferase were more common in the bardoxolone methyl groups. The hypomagnesemia was not present in the majority of patients before or at the time of muscle spasms in patients treated with bardoxolone methyl who complained of them. The transaminase elevations were usually transient, peaking at 2–4 weeks and resolving while the patient continued with the study drug. There were no signs or symptoms of hepatic injury observed.

An amorphous spray dried dispersion formulation was developed to improve the bioavailability of the drug compared to the crystalline formulation. The amorphous formulation was tested in a multicenter, open-label, dose-ranging study in 131 patients with type 2 diabetes mellitus and stage 3b/4 CKD [26]. A linear dose-response trend was identified with a statistically significant increase in eGFR from baseline to days 29 (primary endpoint) and 85 (secondary endpoint) noted in all dose groups both individually and combined. The doses were well tolerated and no new safety signals were identified. The transaminase elevations followed a similar, consistent pattern noted in the previous clinical studies using the crystalline formulation. The results of this study, and subsequent pharmacokinetic and pharmacodynamic dose-exposure modeling, were utilized to identify the dose (20 mg) that best balanced safety and efficacy. The 20-mg dose of the amorphous spray dried dispersion formulation is currently being utilized in the ongoing phase 3 trial of patients with type 2 diabetes mellitus and stage 4 CKD with the composite primary endpoint of progression to end-stage renal disease or cardiovascular death [27].

Safety Study of Bardoxolone Methyl in Patients with Type 2 Diabetes Mellitus and End-Stage Renal Disease Treated with Peritoneal Dialysis

The previous and ongoing clinical trials with bardoxolone methyl have excluded CKD patients with eGFR <15 ml/min/1.73 m^2. The objective of this prospective double-blind placebo-controlled trial is to evaluate the safety profile of 20 mg amorphous formulation of bardoxolone methyl given daily for 6 months to patients with type 2 diabetes mellitus and ESRD on PD. In addition, the study will explore the effects of bardoxolone methyl on RRF in this population (PD Study: clinicaltrials.gov NCT pending).

Study Design and Objectives

Forty-five patients with type 2 diabetes mellitus and ESRD on PD will be randomized to receive 20 mg of bardoxolone methyl or placebo once daily for 6 months on a 2:1 allocation stratified by study site. The study will consist of a 45-day screening period, 6 months of study drug administration, and a 1-month post-treatment visit. RRF, defined as the mean of the urea and creatinine clearances on a 24-hour urine collection normalized to 1.73 m^2 body surface area will be measured twice during the screening period to provide a baseline value, monthly after study randomization, and again at the post treatment visit.

The primary objective of the study is to assess the safety and pharmacokinetic profile of bardoxolone methyl in patients with type 2 diabetes mellitus and ESRD on PD. The secondary objective is to assess the effect of bardoxolone methyl on of RRF at 6 months compared to the baseline established during the screening visits.

Inclusion and Exclusion Criteria

To be eligible for the study, patients must have been on PD for more than 3 months and have a documented RRF ≥25 liters/week/1.73 m^2 (2.5 ml/min/1.73 m^2) in the 4 months prior to screening. The patients must also have stable RRF ≥25 l/week/1.73 m^2 documented during both screening visits. Selected inclusion and exclusion criteria are listed in table 1.

Study Procedures

When enrolled in the study, patients will be managed according to local standard of care. At each monthly visit, patients will report adverse events that will be categorized by intensity and relationship to study drug. Patients will receive monthly laboratory measurements, and a single central laboratory will perform all analyses. Peritoneal equilibration testing will be performed at study randomization and again at 3 and 6 months. Pharmacokinetic profiling over the first 24 h after study drug administration will occur in the first 8 patients enrolled in the study, and plasma study drug levels will be collected monthly in all patients.

Early Study Termination

Patients who discontinue study drug because of an adverse event, and those who discontinue study drug because they received an organ transplant or changed modality to hemodialysis will then undergo a post-treatment visit. If a patient's RRF improves sufficiently and a clinical decision is made to discontinue PD, study drug will be continued for the remainder of the 6-month treatment period. The patient will continue monthly in-person visits and study assessments, as well as the post-treatment visit 30 days after discontinuation of study drug.

Sample Size and Intention-to-Treat Analysis

The sample size was calculated under assumptions regarding the secondary efficacy outcome of a mean change from baseline RRF at 6 months. Allowing for a 25% drop out rate and a study design consisting of 7 repeated measures with a first-order autoregressive model covariance, where the standard deviation in measuring RRF is 8 liters/week/1.73 m^2, the correlation between observations on the same subject is 0.9 and the alpha level is 0.05, group samples sizes of 11 in the placebo group and 22 in the bardoxolone methyl group achieve approximately 85% power to detect a difference in RRF of 8 liters/week/1.73 m^2. Analyses of the efficacy data will be based on the intent to treat population, which will include all patients randomized into the study. Safety analyses will include patients receiving any dose or duration of study drug following enrollment.

Table 1. Inclusion and exclusion criteria

Inclusion criteria

The following criteria must be met for inclusion in the study:

1 Adult patients with type 2 diabetes mellitus and ESRD who have been treated with peritoneal dialysis for longer than 3 months, with RRFunction (mean of urea and creatinine clearance) ≥ 25 liters/week/1.73 m^2 in the 4 months prior to screen visit A, and at both screen visits A and B.

2 Patients must have a mean systolic blood pressure, on three readings at both screen visits A and B, ≤160 mm Hg and ≥90 mm Hg. Patients must have a mean diastolic blood pressure, on three readings at both Screen visits A and B, ≤100 mm Hg and ≥40 mm Hg.

3 Willing to practice methods of birth control (both males who have partners of childbearing potential and females of childbearing potential) during screening, while taking study drug and for at least 30 days after the last dose of study drug is ingested.

4 Patients must be willing and able to give written informed consent to participate in the study. They must provide consent for access to medical data according to appropriate local data protection legislation and allow authorization to access medical records that describe events captured in the endpoints. Patients must be willing and able to cooperate with all aspects of the protocol.

Exclusion criteria

Patients with any of the following conditions must be excluded from the study:

1 Hepatitis B surface antigen-positive status; hepatitis C antibody-positive being treated with antiviral therapy, or cirrhosis of the liver.

2 Known history of amyloidosis or light chain nephropathy, autosomal dominant polycystic kidney disease.

3 Hemoglobin A1c level > 11.0% (97 mmol/mol) in the 4 months prior to screening.

4 A serum magnesium level less than 1.4 mEq/l on either screen A or screen B laboratory test results.

5 Total bilirubin, aspartate transaminase, or alanine transaminase level greater than the upper limit of normal or alkaline phosphatase level greater than two times the upper limit of normal on either the screen A or screen B laboratory test results.

6 Recently active cardiovascular disease defined as:
- Unstable angina pectoris within 12 weeks before study randomization.
- Myocardial infarction, coronary artery bypass graft surgery, or percutaneous transluminal coronary angioplasty/stent within 12 weeks before study randomization.
- Cerebrovascular accident, including transient ischemic attack within 12 weeks before study randomization.
- History of hospitalization for congestive heart failure or pulmonary edema within 12 weeks before study randomization.
- Known severe obstructive valvular heart disease or severe obstructive hypertrophic cardiomyopathy.
- Known 2° or 3° AV block not successfully treated with a pacemaker.
- Known history of resuscitated sudden cardiac death.
- Known history of an automatic implantable defibrillator.
- Rate-corrected QT interval (QT_c) greater than 0.50 seconds on an ECG obtained during screening.

7 Currently active systemic lupus erythematosus.

8 Systemic immunosuppression for more than 15 days, cumulatively, within 12 weeks before study randomization or anticipated need for more than 15 cumulative days of therapy during the study.

9 History or planned organ transplant.

10 Clinically significant infection requiring intravenous administration of antibiotics or hospitalization within 12 weeks before study randomization. In a patient who has been on peritoneal dialysis for ≥6 months, two or more episodes of peritonitis in the 6 months before study randomization. In a patient who has been on peritoneal dialysis for <6 months, one episode of peritonitis before study randomization.

11 Diagnosis or treatment of a malignancy in the past 5 years, excluding nonmelanoma skin cancer and carcinoma in situ of the cervix.

12 Diagnostic or interventional procedure that required intravenous administration of an iodinated contrast agent or gadolinium within 12 weeks before study randomization.

Discussion

The previous and current studies of bardoxolone methyl therapy in patients with type 2 diabetes mellitus and CKD have not enrolled subjects with a baseline eGFR <15 ml/min/1.73 m^2. Nrf2 expression is ubiquitous and multiple biochemical and physiological changes can be seen with bardoxolone methyl therapy. While there is no reason to anticipate any untoward effects from these changes in patients with type 2 diabetes mellitus and stage 5 CKD on dialysis, it is important to prospectively evaluate the safety and pharmacokinetic profile of bardoxolone methyl therapy in a population downstream from those being studied in BEACON.

The data from this proposed study may provide additional insight into the effects seen in previous studies of bardoxolone methyl. For example, previous studies have shown that hypomagnesemia occurs more frequently in patients taking bardoxolone methyl compared to placebo [24, 25]. Evaluating whether hypomagnesemia occurs with bardoxolone methyl in patients with ESRD will help narrow the potential causes since renal losses of magnesium are less likely in this population.

Finally, this proposed study will provide guidance for future studies in the ESRD population. If bardoxolone methyl is found have a similar safety profile in this population as earlier stages of CKD, and is shown to maintain or improve RRF, further consideration may be given to conducting additional clinically meaningful studies in a PD population.

References

1 Capusa C, Stoian I, Rus E, et al: Does dialysis modality influence the oxidative stress of uremic patients? Kidney Blood Press Res 2012;35:220–225.

2 Aroeira LS, Lara-Pezzi E, Loureiro J, et al: Cyclooxygenase-2 mediates dialysate-induced alterations of the peritoneal membrane. J Am Soc Nephrol 2009;20:582–592.

3 Bargman JM, Thorpe KE, Churchill DN: Relative contribution of residual renal function and peritoneal clearance to adequacy of dialysis: a reanalysis of the CANUSA study. J Am Soc Nephrol 2001;12:2158–2162.

4 Khaira A, Mahajan S, Kumar A, et al: Oxidative stress, endothelial function, carotid artery intimal thickness and their correlates among chronic peritoneal dialysis patients. Indian J Nephrol 2011;21:264–269.

5 Misra M, Khanna R: Peritoneal dialysis in diabetic end-stage renal disease; in Khanna R, Kredict RT (eds): Nolph and Gokal's Textbook of Peritoneal Dialysis. Berlin, Springer Science, 2009, pp 781–802.

6 De Vriese AS: The John F. Maher Recipient Lecture 2004: rage in the peritoneum. Peritoneal Dialysis Intern 2005;25:8–11.

7 Nakamura S, Tachikawa T, Tobita K, et al: Role of advanced glycation end products and growth factors in peritoneal dysfunction in CAPD patients. Am J Kidney Dis 2003;41:S61–S67.

8 Schwenger V, Morath C, Salava A, et al: Damage to the peritoneal membrane by glucose degradation products is mediated by the receptor for advanced glycation end-products. J Am Soc Nephrol 2006;17:199–207.

9 Gonzalez-Mateo GT, Aroeira LS, Lopez-Cabrera M, et al: Pharmacological modulation of peritoneal injury induced by dialysis fluids: is it an option? Nephrol Dial Transplant 2012;27:478–481.

10 Singhal MK, Bhaskaran S, Vidgen E, et al: Rate of decline of residual renal function in patients on continuous peritoneal dialysis and factors affecting it. Perit Dial Int 2000;20:429–438.

11 Jansen MA, Hart AA, Korevaar JC, et al: Predictors of the rate of decline of residual renal function in incident dialysis patients. Kidney Int 2002;62:1046–1053.

12 Maiorca R, Brunori G, Zubani R, et al: Predictive value of dialysis adequacy and nutritional indices for mortality and morbidity in CAPD and HD patients. A longitudinal study. Nephrol Dial Transplant 1995;10:2295–2305.

13 Bargman JM, Thorpe KE, Churchill DN, CANUSA Peritoneal Dialysis Study Group: Relative contribution of residual renal function and peritoneal clearance to adequacy of dialysis: a reanalysis of the CANUSA study. J Am Soc Nephrol 2001;12:2158–2162.

14 Paniagua R, Amato D, Vonesh E, et al: Effects of increased peritoneal clearances on mortality rates in peritoneal dialysis: ADEMEX, a prospective, randomized, controlled trial. J Am Soc Nephrol 2002;13:1307–1320.

15 van der Wal WM, Noordzij M, Dekker FW, et al: Full loss of residual renal function causes higher mortality in dialysis patients; findings from a marginal structural model. Nephrol Dialysis Transplant 2011;26:2978–2983.

16 Clinical Practice Guidelines for Peritoneal Adequacy, Update 2006. Am J Kidney Dis 2006;48:S91–S97.

17 Kendrick J, Teitelbaum I: Strategies for improving long-term survival in peritoneal dialysis patients. Clin J Am Soc Nephrol 2010;5:1123–1131.
18 Dinkova-Kostova AT, Liby KT, Stephenson KK, et al: Extremely potent triterpenoid inducers of the phase 2 response: correlations of protection against oxidant and inflammatory stress. Proc Natl Acad Sci USA 2005;102:4584–4589.
19 Willoughby DA, Moore AR, Colville-Nash PR: Cyclopentenone prostaglandins-new allies in the war on inflammation. Nat Med 2000;6:137–138.
20 Yoh K, Itoh K, Enomoto A, et al: Nrf2-deficient female mice develop lupus-like autoimmune nephritis. Kidney Int 2001;60:1343–1353.
21 Hirayama A, Yoh K, Nagase S, et al: EPR imaging of reducing activity in Nrf2 transcriptional factor-deficient mice. Free Radic Biol Med 2003;34:1236–1242.
22 Li J, Stein TD, Johnson JA: Genetic dissection of systemic autoimmune disease in Nrf2-deficient mice. Physiol Genomics 2004;18:261–272.
23 Ma Q, Battelli L, Hubbs AF: Multiorgan autoimmune inflammation, enhanced lymphoproliferation, and impaired homeostasis of reactive oxygen species in mice lacking the antioxidant-activated transcription factor Nrf2. Am J Pathol 2006;168:1960–1974.
24 Pergola PE, Krauth M, Huff JW, et al: Effect of bardoxolone methyl on kidney function in patients with T2D and Stage 3b-4 CKD. Am J Nephrol 2011;33:469–476.
25 Pergola PE, Raskin P, Toto RD, et al: Bardoxolone methyl and kidney function in CKD with type 2 diabetes. N Engl J Med 2011;365:327–336.
26 Pergola PE, Grossman EB, Krauth M, Ruiz S, Meyer CM: Results from a phase 2 study of an amorphous spray-dried dispersion (SDD) formulation of bardoxolone methyl. Abstract and Poster World Congress of Nephrology, Vancouver, 2011.
27 Bardoxolone Methyl Evaluation in Patients with Chronic Kidney Disease and Type 2 Diabetes (BEACON): NCT01351675. Date Accessed: February 8, 2012; http://clinicaltrials.gov/ct2/show/NCT01351675?term=NCT01351675&rank=1.

David G. Warnock, MD
Room 636 ZRB, UAB
1530 3rd Avenue South
Birmingham, AL 34294–0007 (USA)
Tel. +1 205 934 9509, E-Mail dwarnock@uab.edu

Ronco C, Rosner MH, Crepaldi C (eds): Peritoneal Dialysis – State-of-the-Art 2012.
Contrib Nephrol. Basel, Karger, 2012, vol 178, pp 164–168

Assessment of Fluid Status in Peritoneal Dialysis

Graham Woodrow[a] · Claudio Ronco[b]

[a]Renal Unit, St James's University Hospital and University of Leeds, Leeds, UK; [b]Department of Nephrology, International Renal Research Institute, San Bortolo Hospital, Vicenza, Italy

Abstract

Fluid management is recognized as a basic component of management of patients on dialysis. Fluid overload is an important adverse factor in patient outcomes, and the negative effects of fluid depletion, including on residual renal function, are also increasingly being recognized. The complexities of fluid distribution in renal failure need to be understood to inform assessment of hydration. Clinical assessment of hydration is insensitive to abnormalities in hydration. BIA is the most promising technique for objective assessment of fluid status, but it is essential that the underlying principles and limitations are understood, and that results from BIA are utilized in conjunction with clinical assessment rather than in isolation.

Fluid management is one of the basic and essential roles of renal replacement therapy in patients with end-stage renal failure. Abnormalities of body fluid content have a critical interaction with the cardiovascular system and residual renal function. Control of fluid status may be one of the most important factors impacting on patient outcomes in dialysis patients, which can be modified by available treatment strategies.

Volume overload in dialysis patients is associated with hypertension, left ventricular hypertrophy, dilatation and dysfunction, which are strongly associated with mortality and reduced survival. Fluid overload may also commonly lead to adverse patient symptoms including edema and dyspnea. However, fluid depletion is increasingly recognized to also have adverse consequences. Fluid depletion is an important factor associated with rate of decline in residual renal function in peritoneal dialysis (PD), which is of great significance given the relationship of preserved residual renal function to better survival in PD patients. Achieving excess fluid removal by PD may involve exposing the patient to unnecessary hypertonic glucose dialysate, with the associated unwanted adverse metabolic effects and impact on the peritoneal membrane. Excess fluid removal may also actually have an adverse cardiovascular effect, potentially through effects on coronary perfusion and peripheral vascular resistance.

With current techniques in PD including the appropriate use of APD, icodextrin dialysate and diuretics, combined with controlled fluid and dietary sodium intake, it is possible to achieve adequate fluid removal to prevent fluid excess in the majority of PD patients. Two key aspects of fluid management in clinical practice in PD are how to assess fluid status, preferably in an objective and accurate manner, and secondly

Table 1. Body water distribution

Total body water	
Intracellular fluid	reflects body cell mass, not hydration reduced in wasting
Extracellular fluid	
Intravascular	affects tissue perfusion, blood pressure
Extravascular	excess leads to edema

to define what the desirable state of hydration actually is.

Normal Body Fluid Content

Body water is distributed between different compartments, which are crucial to assessing and understanding abnormalities of fluid status and assessment methods in clinical practice (table 1).

Importantly, the volumes of these water compartments may vary independently of each other, so it is important to consider which aspects are being assessed by particular techniques for determining hydration.

An additional challenge in patients with advanced renal disease is the presence of pathological factors that may affect the relationship between these different water compartments. These include the presence of cardiorespiratory disease, reduced oncotic pressure (especially in PD patients who tend to have relatively reduced serum albumin levels), malnutrition and wasting, altered autonomic nervous system function and vascular tone and vascular permeability. This means that it may be desirable to assess fluid status from various aspects reflecting differing compartments to gain a detailed picture rather than a single gold standard being possible. Recent studies have suggested that in PD patients, there may be a relative excess of extravascular compared with intravascular water, potentially related to lower serum albumin in PD patients [1], and that factors other than fluid content may play a role in fluid distribution and edema [2]. Thus, patients on PD with normal intravascular volume may tend to have increased extravascular volume and thus increased total ECW volume.

Assessment Techniques

Assessment by clinical examination is imprecise, and may be insensitive to significant abnormalities of hydration. Significant fluid excess for example may be hidden or manifest as hypertension alone. This has led to the search for more sophisticated and objective measurement techniques. However, clinical examination may provide important information in an individual patient, and may reflect aspects not assessed by other methodology (such as features of cardiovascular dysfunction) and so examination findings should be used in conjunction with other methodology rather than being discarded. Blood pressure is a crucial parameter which should be incorporated into any assessment of fluid status and clinical management decision. Chest X-ray allows measurement of cardiac diameter and sometimes detection of subclinical fluid excess and has been used in monitoring fluid status and determining target weight, though aggressive fluid removal in the setting of cardiac dysfunction by this approach may accelerate residual function loss [3].

Measurement of inferior vena cava (IVC) diameter by ultrasound has been investigated as a measure of hydration. The diameter and 'collapsibility' of the inferior vena cava has been shown to reflect fluid status in PD patients, though may have only modest sensitivity for detecting important changes in fluid status in individual subjects. Natriuretic peptides such as ANP, BNP and NT-proBNP are produced by the heart, and blood concentrations have been shown to reflect hydration. They are attractive as a marker reflecting intravascular filling which can be determined from a blood test. However, concentrations are affected by renal failure leading to wide variations in concentrations in dialysis patients, and also may vary due to a direct effect of cardiac disease. Thus, at present, they cannot be used to 'diagnose' the state of hydration in an individual patient.

Bioelectrical Impedance Analysis

Bioelectrical impedance analysis (BIA) is a technique that has become increasingly prominent in the renal literature, and is now increasingly making the transition to being used in the clinical setting. It is important to appreciate that BIA actually refers to a group of differing technologies, and that commercially produced systems may have their own individual unique algorithms for estimating body water volumes. Thus, limitations of the accuracy, nature and validity of the information produced by BIA may be quite different between different systems and methodologies.

BIA involves passage of an AC electrical current through the body and measuring the resulting impedance. The underlying assumption is that the electrical current is conducted by body water, and thus impedance is inversely related to total body water content. Body mass can be split into body fat and fat-free compartments. Water content is present as the dominant component of the fat free compartment (in normal man is believed to be 73% of fat-free mass). Thus, impedance also reflects fat-free mass, whilst theoretically fat is anhydrous and so does not contribute to conduction of the current and thus is not directly reflected in impedance. Earliest techniques used single-frequency BIA (with current frequency 50 kHz). Total body water was estimated by predictive equations, typically including the term height^2/impedance. These provide moderately accurate estimates of total body water. However, there are significant potential errors in individual patients.

There are important underlying assumptions of BIA which do not hold true and contribute to potential error. One of the most important is that the body acts as a uniform electrical conductor. Clearly, the body is closer to a series of cylinders of different length and cross-sectional area, in series. The limbs, having smaller cross-sectional area and greater length than the trunk, actually account for the majority of whole body impedance, with the technique being relatively insensitive to the significant component of body mass within the trunk. Segmental BIA, with measurements of impedance of individual segments has been developed to overcome this, but clearly even the limbs and trunk individually are not uniform in cross-sectional area or composition, limiting the improvement in estimating whole body composition from this approach.

An important clinical limitation of the original BIA approach for measuring body composition, is that total body water (TBW) is of limited clinical value in assessing hydration in patients with complex combinations of disordered hydration and nutrition. For example, clinicians are familiar with the dialysis patient with stable body weight masking simultaneous fluid excess and wasting. In this situation, TBW may be stable, whilst extracellular water (ECW), reflecting hydration, is increased, but intracellular water (ICW), reflecting body cell mass, is reduced. Thus, it would be of far greater value, for both fluid and nutritional assessment, to be able to determine ECW and ICW separately, rather than just estimating TBW.

Fortunately, there are a couple of approaches which allow BIA to distinguish between ECW and ICW. Single frequency impedance actually comprises a major resistance component, and smaller reactance component. The relationship between these components can be plotted on an 'RXc graph', and changes in the relationship between these components reflects the relative contributions of ECW and ICW, in the 'phase angle' [4]. Following changes in the resistance/reactance vector on the graph reflects the relative changes in ECW and ICW, and some normal population ranges for these variables have been described.

The passage of an AC electrical current also varies according to the current frequency. At low frequencies, the current passes largely through the ECW space, with the capacitance effect of cell membranes preventing penetration of the intracellular space. With increasing frequency of the current, there is increasing passage of the current through the ICW as well as ECW compartments. Multifrequency BIA techniques utilize this property to distinguish between ECW and ICW volumes. Some methods use measurements at a few lower and higher frequency currents. Bioimpedance spectroscopy is a widely used method which involves measurements at a large number of frequencies across a wide range, allowing by mathematical modeling, the derivation of the theoretical values at 0 frequency (reflecting just ECW) and infinite frequency, reflecting true TBW [5].

BIA is a simple to perform, portable and non-invasive technique that is very suitable for performing measurements in the clinical setting, including the hospital clinic and dialysis unit settings and in the patient's home [6]. BIA needs to be performed according to standard procedures, with attention to electrode position and contact, and usually the patient should lie flat for 5 min before performing the reading due to the effect of posture (although there are some commercial systems designed for the standing subject). A valuable feature of BIA is the high precision of measurement, making it a potentially valuable tool for repeat measurements over time, for longitudinal monitoring and detection of changes in hydration and body composition over time.

Expressions of Hydration and Defining Ideal Dry Weight

One challenging issue is converting measures of ECW to expressions of 'hydration' relevant to the individual, to take account of variation in body size and body composition. A widely used approach has been to express ECW divided by ICW or TBW, as a way of normalizing to body size. An attraction is that this is an easily derived ratio from BIA devices that allow assessment of ECW separate from ICW. Normal ranges for the population have been derived to determine the normality of results in terms of standard deviations from the population mean [7]. However, a limitation is that the ratio reflects both the numerator and the denominator. Thus elevated ECW/ICW or ECW/TBW may well reflect overhydration with increased ECW, but also could be due to reduced ICW in the patient with wasting (which also reduces total TBW), or a combination of overhydration and wasting [8]. An alternative approach is to normalize ECW to other measures of body size such as height.

A recent development has been the development of a novel model of body composition, which defines the amount of water that should be present in the different compartments according to body composition theory, with any excess or deficit being designated as the volume of overhydration (or depletion) compared with ideal [9]. Initial clinical studies in groups of patients on hemodialysis, and more recently PD, suggest that this may have useful application in assessing hydration in patients with end-stage renal disease [10–12].

However, some caution is required in applying the results of BIA to the clinical management and determination of ideal dry weight. Even with sophisticated models of body composition, there would be expected to be some variation in normality and some potential error in actual measurement due to measurement error. Clinical experience suggests that in some patients even modest change in dry weight or fluid removal can have a significant clinical effect, so erroneous changes in dry weight could have clinically important effects. The other limitation of BIA is that in the complex patients on dialysis, the 'ideal' ECW volume may not be the 'normal' ECW volume defined for a healthy individual by body composition analysis. Thus, if PD patients have relative extravascular fluid increase, normalizing ECW will lead to depleted intravascular volume, with potential effects of loss of residual renal function and hypotension. Also, in the presence of cardiorespiratory disease, the clinically optimal ECW volume may differ from normal body composition. In some patients fluid removal could be limited by hypotension, others needing greater fluid removal to prevent pulmonary edema due to left ventricular dysfunction. Thus, it is imperative that techniques such as BIA should be used in conjunction with blood pressure and clinical and other information rather than as a 'gold standard' to be applied to fluid adjustment in isolation.

Conclusion

Fluid management is an important aspect of management of patients on dialysis and may have a significant impact on outcomes. An important challenge is striking a balance between the potentially adverse effects of fluid overload and deletion. Assessment of hydration and determination of ideal hydration remains a challenge. BIA represents a potentially valuable tool in monitoring change in fluid state and body composition. BIA may be useful in combination with clinical assessment in adjusting target weight. The results of further studies are required to define the use of BIA in clinical practice and impact on management and outcomes in dialysis patients.

References

1 John B, Tan BK, Dainty S, Spanel P, Smith D, Davies SJ: Plasma volume, albumin, and fluid status in peritoneal dialysis patients. CJASN 2010;5:1463–1470.
2 Tang W, Tian X, Xin-Hong L, Ya-Jun L, Wang T: Factors contributing to formation of oedema in volume overloaded continuous ambulatory peritoneal dialysis patients. Perit Dial Int 2011;31:160–167.
3 Aşci G, Özkahya M, Duman S, Erten S, Ok E: Volume control associated with better cardiac functions in long-term peritoneal dialysis patients. Perit Dial Int 2006;26:85–88.
4 Piccoli A, Rossi B, Pillon L, Bucciante G: A new method for monitoring body fluid variation by bioimpedance analysis: the RXc graph. Kidney Int 1994;46:534–539.
5 Matthie J, Zarowitz B, DeLorenzo A, et al: Analytic assessment of the various bioimpedance methods used to estimate body water. J Appl Physiol 1998;84:1801–1816.
6 Woodrow G, Devine Y, Cullen M, Lindley E: Application of bioelectrical impedance to clinical assessment of body composition in peritoneal dialysis. Perit Dial Int 2007;27:496–502.
7 Lindley E, Devine Y, Hall L, Cullen M, Cuthbert S, Woodrow G, Will E, Lopot F: A ward based procedure for assessment of fluid status in peritoneal dialysis patients using bioimpedance spectroscopy. Perit Dial Int 2005;25(suppl 3):S46–S48.
8 Woodrow G, Oldroyd B, Wright A, Coward A, Truscott JG: Effect of normalisation of ECW volume as a marker of hydration in PD patients and controls. Perit Dial Int 2005;25(suppl 3):S49–S51.
9 Chamney PW, Wabel P, Moissl UM, et al: A whole body model to distinguish excess fluid from the hydration of major body tissues. Am J Clin Nutr 2007;85:80–89.
10 Devolder I, Verleysen A, Vijt D, Vanholder R, Van Biesen W: Body composition, hydration, and related parameters in hemodialysis versus peritoneal dialysis patients. Perit Dial Int 2010;30:208.
11 Van Biesen W, Williams JD, Covic AC, et al: Fluid status in peritoneal dialysis patients: The European body composition monitoring (EuroBCM) study cohort. PLoS ONE 2011;6:e17148.
12 Wabel P, Moissl U, Chamney P, et al: Towards improving cardiovascular management: the necessity of combining blood pressure and fluid overload. Nephrol Dial Transplant 2008;23:2965–2971.

Dr. Graham Woodrow
Renal Unit, St James's University Hospital
Beckett Street
Leeds LS9 7TF (UK)
Tel. +44 113 2066247, E-Mail Graham.Woodrow@leedsth.nhs.uk

Ronco C, Rosner MH, Crepaldi C (eds): Peritoneal Dialysis – State-of-the-Art 2012.
Contrib Nephrol. Basel, Karger, 2012, vol 178, pp 169–173

Fluid Transport and Homeostasis in Peritoneal Dialysis

Josep Teixidó Planas

Hospital Universitari Germans Trias i Pujol, Nephrology Department, Badalona, Spain

Abstract

Ultrafiltration failure is one of the main concerns for patients on long-term peritoneal dialysis. According to the three-pore model of peritoneal transport, peritoneal water flows via four pathways: ultrasmall pores, small pores, large pores and through peritoneal or lymphatic reabsorption. New methods that allow clinicians to identify the mechanisms behind disturbances in water transport can be applied in clinical practice. Small pore transport and free water transport can be estimated after a short 1-hour dwell with a glucose solution, without the need for an intraperitoneal volume marker. Until now, peritoneal reabsorption has been calculated using indirect and complicated methods. However, a simple, standardized method that is useful in clinical practice is needed. Ultrafiltration failure may be caused by rapid solute transport, slow solute transport, high peritoneal reabsorption and decreased free water transport (aquaporin failure). This article briefly discusses the clinical significance of disturbances in ultrafiltration, possible improvements in treatment options, and how to achieve or maintain fluid homeostasis.

Water transport in peritoneal dialysis (PD) is a crucial factor in the management of patients on peritoneal dialysis. An increasing number of patients experience ultrafiltration failure while undergoing PD, and this could play a key role in technical failure and in decreased patient survival. Ultrafiltration failure is likely due to various mechanisms that are poorly understood in clinical practice. Over the past few years, however, new methods have been developed to estimate free water transport and small pore ultrafiltration, allowing a better understanding of these mechanisms. According to the three-pore model of peritoneal transport, water flows through four pathways or channels: ultrasmall pores, small pores, large pores and through peritoneal reabsorption by lymphatics or capillaries. The calculation of water transport through the different channels enables clinicians to identify disturbances in ultrafiltration in individual patients and to apply the appropriate treatment in order to maintain fluid homeostasis.

Water Pathways in PD

Small Pores

According to the three-pore model, small pores are the clefts or gaps located between endothelial cells in the peritoneal capillaries. They account for approximately 95% of hydraulic transport, and are responsible for transporting small solute, including sodium, through convection [1].

Ultrasmall Pores

AQP-1, an aquaporin found in endothelial capillaries and postcapillary venules of the peritoneum, allows the accommodation of a single water molecule and corresponds perfectly to the ultrasmall pores described in the three-pore model. In addition, ultrasmall pores explain sodium sieving (the dissociation between sodium and water transport during the first part of a peritoneal dwell) when using glucose as a crystalloid osmotic agent [2]. Studies conducted in knockout mice (Aqp1–/–) have shown a significant decrease in osmotic driven water transport compared with Aqp1+/+ mice, and that mice lacking APQ1 show about a 50% decrease in ultrafiltration with hypertonic dialysate. AQPs are also involved in cell migration, wound healing and tumour growth and dissemination [2].

Water transport through AQP1 is directly correlated with the osmotic gradient, while small pore water transport is correlated with only high osmotic gradients. Therefore, during the second or third part of a peritoneal dwell, other nonosmotic forces play a role in maintaining ultrafiltration [3].

Large Pores

These pores are thought to correspond to capillary or venular interendothelial gaps and only account for 5–6% of the peritoneal ultrafiltration fraction. As such, they are currently excluded from water transport calculations.

Peritoneal Reabsorption

In recent years, it has become clear that peritoneal reabsorption is not only, or mainly, a lymphatic reabsorption. Capillaries or venules contribute primarily to interstitial reabsorption. As such, water flows to or from the peritoneum according to pressure gradients during different time points of the dwell [4].

Methods Used to Estimate Water Transport

Two recent reviews provide an overview of the methods used to test peritoneal membrane function [5, 6].

The original peritoneal equilibration test (PET), developed by Twardoski in 1987 and performed using a 2.27% glucose solution, does not provide enough information to fully discriminate between the mechanisms behind ultrafiltration failure.

The standardized peritoneal analysis (SPA) [7], which uses a 3.86% glucose solution, yields more information on small solute transport, protein transport, free water transport, small pore ultrafiltration, large pore ultrafiltration and lymphatic reabsorption. However, when using this test, a macromolecular marker (dextran, RISA) is needed in order to calculate intraperitoneal volume and reabsorption. As such, it is not applicable in a great majority of peritoneal units.

The SPA estimates small pore water transport by calculating the amount of sodium transferred to the peritoneal cavity at different time points, dividing it by membrane sodium concentration (Na plasma + Na peritoneal/2) after subtracting diffused sodium; this calculates convective water transport by small pores. The water volume calculated can be deduced from the total ultrafiltration volume at the same time points of the dwell, to estimate the amount of free water transport [7].

The Mini-PET [6], which uses a 3.86% glucose solution, only takes one hour to perform and calculates the net ultrafiltration directly, without a volume marker. As such, it is applicable in any peritoneal unit. However, it does not provide much more information, and small solute transport at 60 min has not been confirmed to be equivalent to the standard 4-hour PET.

Venturoli and Rippe [8] compared the SPA method and the Mini-PET method using the three-pore model. The authors found that while the Smit method is more accurate all along the dwell, La Milia's method is more applicable, although it underestimates free water transport by approximately 20%. The latter could be considered a new tool to estimate water transport, and is more precise than sodium sieving.

The inclusion of a complete peritoneal drainage at 60 min followed by reinfusion of the effluent in a standard 4-hour PET did not show significant differences in solute transport or ultrafiltration compared to the standard 4-hour PET. This combined PET estimates free water transport and small pore water transport without a volume marker.

The Double Mini-PET (Mini-PET 1.36% glucose solution followed by Mini-PET 3.86% glucose solution) allows the calculation of osmotic conductance, or the membrane's response to a given crystalloid osmotic gradient. A worsening in osmotic conductance is a sign of AQP-1 damage and serious impairment of the peritoneal membrane, which could result in encapsulating peritoneal sclerosis (EPS) [6].

Until now, peritoneal reabsorption has been calculated using indirect methods, using the disappearance of volume marker corrected with the coefficient K_e, or by assessing the difference between the night dwell and the PET dwell. We propose an extended peritoneal test from 4 to 8 h, reinfusing the effluent to calculate the reabsorption when the glucose osmotic gradient has disappeared. A preliminary study has yielded consistent results, and this could be a standardized method.

Disturbances in Water Transport

Ultrafiltration failure accounts for approximately 30% of cases of technical failure in patients on long-term PD. In searching for the cause of ultrafiltration failure, one must look at peritoneal injury as a result of the catheter or as a result of the peritoneal solution, such as epithelial mesenchymal transition [9] or other basic changes in capillaries, interstitium or mesothelium, which can result in interstitial fibrosis, neoangiogenesis and lymphatic disturbances. These processes can lead to AQP-1 damage and contribute to impairments in water homeostasis. Moreover, genetic factors may be involved: polymorphisms have been found in VEGF, IL-6, RAGE, eNOS and in plasminogen activating factor-1.

Patients on peritoneal dialysis are frequently hypoalbuminemic, retain sodium and water, have cardiovascular overload and are at an increased risk for death. This physiopathological process could be accelerated when residual renal function declines and when ultrafiltration failure occurs.

Disturbances in water homeostasis, therefore, could decrease patient survival and increase technical failure. A daily ultrafiltration of <1 liter/24 h together with age and serum albumin have been found to be independent predictors of mortality, while ultrafiltration independently predicted technical failure in a recent cohort study.

Mechanisms of Ultrafiltration Failure

Now that we can better distinguish some of the mechanisms behind water transport impairment using the methods mentioned above, we can classify disturbances in ultrafiltration as rapid solute transport, slow solute transport, high peritoneal reabsorption and aquaporin failure.

In using the SPA in 154 patients on PD, Smit et al. [7] identified 53 patients with ultrafiltration failure. The causes (mechanisms) they found were high mass transfer area coefficient (MTAC), 37 (70%); low MTAC, 0; high effective lymphatic absorption rate (ELAR), 30 (56.4%), and an absent dip in sodium, 14 (26.4%). Most patients have more than one mechanism of ultrafiltration failure. In another study, the authors found similar results.

In two subsequent studies, the same authors showed that in the early years of PD (2 years) ultrafiltration impairment is related to fast solute transport and high lymphatic reabsorption, while in later years (>2 or >4 years) a decrease in osmotic conductance plays a role. This is probably due to aquaporin damage as a sign of critical peritoneal injury.

Sampimon et al. [10] compared 11 patients on PD who were diagnosed of encapsulating peritoneal sclerosis (EPS) with 31 controls on PD to try to elucidate what precedes EPS. They observed (1) that patients who developed EPS were younger and the duration of PD was longer, (2) that peritoneal small solute transport showed significant inverse U-shaped trends before the diagnosis of EPS, (3) a progressive decrease in ultrafiltration, and a more pronounced decrease in free water transport, and (4) a lower appearance rate of CA-125 and a higher appearance rate of IL-6, which combined showed a sensitivity of 70% and a specificity of 89%.

Lambie et al. [11] studied 9 patients with EPS among 690 patients on PD with the same objective described above. They found similar observations prior to a diagnosis of EPS: (1) an increase in small solute transport, (2) ultrafiltration capacity was significantly worse 2 years prior to stopping dialysis, (3) glucose exposure was significantly higher in the five years preceding EPS, and (4) a higher exposure to the osmotic agent icodextrin. These changes suggest reduced osmotic conductance in patients with EPS.

Asghar and Davies [12] conducted a study in 8 stable PD patients by using two PETs (1.36 and 3.86% glucose) lasting for 4 h and using ^{125}I-albumin as a volume marker. They found some very interesting observations: (1) during the first part of a 3.86% dwell, small pore ultrafiltration positively correlated with solute transport, (2) transcellular ultrafiltration showed a stronger negative correlation with small solute transport over the whole dwell, and (3) the rate of fluid reabsorption strongly correlated to the solute transport rate, indicating that patients with high transport absorbed fluid more rapidly.

The important observation, therefore, is that in the predominant reabsorption phase, mainly seen with a low glucose concentration (1.36%), water flows back (back-filtration) primarily through small pores, making them a two-way channel, and thus confirming the predictions of the three-pore model [13].

Can We Prevent Ultrafiltration Failure?

Studies assessing new peritoneal solutions suggest less peritoneal damage and better preservation of peritoneal function.

Studies in rats using a combined solution of glycerol, amino acids and dextrose showed similar solute transport, ultrafiltration and better preservation of peritoneal morphology, compared with conventional solutions with GDPs.

L-Carnitine can be used as an osmotic agent in peritoneal solutions. Endothelial cell cultures with L-carnitine show increased AQP-1 expression, improved viability and less apoptosis. A combination of glucose 1.5% and L-carnitine 0.25%, administered in 4 CAPD patients, was well tolerated and resulted in high ultrafiltration.

In rats treated with conventional solutions, celecoxib inhibited Cox-2 and drastically reduced PGE2 levels, angiogenesis, lymphangiogenesis, fibrosis, milky spot formation and completely prevented ultrafiltration failure. In the clinical setting, COX-2 inhibitors are associated with cardiovascular side effects, making them difficult to use. However, this could be a new strategy to explore to prevent peritoneal damage and the resulting ultrafiltration failure [14].

Other researchers have attempted to enhance free water transport: (1) glucose exposure enhanced AQP1 biosynthesis in a time- and dose-dependent manner; (2) high doses of corticoesteroids enhanced AQP-1 expression in rats; (3) after renal transplantation in 3 patients on PD treated with high-dose methylprednisolone, a twofold increase in sodium sieving and ultrasmall pore ultrafiltration was found, suggesting that glucocorticoids have an effect on APQ-1, mediated by the promoter of the AQP-1 gene, and (4) some studies suggest aryl sulfonamide derivatives can act as AQP agonists, enhancing water transport across the membrane [2].

Achieving or Maintaining Fluid Homeostasis

The first treatment option to improve fluid status and hypertension is salt and water restriction. However, although this is a clinician's best advice, it is difficult for patients to accept and adhere to this option.

Automated peritoneal dialysis may obtain acceptable results in rapid transporters.

Also in rapid transporters and in patients who develop ultrafiltration failure mainly because of disturbances in free water transport, icodextrin may recuperate ultrafiltration and improve patient survival and prevent technical failure in the short term.

Studies on low sodium solutions have provided a good outlook for the future, although results have to be confirmed in larger clinical studies. In this field, some observations of published studies must be considered: (1) patient overhydration does not necessarily aid in maintaining residual renal function, as would be expected, (2) overhydration does not change the plasma volume, so attempts to reduce extracellular fluid may cause plasma volume shrinkage and residual renal function impairment, (3) in studies maintaining a strict fluid balance, patients have a lower cardiovascular risk profile and decreased left ventricular hypertrophy and it would therefore be better to avoid overhydration by using some hypertonic glucose concentrations, if sodium balance is under control, and (4) this must be counterbalanced by the risk of increasing membrane injury by the glucose solutions.

Conclusions

New practical methods exist to better control disturbances in water transport by calculating free water transport, small pore water transport and the peritoneal reabsorption rate. All peritoneal water pathways have to be considered in individual patients. Understanding these disturbances in individual patients will allow clinicians to more appropriately apply available treatment options in PD.

References

1 Rippe B, Venturoli D: Simulations of osmotic ultrafiltration failure in CAPD using a serial three-pore membrane/fiber matrix model. Am J Physiol Renal Physiol 2007;292:F1035–F1043.

2 Devuyst O, Yool AJ: Aquaporin-1: new developments and perspectives for peritoneal dialysis. Perit Dial Int 2010;30:135–141.

3 Parikova A, Smit W, Zweers MM, Struijk DG, Krediet RT: Free water transport, small pore transport and the osmotic pressure gradient. Nephrol Dial Transplant 2008;23:2350–2355.

4 Rippe B: Free water transport, small pore transport and the osmotic pressure gradient three-pore model of peritoneal transport. Nephrol Dial Tranplant 2008;23:2147–2153.

5 van Biesen W, Heimburger O, Krediet R, Rippe B, La Milia V, Covic A, Vanholder R, ERBP Working Group on Peritoneal Dialysis: Evaluation of peritoneal membrane characteristics: clinical advice for prescription management by the ERBP working group. Nephrol Dial Transplant 2010;25:2052–2062.

6 La Milia V: Peritoneal transport testing. J Nephrol 2010;23:633–647.

7 Smit W, van Dijk P, Langedijk MJ, Schouten N, van den Berg N, Struijk DG, Krediet RT: Peritoneal function and assessment of reference values using a 3.86% glucose solution. Perit Dial Int 2003;23:440–449.

8 Venturoli D, Rippe B: Validation by computer simulation of two indirect methods for quantification of free water transport in peritoneal dialysis. Perit Dial Int 2005;25:77–84.

9 Aroeira LS, Aguilera A, Sánchez-Tomero JA, Bajo MA, del Peso G, Jiménez-Heffernan JA, Selgas R, López-Cabrera M: Epithelial to mesenchymal transition and peritoneal membrane failure in peritoneal dialysis patients: pathologic significance and potential therapeutic interventions. J Am Soc Nephrol 2007;18:2004–2013.

10 Sampimon DE, Coester AM, Struijk DG, Krediet RT: The time course of peritoneal transport parameters in peritoneal dialysis patients who develop encapsulating peritoneal sclerosis. Nephrol Dial Transplant 2011;26:291–298.

11 Lambie ML, John B, Mushahar L, Huckvale C, Davies SJ: The peritoneal osmotic conductance is low well before the diagnosis of encapsulating peritoneal sclerosis is made. Kidney Int 2010;78:611–618.

12 Asghar RB, Davies SJ: Pathways of fluid transport and reabsorption across the peritoneal membrane. Kidney Int 2008;73:1048–1053.

13 Rippe B, Venturoli D: Fluid loss from the peritoneal cavity by backfiltration through the small pores of the three-pore model. Kidney Int 2008;73:985–986.

14 Fabbrini P, Schilte MN, Zareie M, ter Wee PM, Keuning ED, Beelen RH, van den Born J: Celecoxib treatment reduces peritoneal fibrosis and angiogenesis and prevents ultrafiltration failure in experimental peritoneal dialysis. Nephrol Dial Transplant 2009;24:3669–3676.

Josep Teixidó Planas, PhD
Hospital Universitari Germans Trias i Pujol, Nephrology Department
Ctera. Canyet s/n
ES–08916 Badalona (Spain)
Tel. +34 93 497 88 98, E-Mail jteixido@acmcb.es

Ronco C, Rosner MH, Crepaldi C (eds): Peritoneal Dialysis – State-of-the-Art 2012.
Contrib Nephrol. Basel, Karger, 2012, vol 178, pp 174–181

Bioimpedance and Brain Natriuretic Peptide in Peritoneal Dialysis Patients

Carlo Crepaldi[a,b] · Elena Iglesias Lamas[b] · Francesca Katiana Martino[a,b] · Maria Pia Rodighiero[a,b] · Elisa Scalzotto[b] · Marzena Wojewodzka-Zelezniakowicz[b] · Mitchell H. Rosner[c] · Claudio Ronco[a,b]

[a]Department of Nephrology Dialysis and Transplantation, [b]International Renal Research Institute (IRRIV), San Bortolo Hospital, Vicenza, Italy; [c]Department of Medicine, University of Virginia Health System, Charlottesville, Va., USA

Abstract

Assessment of ideal body weight in peritoneal dialysis (PD) patients is important for clinical practice. Fluid overload may produce hypertension, reduced arterial distensibility, left ventricular hypertrophy. All these are risk factors for mortality in PD patients: cardio- and cerebrovascular events are the main causes of morbidity and mortality in PD population. Nowadays, a clear and widely accepted definition of ideal body weight in PD patients does not exist. Probably the ideal body weight is the weight at which the extracellular volume is normal. Many different tools have been used to assess the hydration status in dialysis patients. Ultrasonic evaluation of inferior vena cava diameter only assesses intravascular volume, and is also influenced by diastolic dysfunction and is thus a reflection of preload and not of tissue hydration. Direct measurement of extracellular and total body water by dilution methods is considered as the golden standard, but these techniques are laborious and expensive. Parameters, such as brain natriuretic peptide (BNP) or NT-proBNP can reflect changes in hydration status and may help the nephrologist to estimate it. Natriuretic peptides are influenced both by preload and ventricular abnormalities and in patients with renal failure accumulation can occur. Bioimpedance is an accurate, reproducible, not expensive and not invasive technique that permits a good evaluation of hydration status in PD and can drive the nephrologist in his clinical choices. Clinical evaluation, strict control of body weight, diuresis, sodium and fluids intakes, bioimpedance monitoring and serum levels of natriuretic peptides may all together help us to maintain the PD patient euvolemic.

A definition of dry body weight in peritoneal dialysis (PD) patients remains unclear. At the moment, there is no reliable and widely accepted definition of dry body weight in PD patients. The concept of dry body weight is extensively used in hemodialysis (HD) patients. It can be defined as 'the weight at the end of a hemodialysis session, at and below which the patient is free of edema, is normotensive until the next dialysis and has no symptomatic complaints during hemodialysis'. At dry weight, the extracellular volume is at or near normal, but not less than normal. Because of the continuous nature of renal replacement treatment in PD, the determination of dry weight is much more difficult. Thus, determination of dry weight must rely on methods to assess the extracellular volume [1].

Is well known that euvolemia is a predictor of outcome in PD patients. Volume overload is related to cardiac dysfunction and mortality

[2]. Objective tools for estimating dry weight are necessary. Several methods have been proposed for dry weight assessment; these include natriuretic peptides, ultrasound measurement of inferior vena cava diameter and collapsibility on inspiration and intradialytic relative blood volume change. Unfortunately, these methods suffer from several shortcomings, such as poor specificity (natriuretic peptides), operator dependence (inferior vena cava diameter measurements) and poor correlation with extracellular volume (continuous blood volume measurement) [3]. Bioelectrical impedance analysis has been recognized as a noninvasive and simple technique for the assessment of hydration status and may offer unique advantages for the PD patient.

Preservation of residual renal function and reduced early mortality rates are likely to reflect the relative ease with which euvolemia can be achieved in PD patients. Yet, there is concern that these patients are frequently fluid loaded, fuelled by the problems of ultrafiltration failure and worse survival observed in anuric patients with low fluid removal. In reality, the proportion of PD patients that are overhydrated is not dissimilar to HD but the challenges in achieving euvolemia might be different [4].

The system of natriuretic peptides ANP, BNP and CNP play an important role in enhancing the excretion of sodium and water in the kidneys, relaxing of vascular smooth muscle cells and counteracting of the human vasoconstrictor system. Effects in heart include lowering of cardiac preload and afterload and improved myocardial perfusion with coronary vasodilation. A great number of studies have demonstrated the practicability and importance of BNP (BNP and NT-proBNP) testing in various cardiac pathologies including prediction of left ventricular abnormalities in the general population, recognizing cardiac ischemia, and diagnosing, predicting prognosis and monitoring therapy of heart failure. To date, interpretation of BNP levels in PD patients is limited to the areas of hydration status assessment and optimal dry weight determination [5].

Fluid Overload, Hypertension and Cardiovascular Abnormalities in Peritoneal Dialysis Patients

In patients with end-stage renal disease, cardiovascular disease is by far the most common cause of death. Cardiac abnormalities, such as left ventricular hypertrophy (LVH), are strongly related to morbidity and mortality. Several studies have shown a relation between fluid overload, hypertension, and cardiac abnormalities in HD patients, despite the fact that interpretation of these data is complicated by the continuously changing fluid status in these patients. Moreover, abnormalities of the large capacitance arteries, resulting in reduced arterial distensibility and compliance, were also found to be related to both systolic hypertension and changes in cardiac structure. In contrast, few detailed data exist on the fluid status of PD patients [7], or on the relation between fluid status, blood pressure (BP), and structural cardiovascular abnormalities in this population. Various authors have suggested a theoretical benefit for PD due to the continuous removal of fluid and the fact that residual diuresis is often better maintained. However, this may not be the case as a recent study even suggested that PD patients are actually more overhydrated than HD patients [8]. Recent large-scale studies based on dialysis registries have shown that after appropriate statistical adjustment survival in patients on PD is substantially similar to that in HD patients [9]. This may suggest that extracellular volume control is suboptimal in these patients. Maintaining extracellular fluid and salt balance is a major challenge in dialysis patients, and particularly so in PD patients with minimal or no residual renal function. Early experience, generally based on patients with a short duration of treatment, suggested that PD provided a more effective management of hypertension and extracellular volume overload. Other studies, including patients treated for longer periods, seem to indicate the opposite. Hypertension appears to be controlled better by HD than by PD in ESRD patients. The gain in body weight observed with PD treatment may reflect an increase in total body fluid volume which may partly explain why hypertension is less adequately controlled during PD than during HD treatment [10]. An Italian multicentric study on 504 PD patients has demonstrated that hypertension is a dramatic, unsolved problem in uremic patients treated with PD, and casts doubts on the effectiveness of our current PD strategies and pharmacological management of hypertension [11].

A study including all adult 24,587 Australian and New Zealand patients commencing dialysis between January 1, 1997 and December 31, 2007 (first treatment PD n = 6,521; HD n = 18,066) demonstrated that the hazard of death from cardiovascular disease (CVD) in PD patients was not significantly different from that in HD patients in the first year of treatment with an increased risk of death from CVD after 2 years of treatment. A possible explanation of this observation may be the progressive reduction of residual renal function (RRF) along with a suboptimal volume and blood pressure [12].

Interestingly, the definition of dry body weight is different in HD and in PD patients. Dry body weight in HD can be defined as the weight below which the patient is free of edema, normotensive, and without systemic complaints during dialysis [13]. Currently, for PD patients there is no such definition of dry body weight. Krediet [13] defines the dry weight in PD as the weight associated with a normal extracellular volume (ECW). But still the definition of the ECW is related to the method used for estimate it. Evaluation of ECW can be performed by sodium bromide dilution (ECW(NaBr)) and total body potassium (TBK; whole-body (40) K counting) to total body water (TBW; isotope dilution) methods (ECW(TBK-TBW) [14]. These techniques are performed very seldom due to high costs and are not available for everyday use. A useful, alternative technique may be bioimpedance, which permits noninvasive, extracellular, intracellular and total body water measurements.

Bioimpedance

Bioelectrical impedance (BIA) is generated in soft tissue as an opposition to the flow of an injected alternate current and is measured from skin electrodes that are placed on hand and foot (whole body analysis) or on segments and regions of the body (segmental, regional analysis). Bioimpedance techniques are based on this principle: impedance (*Z*) denotes the opposition to injected alternating and/or direct electric current; *Z* has two components: resistance (R; x-axis) and reactance (Xc; y-axis). Resistance is the opposition to the flow of direct and alternating electric current and reactance is the opposition to the passage of alternating current. Resistance and reactance decrease with higher frequencies of the alternating current. The size of the body fluid component is largely reflected in the resistance, whereas reactance might represent the cell membrane area.

Bioimpedance may be single-frequency or multifrequency. With the single-frequency bioimpedance devices the optimal performance of the method is obtained with the standard, single frequency, 50 kHz current that allows impedance measurements with the best signal to noise ratio. The last generation of multifrequency bioimpedance devices measures total-body impedance to an alternating electrical current (0.2 mA) at 50 different frequencies (5–1,000 kHz). Bioimpedance spectroscopy (BIS) uses physiological modeling and mixture equations (Cole-Cole plot and Hanai formulae) to first determine the electrical resistance of ECW and ICW and then calculate the volumes of these respective compartments. BIS has the ability to provide relatively accurate ECV, ICV, TBW and muscle mass measurements. The bioelectrical impedance vector analysis (BIVA) is a single-frequency bioimpedance that generates a vector on a resistance/height-reactance/height graph. The RXc graph is a probability chart that classifies and ranks individual vector according to the distance from the mean value of a reference population. The BIVA may define the hydration status of a patient even not knowing the weight of the patient [4].

Bioimpedance analysis techniques have been considered as a potential tool to measure extracellular body fluid volume noninvasively. Although bioimpedance analysis has been used in clinical studies for more than 20 years, the knowledge of the electrical properties of body tissues is still evolving and the technology has shown continued improvement [15].

After years of bioimpedance analysis (BIA) research in dialysis patients, this technique is now increasingly used clinically. BIA as a means to determine extracellular volume (ECV) and/or intracellular volume (ICV) has been validated by applying dilution methods as the gold standard.

Body composition analysis by BIA has been compared to magnetic resonance imaging (MRI) and appropriate regression models have been developed to estimate fat and muscle content. The clinical use of BIA is currently focused on two major fields, firstly the management of extracellular fluid (dry weight) and secondly the assessment of nutritional status [3].

As excess fluid accumulates mainly in the extracellular space, the ratios of ECW to body surface area, ECW/ICW, and ECW/TBW have all been used to assess fluid status in PD patients. The proportion of ECW also varies with body composition as water in adipose tissue is mainly extracellular (whereas in lean tissue it is mainly intracellular) [16]. Lopot et al. [17] determined the optimal dry weight of HD patients using deviation of ECW/TBW from the ratio in age-matched normal controls, allowing for the change in body composition with age. The ECW/TBW ratio measurements were made using a four electrode, wrist to ankle, multifrequency bioimpedance spectroscope. Measurements were used to generate age- and gender-related ECW/TBW distributions and define the mean ratio as a function of age:

For males: ECW/TBW (%) = 40.02 + 0.0714 × age.

For females: ECW/TBW (%) = 43.28 + 0.0470 × age.

The ECW/TBW ratio was then expressed as a 'hydration score', i.e. the number of standard deviations a patient's ECW/TBW ratio was from the mean for normal controls of their age and gender. Interventions (increased use of high glucose or icodextrin bags and/or advice on fluid intake) were made if patients had a hydration score greater than +2.0.

Since the end of 2007, a new multifrequency bioimpedance spectroscopy device: the Body Composition Monitor (BCM, Fresenius Medical Care, Bad Homburg, Germany) has been available. The BCM expresses the body weight in terms of lean tissue mass (LTM – mainly muscle), adipose tissue mass (ATM – mainly fat) and overhydration (OH). Each of these compartments has a specific composition and contains a known quantity of water per mass of tissue. OH is almost 100% extracellular water, whereas the water of LTM and ATM consist of differing proportion of extracellular and intracellular water in addition to solid components. Excess fluid (a positive OH) represents an expansion of only the extracellular water, whereas ICW remains unchanged. The excess fluid may reside within adipose tissue or lean tissue raising the hydration of the respective tissue above the 'normal' values (e.g. edema). Alternatively, excess fluid may simply appear as a distinct compartment without altering the hydration of the major tissues (e.g. ascites, pleural effusion). A single-center study has recently found that clinically relevant OH, as defined by the BCM, is prevalent in 37.4% of 79 prevalent continuous ambulatory PD (CAPD) patients. This study showed that the OH/ECW ratio was also correlated with the left ventricular mass index (LVMi) in the studied population [18].

The EuroBCM study is a large multicenter study of hydration status and its associated factors in PD patients in Europe allowing comparison to a healthy reference population [2]. Fluid overload was a frequent finding in PD patients as compared to a healthy reference population, but comparable to that reported in HD patients. Absolute Δtissue hydration (AΔTH) was derived from the impedance data based on a physiologic tissue model [18, 19]. Absolute Δtissue hydration represents the difference between the amount of ECW in the tissue as actually detected by the BCM and the amount of water present in tissue, as predicted by physiological models under normal physiological (normohydrated) conditions [19]. Of note, AΔTH has no direct relation to circulating volume. Underhydration (AΔTH <10th percentile), normohydration and overhydration (AΔTH >90th percentile), as defined by the 10th and 90th percentile of values obtained in the normal population were present in 6.7, 39.9 and 53.4% of the EuroBCM cohort. Fluid overload and severe fluid overload, as defined by a relative Δtissue hydration (AΔTH/ECW) above 7% or above 15% were present in 53.4 and 25.2% of the study population. In the large cohort of the EuroBCM PD study, a substantial portion of patients were fluid overloaded by more than 1.1 liters, the 90th percentile of absolute Δtissue hydration in the normal reference population [2].

Natriuretic Peptides

Natriuretic peptides are a group of hormones with similar chemical structure and biological actions. They constitute an important part of the vasodilatatory system in human physiology with diversified effects on heart, kidneys, vascular tree and central nervous system. A-type natriuretic peptide (ANP) was the first one discovered in the beginning of the 1980s, followed by characterization of B-type (BNP) and C-type (CNP) natriuretic peptides approximately 20 years ago. Later, similar peptides with effects on blood pressure and fluid homeostasis have been identified, namely dendroaspis (D-type) natriuretic peptide, urodilatin and guanylin, and uroguanylin [20]. The common physiological effects of natriuretic peptides include enhanced excretion of sodium and water in the kidneys, relaxation of vascular smooth muscle cells and counteraction of the human vasoconstrictor system (sympathetic nervous system, renin-angiotensin-aldosterone system, endothelin and vasopressin) resulting in natriuresis, diuresis and vasodilation. Renal effects are achieved by dilatation of afferent and constriction of efferent arterioles with subsequent increase in renal glomerular filtration and filtered sodium fraction. Effects in heart include lowering of cardiac preload and afterload and improved myocardial perfusion with coronary vasodilation [6, 20].

B-type natriuretic peptide (BNP) is a cardiac hormone synthesized as a prepro 134-mer protein in atrial and ventricular myocytes. Processing by secretase(s), likely furin, generates a 108-mer (proBNP) which is further processed to a 76-mer N-terminal fragment (NT-proBNP) and the active 32-residue hormone (BNP) [21]. Whereas ANP is stored in granules and can be released immediately after stimulation, only small amounts of BNP are stored in granules and rapid gene expression with de novo synthesis of the peptide is the underlying mechanism for the regulation of BNP secretion. BNP is cleared from plasma by binding to the natriuretic peptide receptor type C (NPR-C) and through proteolysis by neutral endopeptidases. In contrast, NT-proBNP is mainly cleared by renal excretion. The half-life of BNP is 20 min whereas NT-proBNP has a half-life of 120 min, which explains why NT-proBNP serum values are approximately six times higher than BNP values, even though both molecules are released in equimolar proportions. BNP and NT-proBNP have emerged as powerful biomarkers in various cardiovascular diseases. Both markers can be detected in serum plasma using commercially available assays. The diagnostic performance of BNP and NT-proBNP is comparable and there is no meaningful difference between them. They reflect hemodynamic myocardial stress independent of the underlying pathology, thus they are not specific for a distinct pathology such as heart failure but for cardiovascular diseases in general. Their particular strength is to rule out heart failure in patients presenting to the emergency department with shortness of breath. They provide strong and independent prognostic information in patients with heart failure, stable coronary artery disease, acute coronary syndromes, and valvular aortic stenosis. There are some data available to suggest that BNP and NT-proBNP values might assist in deciding upon the optimal treatment of patients with heart failure, but to date there are no data to support the use of these markers for reaching therapeutic decisions in patients with coronary artery disease or valvular heart disease [22].

BNP measurement has become a routine in cardiovascular disorders where often reduced myocardial performance goes together with an overhydration status. The same scenario may be encountered in dialysis patients where overhydration status is linked with cardiomyopathy.

In nephrology, the use of BNP as marker of hydration status is more recent and many questions regarding its usefulness for assessment of dry weight remain. For example, establishing dry weight for PD patients using information provided by BNP has not been successful. Lee et al. [23] found no differences in ECW% and no link between ECW% and serum NT-pro-BNP levels. Therefore, it may be that serum NT-pro-BNP levels in CAPD patients do not provide objective information with respect to hydration status. However, this study found that serum NT-pro-BNP levels correlated with LVMI and LV ejection fraction in CAPD patients. These observations suggest that, while the serum NT-pro-BNP concentration may not be a useful clinical marker for extracellular fluid volume load, it may be useful for evaluating LV hypertrophy and left LV dysfunction in CAPD patients.

Significant rises in BNP concentration has been observed in patients on chronic dialysis. Renal insufficiency by itself does not appear to explain the plasma BNP levels. General consensus exists that BNP is related to the stretching of myocardial fibers following volume overload. However, since BNP levels remain elevated after significant fluid loss after each dialysis session in both HD as well as CAPD patients, other factors must also be involved in the persistent elevations of BNP values [24]. However, BNP levels may have utility in the assessment of extracellular volume. For example, Bavbek et al. [25] have found that treatment with APD is associated with higher plasma BNP levels and LVMI compared to CAPD. This may be the result of chronic fluid retention caused by lower ultrafiltration in the studied APD population. Furthermore, several large scale studies have convincingly shown that elevations in both BNP and NT-proBNP provide strong negative prognostic information (death, cardiovascular death, readmission or cardiac events) in patients with heart failure or asymptomatic left ventricular dysfunction [26]. BNP could be considered as a potential marker of volume overload in PD patients with elevated ECW/TBW bioimpedance without overt cardiac disease [27]. In the ADEMEX study there was a direct correlation between NT-proBNP and systolic BP and an inverse correlation between NT-proBNP and both urine volume and GFR. The value of baseline natriuretic peptides in predicting outcomes was explored by defining the population on the basis of median values of the respective natriuretic peptides (above or below the median value for the parameter of interest). NT-proBNP had a significant effect on overall survival (all-cause mortality; $p < 0.001$) that was independent of whether patients were on the control prescription (control) or the enhanced treatment (treatment). The same was true of the effects of NT-proBNP on cardiovascular mortality independent of the treatment assignment ($p < 0.001$). Cardiovascular mortality was defined as death due to any cardiac or cerebrovascular disease or event. The findings of this study can be summarized as follows: plasma levels of cardiac natriuretic peptides are elevated in patients on PD; the levels observed correlate with the level of residual renal function and systolic BP; NT-proBNP [but neither proANP(1–30) nor proANP(31–67) nor proANP(1–98)] is a powerful predictor of total as well as cardiovascular mortality [28, 29].

Conclusions

Determination of body hydration is a significant problem in PD patients. In practice, clinical evaluation is usually used to estimate the ultrafiltration target, since accurate knowledge of dry weight is lacking. Several methods have been proposed for nonclinical dry weight assessment; these include natriuretic peptides, measurement of inferior vena cava diameter and collapsibility on inspiration by ultrasound and intradialytic relative blood volume change. Unfortunately, these methods suffer from several shortcomings, such as poor specificity (natriuretic peptides), operator dependence (inferior vena cava diameter measurements) and poor correlation with extracellular volume (continuous blood volume measurement). Whole-body bioimpedance spectroscopy in combination with a physiologic tissue model provides for the first time an objective target which can be used for clinical management of fluid balance. Many studies indicate that achieving optimal fluid status is likely to have a profound impact on reducing mortality. Is ongoing a multicenter, prospective, noninterventional, observational study to assess hydration status of incident PD patients and its evolution over the following 4 years. The objective is also a longitudinal follow-up of additional patient outcomes in PD, e.g. residual renal function, transport status, nutritional status and dialysis prescription overtime, and their relation to hydration status and body composition parameters evaluated by bioimpedance spectroscopy (IPOD-PD Study). The use of bioimpedance and BNP together probably permits a better assessment of fluid status in PD patients. The value of this approach has not been clearly demonstrated in PD patients and will require further study. Some studies have shown that the combined BIVA/BNP measurement as a driving diagnostic tool for fluid removal therapy may represent a significant advance in the management of patients with acute decompensated or chronic heart failure [30–32].

References

1 Krediet RT, Smit W, Coester AM, et al: Dry body weight and ultrafiltration targets in peritoneal dialysis. Contrib Nephrol. Basel, Karger, 2009, vol 163, pp 90–95.
2 Van Biesen W, Williams JD, Covic AD, et al: Fluid status in peritoneal dialysis patients: The European Body Composition Monitoring (EuroBCM) Study Cohort. PLoS One 2011;6:e17148.
3 Kotanko P, Levin NW, Zhu F: Current state of bioimpedance technologies in dialysis. Nephrol Dial Transplant 2008;23:808–812.
4 Piccoli A, Pastori G, Guizzo M, et al: Equivalence of information from single versus multiple frequency bioimpedance vector analysis in hemodialysis. Kidney Int 2005;67:301–313.
5 Tan BK, Chan C, Davies SJ: Achieving euvolemia in peritoneal dialysis patients: a surprisingly difficult proposition. Semin Dial 2010;23:456–461.
6 Haapio M, Honkanen E, Ronco C: Brain natriuretic peptide in peritoneal dialysis patients. Contrib Nephrol. Basel, Karger, 2009, vol 163, pp 110–116.
7 Konings C, Kooman JP, Schonck M, et al: Fluid status, blood pressure and cardiovascular abnormalities in PD patients. Perit Dial Int 2002;22: 477–487.
8 Enia G, Mallamaci F, Benedetto FA, et al: Long-term CAPD patients are volume expanded and display more severe left ventricular hypertrophy than haemodialysis patients. Nephrol Dial Transplant 2001;16:1459–1464.
9 Vonesh E, Moran J: Mortality in end-stage renal disease. A reassessment of differences between patients treated with hemodialysis and peritoneal dialysis. J Am Soc Nephrol 1999;10:354–365.
10 Velasquez MT, Lew SQ, Von Albertini B, et al: Control of hypertension is better during hemodialysis than during continuous ambulatory dialysis in ESRD patients. Clin Nephrol 1997;48: 341–345.
11 Cocchi R, Degli Esposti E, Fabbri A, et al: Prevalence of Hypertension inpatients on peritoneal dialisi: results of an Italian multicnete study. Nephrol Dial Transplant 1999;14:1536–1540.
12 Johnson DW, Dent H, Hawley CM, et al: Association of dialysis modality and cardiovascular mortality in incident dialysis patients. Clin J Am Soc Nephrol 2009;4:1620–1628.
13 Krediet RT: Dry Body weight: water and sodium removal targets in PD. Contrib Nephrol. Basel, Karger, 2006, vol 150, pp 104–110.
14 Silva AM, Heymsfield SB, Gallagher D, et al: Evaluation of between-methods agreement of extracellular water measurements in adults and children. Am J Clin Nutr 2008;88:315–323.
15 Zhu F, Wystrychowski G, Kitzler T, et al: Application of bioimpedance techniques to peritoneal dialysis. Contrib Nephrol. Basel, Karger, 2006, vol 150, pp 119–128.
16 Lindley E, Devine Y, Hall L: A ward-based procedure for assessment of fluid status in peritoneal dialysis using bioimpedance spectroscopy. Perit Dial Int 2005;25(S3):S46–S48.
17 Lopot F, Nejedly B, Novotna H, et al: Age-related extracellular to total body water volume ratio (ECV/TBW) – can it be used for 'dry weight' determination in dialysis patients? Application of multifrequency bioimpedance measurement. Int J Artif Organs 2002;25:762–769.
18 Chamney PW, Wabel P, Moissl UM: A whole-body model to distinguish excess fluid from the hydration of major body tissues. Am J Clin Nutr 2007;85:80–89.
19 Wang J, Pierson R: Disparate hydration of adipose and lean tissue requires a new model for body water distribution in man. J Nutr 1976;106:6.

20 Woodard GE, Rosado JA: Recent advances in natriuretic peptide research. J Cell Mol Med 2007;11:1263–1271.
21 Crimmins DL, Kao JL: A glycosylated form of the human cardiac hormone pro B-type natriuretic peptide is an intrinsically unstructured monomeric protein. Arch Biochem Biophys 2008;475:36–41.
22 Weber M, Hamm C: Role of B-type natriuretic peptide (BNP) and NT-PROBNP in clinical routine. Heart 2006;92:843–849.
23 Lee JA, Kim DH, Yoo SJ, et al: Association between serum N-terminal pro-brain natriuretic peptide concentration and left ventricular dysfunction and extracellular water in continuous ambulatory peritoneal dialysis patients. Perit Dial Int 2006;26:360–365.
24 Akiba T, Tachibana K, Togashi K, et al: Plasma human brain natriuretic peptide in chronic renal failure. Clin Nephrol 1995;44(suppl 1):S61–S64.
25 Bavbek N, Akay H, Altay M, et al: Serum BNP concentration and left ventricular mass in CAPD and automated peritoneal dialysis patients. Perit Dial Int 2007;27:663–668.
26 Sav T, Inanc MT, Dogan A, et al: Two daytime icodextrin exchanges decrease brain natriuretic peptide levels and improve cardiac functions in continuous ambulatory peritoneal dialysis patients. Nephrology 2010;15:307–312.
27 Papakrivopoulou E, Lillywhite S, Davenport A: Is N-terminal probrain-type natriuretic peptide a clinically useful biomarker of volume overload in peritoneal dialysis patients? Nephrol Dial Transplant 2012;27:396–401.
28 Paniagua R, Amato D, Mujais S, et al: Predictive value of brain natriuretic peptides in patients on peritoneal dialysis: results from the ADEMEX Trial. Clin J Am Soc Nephrol 2008;3:407–415.
29 McCormick BB, Bargman JM: The implications of the ADEMEX study for the peritoneal dialysis prescription: the role of small solute clearance versus salt and water removal. Curr Opin Nephrol Hypertens 2003;12:581–585.
30 Valle R, Aspromonte N, Milani L, et al: Optimizing fluid management in patients with acute decompensated heart failure (ADHF): the emerging role of combined measurement of body hydration status and brain natriuretic peptide (BNP) levels. Heart Fail Rev 2011;16:519–529.
31 Tuy T, Peacock F: Noninvasive volume assessment in the emergency department: a look at B-type natriuretic peptide and bioimpedance vector analysis. Contrib Nephrol. Basel, Karger, 2011, vol 171, pp 187–193.
32 Tanino Y, Shite J, Paredes OL: Whole body bioimpedance monitoring for outpatient chronic heart failure follow up. Circ J 2009;73:1074–1079.

Dr. Carlo Crepaldi
Department of Nephrology, San Bortolo Hospital
Viale Rodolfi
IT–36100 Vicenza (Italy)
Tel. +39 0444 753650, E-Mail carlo.crepaldi@ulssvicenza.it

Ronco C, Rosner MH, Crepaldi C (eds): Peritoneal Dialysis – State-of-the-Art 2012.
Contrib Nephrol. Basel, Karger, 2012, vol 178, pp 182–188

Role of Peritoneal Dialysis as a Chronic Renal Replacement Therapy in Cardiorenal Patients

C. Pego[a] · A. Rodrigues[a] · C. Ronco[b]

[a]Nephrology Department, CHP-Hospital Santo Antonio, ICBAS and UMIB/University of Porto, Porto, Portugal;
[b]Department of Nephrology, International Renal Research Institute, San Bortolo Hospital, Vicenza, Italy

Abstract

The cardiorenal syndrome (CRS) is a pathophysiological condition characterized by a simultaneous combination of cardiac and renal dysfunction. When diuretic resistance occurs, fluid removal by ultrafiltration (UF) is beneficial. However, in progressive CRS type II multiple hospitalizations for intravenous therapy or extracorporeal UF due to recurrent decompensations have important implications in the deterioration of quality of life and in the use of hospital resources. Peritoneal daily sustained UF appears to be a good therapeutic tool for the chronic ambulatory management of these patients avoiding the risks of a central venous access, aggressive volume shifts and the circulatory stress of the extracorporeal techniques. Controversies on the results of peritoneal dialysis in cardiorenal patients are mostly dependent on therapy skills since individuals with heart failure have a narrower window of tolerance, presenting significant complications even in presence of small deviations from optimal fluid balance. The updated use of volume monitoring tools is recommended. Multifrequency bioimpedance allows detailed information on the total body water overload and, more importantly on the extracellular/intracellular water distribution. This is an instrument that can be longitudinally used to improve the accuracy of clinical judgment concerning volume status. Incremental PD with use of icodextrine besides the promising role of low sodium solutions and bimodal solutions are therapy issues that can improve clinical outcomes of cardio-renal patients under peritoneal dialysis, as a home-based continuous therapy.

Cardiorenal Syndrome Type II: Definition

The cardiorenal syndrome (CRS) is a pathophysiological condition characterized by a simultaneous combination of cardiac and renal dysfunction whereby acute or chronic dysfunction in one organ induces acute or chronic dysfunction in the other organ. The 7th Consensus Conference ADQI [1] established an uniformization of the definition and of the classification of CRS in various subtypes (I–V) allowing a better comprehension of its epidemiology and a potential standardization of the study of this entity. In CRS type II chronic heart disease induces progressive and potentially irreversible renal injury. The increased life expectancy with the advances in the treatment of ischemic and hypertensive heart diseases, but also the common risk factors and pathophysiological mechanisms between heart and renal diseases may explain the increasing incidence of this syndrome [2]. The multicentric study ADHERE [3], which involved 105,388 patients with chronic congestive heart failure, illustrates the magnitude of the problem, since 30% of patients studied presented concomitant chronic renal disease (stages 3–5). Patients with CRS have higher rates of morbidity and mortality [4] with the glomerular filtration rate (GFR) being the most important mortality predictive risk factor [5] which has important therapeutic and prognostic implications making its management a constant challenge throughout the various stages of the disease.

Pathophysiology and the Role of Ultrafiltration in CRS

CRS type II is a progressive disorder and the mechanisms underlying this syndrome are part of a vicious cycle that amplifies and perpetuates the deleterious effects of the primary disease. The starting point of this cycle is the reduction of the cardiac output which has three main effects: arterial underfilling, venous congestion and neuro-hormonal activation (increased activity of the sympathetic nervous system, of the renin-angiotensin-aldosterone axis and increased arginine-vasopressin release). The neuro-hormonal abnormalities contribute to an imbalance between production of vasoconstrictive mediators (epinephrine, angiotensin, endothelin) and of vasodilatory agents (natriuretic peptides, nitric oxide), which leads to renal vasoconstriction, increased proximal tubular sodium and water reabsortion contributing to fluid overload that worsens the congestive heart failure and leads to a further reduction of the cardiac output. In response to the reduced sodium and water delivery at the distal nephron there is an increase in the sensitivity to the aldosterone and a resistance to the atrial natriuretic peptide which could explain the diuretic resistance phenomenon in late stages of the disease. Within these pathophysiological interactions, the development of the renal dysfunction results not only from the hypoperfusion but also from the development of glomerulosclerosis and interstitial fibrosis triggered by the activation of neuro-hormonal systems. During the course of the disease, with the progressive diuretic resistance, the fluid removal by ultrafiltration (UF) seems to be beneficial to these patients, either by extracorporeal techniques or by peritoneal dialysis.

Relevance of Hemofiltration in Acute Exacerbations of CRS Type II

With the progression of the CRS type II and the development of oral diuretic resistance, disease exacerbations become more common with patients requiring frequent hospitalization for optimization and/or correction of extracellular volume status. In patients with diuretic resistance, UF may be the only therapeutic option available. For the acute management of SCR type II exacerbations, extracorporeal UF, particularly hemofiltration (HF), is the more frequently used therapy. The UNLOAD trial showed that peripheral UF is associated with improved extracellular fluid loss, reduced administration of vasoactive drugs and reduced hospital readmissions when compared with intravenous diuretics in patients with acute decompensated heart failure [6].

In the acute setting, peritoneal UF is not as practical as HF because this allows a rapid and effective restoration of the volemic state of the patient and overcomes the logistic difficulties and risks associated with acute use of a peritoneal catheter. However, PD could be a safe option for the long-term ambulatory management of conservative treatment resistant CRS type II patients.

Role of Peritoneal Dialysis in the Management of CRS Type II

In progressive CRS type II multiple hospitalizations for intravenous therapy or extracorporeal UF due to recurrent decompensations have important implications in the deterioration of quality of life and in the use of hospital resources. Peritoneal UF appears to be a good therapeutic tool for the chronic ambulatory management of these patients for several reasons (table 1). Contemporary studies in which CRS type II patients treated with peritoneal dialysis (PD) were included demonstrated well the clinical improvement of cardiac function with NYHA (New York Heart Association) functional class reduction (two functional classes in up to 65% of patients) and a dramatic reduction in hospitalization rates [7–9]. The favorable outcomes of this therapeutic option does not seem to vary with the different PD regimens used, either automated peritoneal dialysis (APD) or continuous ambulatory peritoneal dialysis (CAPD) [7], although most available studies used CAPD modality. The possibility of individualized and incremental steps of PD prescription is one of the advantages, with all the benefits of a home-based therapy, even in patients with severe congestive heart failure without end-stage renal disease [10].

The treatment effectiveness is reflected not only in aspects related with life quality but is also associated with reduced health care costs [8]. Besides the reduced morbidity, in many trials a decreased mortality rate was also evident, a particularly important issue since these patients have very high mortality rates when treated conservatively, with some studies showing improvement in survival rates at 12 months from 25 to 82% [8]. According to some authors improved prognosis is probably related not only with the better volemic control with greater hemodynamic stability in this patients but also with greater preservation of residual renal function and improved clearance of medium molecular weight substances including myocardial depressant mediators and systemic inflammatory mediators [11].

Within treatment regimens, in spite of the allowed variability, icodextrin solution assumes a crucial role because it induces sustained prolonged UF at lower glucose absorption and better systemic metabolic profile [12–14]. In cardiorenal patients, one exchange a day may be sufficient to achieve adequate daily UF, but more often a regimen of two or more exchanges of CAPD are prescribed according to the glomerular filtration rate. APD is also a useful tool and intermittent peritoneal dialysis (IPD) can be considered to target adequate daily UF in patients unable to perform the technique and who need a helper but still maintain good residual glomerular filtration rate. In order to support the events of heart failure exacerbations, it is feasible and increasingly reported the safe use of two icodextrin exchanges [15, 16].

Table 1. Potential benefits and risks of PD as a chronic renal replacement therapy in cardiorenal patients

General PD benefits	Specific PD benefits in CRS	PD risks in CRS
Home-based continuous therapy	Sustained daily ultrafiltration	Lack of capacity for autodialysis
Quality of life	Avoids recurrent circulatory stress	Helper burden
Incremental PD schedules	Avoids myocardial stunning	Peritoneal albumin losses
Vascular access preservation	Avoids peripheral (gut) steal syndrome	Peritoneal infection
Protection of residual renal function	Fewer episodes of hypotension	
Fewer episodes of blood-borne infections		

Controversies in Studies with Cardiorenal Patients

When compared with extracorporeal UF, peritoneal UF appears to be a good therapeutic tool for the chronic ambulatory management of refractory volume overload because of the hemodynamic stability achieved from slow continuous removal of extracellular fluid and by absence of an arteriovenous access that may worsen cardiac dysfunction [17]. In fact, the recurrent circulatory stress of the extracorporeal system is often underestimated, but adversely impacts on patient quality of life and outcomes [18]. Indeed, the dialysis induced myocardial stunning is pointed as a cause of the largely unappreciated dimension of the cardiorenal interaction in patients with end-stage renal disease [19], but it can be avoided under PD schedules [20]. Besides, intradialytic underperfusion of myocardial areas is also associated with the translocation into the circulation of bacterial endotoxin and/or cytokines that escape from a hypoperfused edematous gut and trigger an inflammatory response that interferes with cardiac function through several pathogenic mechanisms [21, 22].

Therefore, daily peritoneal ultrafiltration may offer to cardiorenal patients that which nephrologists are longing to achieve with nocturnal hemodialysis (HD) or more frequent HD schedules [23].

Despite the theoretical advantages of PD compared to HD in patients with chronic cardiac disease, the clinical experiences reported in this risk group are controversial. Both a remote USA registry-based study from Stack et al. [24] and a more recent French registry study [25] concluded that PD was associated with greater mortality in congestive heart failure patients. Which needs to be emphasized is that both studies did not mention or controlled for therapy schedules or adequacy targets. Since both are registry studies this information on therapy skills are lacking but are crucial to validate the results because these risk patients are mainly dependent on how volume control is managed. Notably, it was recognized by Stack et al. [26] that mortality risks in US patients have declined from 1995 to 2005, certainly because of therapy advances.

Additionally, both infection rates and hospitalizations must be taken into consideration. In this sense, PD avoids vascular access related bacteriemias, while hospitalization can also be reduced. Recently, we studied a total of 453 PD patients in our unit from whom 18% had chronic heart disease as baseline comorbidity and the medium follow-up time was 27 ± 24 months. We documented that heart disease, such as age and diabetes, was an independent mortality predictor (HZ 1.6; CI 1.04–2.55, $p = 0.03$), but was not a risk factor for technical failure. The cumulative survival of cardiopathy patients by 24 months was still 71%. When comparing patients with cardiopathy with the others the proportion of patients transferred to HD due to UF inadequacy was similar between groups (29 vs. 22%, p = NS) while the overall rate of peritonitis (0.53 vs. 0.58 episodes/patient-years) and the rate of hospitalization (0.97 vs. 0.9 episodes/patient-years) did not differ significantly. Thus, in our population PD modality was an effective renal replacement option in this group of high-risk patients.

Importance of the Right Hydration Target

The correct understanding of fluid balance requires a clear set of definitions: (1) fluid balance is normally defined by the daily difference in all intakes and outputs; this generally does not include insensible losses, it may not correlate with weight, while it should include dialysis fluid removal. (2) Cumulative fluid balance is defined by the sum of fluid accumulation over a set period of time. This parameter is more important and it is relevant to assess its change over time, the amount and duration of key parameters associated with outcome and finally the response to treatment. (3) Fluid overload is represented by the cumulative fluid balance expressed as a percent of body weight at baseline (hospital admission). A cut-off of 10% has been associated with increased mortality.

Body volume and fluid composition must be considered in conjunction with all the inputs and outputs from the body. Whatever the initial estimate of volume is, in the patient with potential or recognized cardiac problems, continued knowledge of fluid balance is essential to successful fluid management. An accurate measure of body weight is an excellent starting point. In the PD patient, accurate measurement of fluid intake would be required but seldom obtained. While urinary excretion can usually be measured accurately, all other fluid losses are subject to gross error. 'Balance' may often be replaced by estimates of body fluid compartments. This also is difficult

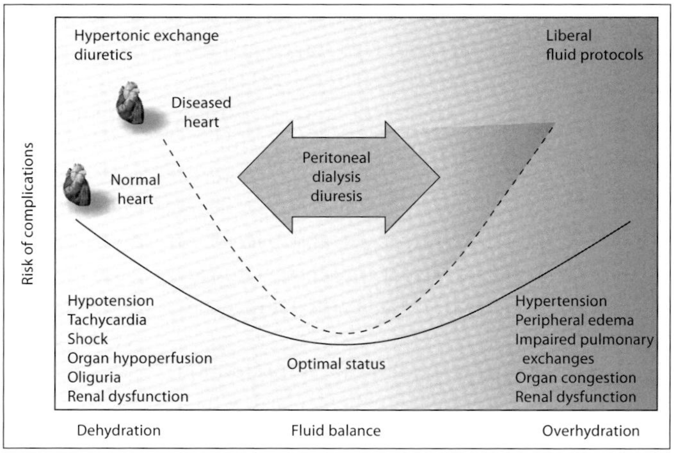

Fig. 1. The importance of fluid balance in cardiorenal patients.

since much excess fluid may be in noncommunicating pools ('third spacing', not directly related to the circulation). New methods of assessing tissue hydration may be useful in this context.

If a fluid optimization is reached, this must be maintained through fluid balance optimization. Considering all the factors described in figure 1, fluid-restrictive protocols with hypertonic exchanges and diuretics may lead to potential dehydration and the risk for complications such as hypotension and loss of residual renal function. On the contrary, fluid liberal protocols may induce various degrees of overhydration with consequent peripheral and pulmonary edema, congestion and worsening of CRS [27]. While the healthy subject presents a certain degree of tolerance and compliance to fluid balance shifts, individuals with heart failure have a narrower window of tolerance, presenting significant complications even in presence of small deviations from optimal fluid balance. The response to fluid removal is dependent on rate of removal, blood volume refilling into the vascular space, cardiovascular compensation, and the initial state of body hydration. Potential errors in the estimation of fluid balance can be from negligible to catastrophic. From these considerations it results clear that a precise definition of the hydration target is quintessential for the stability and the reduction of complications including loss of residual renal function in patients with CRS undergoing treatment with peritoneal dialysis.

Future Strategies to Improve the Role of Peritoneal Dialysis in Cardiorenal Syndrome Patients

Since adequate volume control is the key factor in these risk patients, both new diagnostic and therapeutic strategies should be searched for to improve outcomes of CRS type II patients under PD.

Noteworthy, dietetic sodium restriction and fluid removal have both shown impact on PD patients' mortality. Facing the relevance of volume overload in CRS, ultrafiltration is an utterly important adequacy target. However, the right assessment of dry weight is a major challenge for clinicians.

Hypervolemia is pointed as a frequent deleterious status in both HD and PD, but PD patients are not significantly more overloaded than pre-HD patients [28].

In addition, intermittent fluid removal and rapid UF rates also negatively impact HD patient survival, while sustained continuous UF is beneficial. In cardiorenal patients the equilibrium is harder to achieve because in these patients it may be hazardous to aggressively remove intravascular water. Additionally, in the search for volume control we face the risk of and residual renal function loss (RRF).

In this respect, the updated use of volume monitoring tools is recommended. Pro-brain-natriuretic peptide as an example of congestive heart failure biomarker is of limited clinical use in dialysis patients. Multifrequency bioimpedance, on the other hand, gives detailed information on the total body water (TBW) overload and, more importantly on the extracellular (ECW)/intracellular (ICW) water distribution. This is an instrument that can be longitudinally used to improve the accuracy of clinical judgment concerning volume status. However, there is a complex relationship between volume status, nutrition and inflammation. It deserves to be mentioned that hypoalbuminemic patients, who presented a relative overhydration status according to the bioimpedance ECW:TBW ratio had similar plasma volume as measured by ^{125}I-labeled albumin dilution, and similar absolute total body water quantified with deuterium dilution method in comparison with the control group [29]. This has important clinical consequences since the abnormal body composition observed in hypoalbuminemic patients is indeed associated with excess tissue hydration and not necessarily with increased plasma water. These water distribution peculiarities need to be carefully managed in heart failure patients, who are often hypoalbuminemic and inflamed, to avoid inadequate UF prescription with risk of hypotension and RRF loss.

Concerning therapy issues, in addition to icodextrin and APD already mentioned, both low sodium solutions and bimodal solutions deserve to be highlighted in the portfolio for CRS patients. Compensated low sodium solutions shown to increase the diffusive gradient for sodium removal while similar UF was achieved in comparison with standard solution [30]. This is a promising tool to treat congestive heart failure exarcebations in PD patients, and even as a maintenance therapy to avoid sodium and fluid overload. On the other hand, bimodal solutions, by using a combined crystalloid and colloid PD solution [31], modulate the rate of UF in a long dwell, with a more rapid glucose-derived osmotic UF in the early part of the dwell followed by sustained icodextrin driven UF. In addition, this glucose-sparing strategy also improved sodium removal.

Conclusion

CRS type II has an increasing incidence and although the pathophysiological basis of disease is well established there may be mechanisms and mediators who have not yet been discovered, the functions of which are not well known, that may be therapeutic targets in the future. In these patients, when conservative treatment is exhausted or, instead, when the burden of recurrent exacerbations and hospitalizations is increased, a therapeutic approach must focus sooner or later in UF. If we take into account the particularities of this disease and of these patients, the wide range of current PD therapeutic schemes, the flexibility of PD modality and the advantages of new diagnostic and therapeutic tools, peritoneal UF seems a viable option for the chronic ambulatory management of CRS type II patients.

References

1 House AA, Anand I, Bellomo R, et al: Workgroup statements from the 7th ADQI Consensus Conference. Nephrol Dial Transplant 2010;25:1416–1420.

2 Ronco C, et al: Cardiorrenal syndrome: refining the definition of a complex symbiosis gone wrong. Intens Care Med 2008;34:957–962.

3 Adams KF Jr, Fonarow GC, Emerman CL, et al: Characteristics and outcomes of patients hospitalized for heart failure in the United States: rationale, design, and preliminary observations from the first 100,000 cases in the Acute Decompensated Heart Failure National Registry (ADHERE). Am Heart J 2005; 149:209–216.

4 Fonarow GC, Adams KF Jr, Abraham WT, Yancy CW, Boscardin WJ: Risk stratification for in-hospital mortality in acutely decompensated heart failure: classification and regression tree analysis. JAMA 2005;293:572–580.

5 Hillege HL, Nitsch D, Pfeffer MA, et al: Renal function as a predictor of outcome in a broad spectrum of patients with heart failure. Circulation 2006;113:671–678.
6 Costanzo MR, Guglin M, Saltzberg M: Ultrafiltration is associated with fewer re-hospitalizations than continuous diuretic infusion in patient with decompensated heart failure: results from UNLOAD. J Am Coll Cardiol 2007;49:675–683.
7 Montejo JD, Bajo MA, del Peso G, Selgas R: Papel de la diálisis peritoneal en el tratamiento de la insuficiencia cardíaca refractaria. Nefrologia 2010;30:21–27.
8 Sanchez JE, Ortega T, Rodriguez C, Diaz-Molina B, Martín M, Garcia-Cueto C, Vidau P, Gago E, Ortega F: Efficacy of peritoneal ultrafiltration in the treatment of refractory congestive heart failure. Nephrol Dial Transplant 2010;25:605–610.
9 Gotloib L, Fudin R, Yakubovich M, Vienken J: Peritoneal dialysis in refractory end-stage congestive heart failure: a challenge facing a no-win situation. Nephrol Dial Transplant 2005;20(suppl 7):vii32.
10 Bertoli SV, Ciurlino D, Maccario M, Martino S, Bigatti G, Traversi L, Procaccio M, Buzzi L: Home peritoneal ultrafiltration in patients with severe congestive heart failure without end-stage renal disease Adv Perit Dial 2005;21:123–127.
11 Van Biesen W, Verbeke F, Vanholder R: Cardiovascular disease in haemodialysis and peritoneal dialysis: arguments pro peritoneal dialysis. Nephrol Dial Transplant 2007;22:53–58.
12 Qi H, Xu C, Yan H, Ma J: Comparison of icodextrin and glucose solutions for long dwell exchange in peritoneal dialysis: a meta-analysis of randomized controlled trials. Perit Dial Int 2011;31:179–188.
13 Paniagua R, Ventura MD, Avila-Díaz M, Cisneros A, Vicenté-Martínez M, Furlong MD, García-González Z, Villanueva D, Orihuela O, Prado-Uribe MD, Alcántara G, Amato D: Icodextrin improves metabolic and fluid management in high and high-average transport diabetic patients. Perit Dial Int 2009;29:422–432.
14 Basile C, Chimienti D, Bruno A, Cocola S, Libutti P, Teutonico A, Cazzato F: Efficacy of peritoneal dialysis with icodextrin in the long-term treatment of refractory congestive heart failure. Perit Dial Int 2009;29:116.
15 Sav T, Inanc MT, Dogan A, Oymak O, Utas C: Two daytime icodextrin exchanges decrease brain natriuretic peptide levels and improve cardiac functions in continuous ambulatory peritoneal dialysis patients. Nephrology (Carlton) 2010;15:307–312.
16 Sav T, Oymak O, Inanc MT, Dogan A, Tokgoz B, Utas C: Effects of twice-daily icodextrin administration on blood pressure and left ventricular mass in patients on continuous ambulatory peritoneal dialysis. Perit Dial Int 2009;29:443–449.
17 Cnossen N, Kooman JP, Konings CJ, et al: Peritoneal dialysis in patients with congestive heart failure. Nephrol Dial Transplant 2006;21(suppl 2):ii63–ii66.
18 McIntyre CW: Recurrent circulatory stress: the dark side of dialysis. Semin Dial 2010;23:449–451.
19 Breidthardt T, McIntyre CW: Dialysis-induced myocardial stunning: the other side of the cardiorenal syndrome. Rev Cardiovasc Med 2011;12:13–20.
20 Selby NM, McIntyre CW: Peritoneal dialysis is not associated with myocardial stunning. Perit Dial Int 2011;31:27–33.
21 Ritz E: Intestinal-renal syndrome: mirage or reality? Blood Purif 2011;31:70–76.
22 McIntyre CW, Harrison LE, Eldehni MT, Jefferies HJ, Szeto CC, John SG, Sigrist MK, Burton JO, Hothi D, Korsheed S, Owen PJ, Lai KB, Li PK: Circulating endotoxemia: a novel factor in systemic inflammation and cardiovascular disease in chronic kidney disease. Clin J Am Soc Nephrol 2011;6:133–41.
23 Jefferies HJ, Virk B, Schiller B, Moran J, McIntyre CW: Frequent hemodialysis schedules are associated with reduced levels of dialysis-induced cardiac injury (myocardial stunning). Clin J Am Soc Nephrol 2011;6:1326–1332.
24 Stack AG, Molony DA, Rahman NS, Dosekun A, Murthy B: Impact of dialysis modality on survival of new ESRD patients with congestive heart failure in the United States. Kidney Int 2003;64:1071–1079.
25 Sens F, Schott-Pethelaz AM: Survival advantage of hemodialysis relative to peritoneal dialysis in patients with end-stage renal disease and congestive heart failure. Kidney Int 2011;80:970–977.
26 Stack AG, Mohammed A, Hanley A, Mutwali A, Nguyen H: Survival trends of US dialysis patients with heart failure: 1995 to 2005. Clin J Am Soc Nephrol 2011;6:1982–1989.
27 Ronco C, Kaushik M, Valle R, Aspromonte N, Peacock WF: Diagnosis and management of fluid overload in heart failure and cardio-renal syndrome: the '5B' approach. Semin Nephrol 2012;32:129–141.
28 Devolder I, Verleysen A, Vijt D, Vanholder R, Van Biesen W: Body composition, hydration and related parameters in hemodialysis versus peritoneal dialysis patients. Perit Dial Int 2010;30:208–214.
29 John B, Tan BK, Dainty S, Spanel P, Smith D, Davies SJ: Plasma volume, albumin, and fluid status in peritoneal dialysis patients. Clin J Am Soc Nephrol 2010;5:1463–1470.
30 Davies S, Carlsson O, Simonsen O, Johansson AC, Venturoli D, Ledebo I, Wieslander A, Chan C, Rippe B: The effects of low-sodium peritoneal dialysis fluids on blood pressure, thirst and volume status. Nephrol Dial Transplant 2009;24:1609–1617.
31 Freida P, Issad B, Dratwa M, Lobbedez T, Wu L, Leypoldt JK, Divino-Filho JC: A combined crystalloid and colloid pd solution as a glucose-sparing strategy for volume control in high-transport apd patients: a prospective multicenter study. Perit Dial Int 2009;29:433–442.

Prof. Anabela Rodrigues
Nephrology Department, CHP-Hospital Santo António
Largo Prof. Abel Salazar
PT–4099–001 Porto (Portugal)
Tel. +351222 077 500, E-Mail anabelarodrigues.nefrologia@chporto.min-saude.pt

Ronco C, Rosner MH, Crepaldi C (eds): Peritoneal Dialysis – State-of-the-Art 2012.
Contrib Nephrol. Basel, Karger, 2012, vol 178, pp 189–194

Vascular and Arterial Calcification in Peritoneal Dialysis Patients – State-of-the-Art 2012

E.P. Heymann · H. Penny · D.J.A. Goldsmith

Guy's Campus, King's Health Partners AHSC, London, UK

Abstract

Vascular calcification is a major challenge to the long-term health of many patients with chronic kidney disease, and patients receiving peritoneal dialysis therapy are no exception to this. The mechanisms behind vascular calcification are complex and diverse. There are several different imaging techniques that can be used to interrogate the vasculature in these patients, and the relative merits of these as research and screening tools we discuss. There are some recent epidemiological studies which throw fresh light on the implications of the development or progression of vascular calcification. Finally, an animal model experiment is reported which one day may open up the possibility of a successful therapeutic intervention.

The most common cause of death in dialysis patients is cardiovascular disease (CVD). Much of this turns out to be 'sudden cardiac death' related and not the classical atherosclerotic lesion associated pathologies of acute myocardial infarction, and stroke [1, 2]. It is increasingly accepted that this may be due in part to the presence of excess vascular calcification (VC), particularly in the form of extensive VC, typically presenting as coronary artery calcification (CAC), which can be observed even in very young dialysis patients [3–6]. This may contribute to premature CVD and the markedly increased mortality observed in the dialysis population.

The presence of CAC in the dialysis population is clearly multifactorial and has a complex set of interactions operating [7], but appears to correlate in part with the quantity of ingested calcium-containing oral phosphate binders (OPB) [4]. Such ectopic vascular calcification, however, was commonly noted in patients with renal disease during periods when calcium-containing OPBs were not yet available [6]. This suggests that there are many additional clinical factors also associated with VC and CAC in the dialysis population, though it does not inform us necessarily of the etiological hierarchy of importance in modern-day dialysis patients. Some of these features include increasingly routine use of pharmacologically administered vitamin D therapy, increasing age of dialysis cohorts, and dialysis vintage [8].

Calcium can be deposited into either the medial or intimal layers of the vasculature [7]. Some parts of the vasculature are more susceptible to arteriosclerosis, for example, smaller muscular arteries (e.g. digital). In other territories, atherosclerosis predominates (e.g. ileo-femoral regions). In yet other areas, there can be a mix or blend of these different types of calcification (and it is unwise, we feel, to assume that the drivers and factors for intimal and medial calcifications will be identical), such as the coronary arterial bed. The relationship between adverse cardiovascular outcomes and the particular type of calcium deposition is of considerable relevance: London et al. [9] showed clearly that the presence of VC was detrimental, but that intimal VC was attended by a worse outcome than was medial VC. Intimal calcium deposition, a relatively less common lesion in patients with chronic kidney disease (CKD), is principally associated with atherosclerotic plaques; in patients with normal renal function, such plaques are clearly associated with myocardial infarction and thrombotic events. However, in those with CKD, the association between intimal lesions and these adverse outcomes is less clear [6].

It is clear that of the many different patient populations that are prone to vascular calcification (e.g. diabetics, ageing, coronary disease), patients with CKD, and especially patients on dialysis programs, calcify faster, and much more extensively, than in any other clinical situation save rare congenital syndromes leading to infantile or juvenile arterial calcification [10].

Methods of Detection of Vascular Calcification

Several structural imaging methods are currently available to investigate vascular calcification, such as cardiac CT, planar X-ray, echocardiography and vascular ultrasound [11].

Cardiac CT

Electron beam CT (EBCT) and multislice CT (MSCT) are well-validated, noninvasive imaging methods and are considered the reference standard for assessing CAC and valvular and aortic calcification, with no requirement for contrast administration. CT-based techniques are ideal methodologies for research projects into VC [11].

Both CT-based techniques can be employed accurately to detect and quantify the extent of calcification of the coronary arteries, the aorta and the cardiac valves. Scoring (quantitative) systems such as the Agatston score, the volume score or the mass score are used for inter-scan comparisons [11]. The sum of all scores in each calcified lesion identified along the coronary tree constitutes the total calcium score. CT imaging cannot differentiate between the locations of calcium deposits in the intimal layer from those in the arterial medial layer. Although the total score is believed to reflect the burden of atherosclerosis, there is only a modest correlation between CAC score and the severity of obstructive coronary artery disease in patients with CKD (when assessed conventionally as luminal lesional encroachment); this finding is partly owing to the presence of medial calcification, which increases the overall burden of arterial disease without causing luminal obstruction [12].

When EBCT was first used to quantify the extent of CAC in patients with stage 5D CKD, CAC scores were reported to be much higher in patients on hemodialysis than in healthy individuals as well as patients with known coronary artery disease [13]. Other investigators showed that a progressive decline in renal function is associated with increased prevalence of CAC. The prevalence of CAC was as high as 80–90% in patients with stage 5D CKD [14], whereas the prevalence of CAC was about 40–60% in patients with stages 3–5 CKD [15, 16], indicating that CAC tends to progress and increase dramatically after initiation of dialysis [13].

Limited data are available regarding the ability of CAC to predict outcome in patients with CKD. In 104 patients with stage 5D CKD, Matsuoka et al. [17] reported lower survival in patients with a CAC score greater than the median (median score 200) than in those with a CAC score below the median ($p = 0.01$). Block et al. [16] reported that the presence of a baseline CAC score >400 was a strong predictor of mortality during a 44-month follow-up of a cohort of 129 incident hemodialysis patients after adjustment for age, ethnicity, sex and diabetes mellitus.

Cardiac CT clearly visualizes valvular calcification, which has been associated with an adverse outcome during a follow-up of 4 years. Sequential cardiac CT has been used to follow the progression of vascular calcification to gauge the effects of various treatment options. Studies comparing the impact of various treatments, such as phosphate-binding agents (sevelamer and calcium-based binders), calcimimetics (cinacalcet) and vitamin D, on CAC have shown differential effects, suggesting that both coronary as well as cardiac valvular calcifications may be valid surrogate markers for research into interventions [11].

Aortic arch and descending aortic calcification has been least studied to date but may also be of particular interest, as one would expect that aortic stiffness, a prime determinant of patient-level outcomes [6] would most closely be correlated with aortic mural calcification scores.

Planar X-Ray

Although planar X-ray is mostly qualitative [11], several semiquantitative methods have been developed [18]. The best known of these methods is that proposed by Kauppila's group from the Framingham cohort studies [19] in which AAC visualized on a lateral X-ray of the lumbar spine is given a score of 0–24 based on the number and extent of calcified foci in the aortic segments extending in front of lumbar vertebrae 1 through 4. In the general population, the AAC score was shown to be predictive of cardiovascular events and mortality in two cohorts of the Framingham Heart Study [19]. Bellasi et al. [20] reported a good correlation of the AAC score – estimated by planar lumbar spine X-rays – with the CAC score measured by EBCT in 140 prevalent patients on haemodialysis ($r = 0.7$). Verbeke et al. [21, 22] reported the prognostic value of the AAC score in 1,084 prevalent patients on dialysis during a median follow-up of 2 years. The AAC score was categorized into tertiles: AAC score ≤4 (no or minor calcification); 5–15 (moderate calcification); and ≥16 (heavy calcification). The presence of moderate or heavy calcification was highly predictive of mortality or nonfatal cardiovascular events compared with no or minimal calcification (HR for moderate calcification, 3.682; 95% CI 1.356–9.997; $p = 0.01$, and HR for heavy calcification, 8.64; 95% CI 3.528–21.158; $p < 0.001$). These two studies strongly support the utility of the AAC score for risk stratification of patients with stage 5D CKD for all-cause mortality and cardiovascular events. However, until there is a proven interventional strategy to halt or to reverse arterial calcification in CKD, there are other considerations to take into account before embarking on a routine screening programme of this sort.

Ultrasonography

Ultrasound-based imaging techniques can be used to evaluate vascular disease in patients with CKD and ultrasonography is helpful to assess superficial vessels, such as the femoral and carotid arteries. Vascular calcification detected by means of ultrasound has been associated with abnormal arterial functional properties as well as an adverse cardiovascular outcome. Similar to planar X-ray, ultrasound provides a qualitative or semiquantitative assessment of vascular calcification but the distinction of intimal from medial calcification remains difficult and mostly based on subjective interpretation [11]. Intima-media thickness (not calcification, but a good marker of atherosclerosis in the carotid and coronary arterial beds, and of prognostic relevance) can also be estimated from measurements taken from the common carotid arteries.

Echocardiography

Echocardiography is the gold standard for rapid, bedside noninvasive assessment of ventricular structure and function, as well as cardiac valves. Echocardiography is portable and widely available and gives an accurate estimate of valvular stenosis and/or regurgitation. With this technique, however, valvular calcification can be assessed only qualitatively or subjectively as mild, moderate and severe. Mitral and aortic valve calcifications are much more prevalent in patients on dialysis than in the general population. In fact, mitral calcification has been reported in 10–40% and aortic valve calcification in 25–55% of patients on dialysis [11, 23–24]. Accordingly, calcification of one or two valves has been associated with an adverse cardiovascular outcome and high mortality in patients on dialysis, independent of atherosclerotic vascular disease history [11, 23–24].

Recent Clinical Studies and Findings – Focusing on Peritoneal Dialysis

In a recent report from Korea [25], 184 dialysis patients (age 58.6 ± 12.7 years, 46% male, 32% peritoneal dialysis; PD) were enrolled into a study examining de novo VC in incident dialysis. The extent and progression of aortic arch calcification (AoAC) was estimated from chest X-rays taken before initial dialysis therapy, and every subsequent year thereafter. Patients were divided into two groups based on the presence or absence of AoAC progression and clinical and biochemical parameters were compared. The mean duration of follow-up was 2.7 ± 1.0 years. Seventy-six patients (41.3%) had AoAC before initial dialysis, with a mean AoAC score of 13.0 ± 20.4%. Half of the patients (50%) had progressive AoAC. Age >65 years ($p = 0.003$), dialysis duration ($p = 0.004$), diabetes ($p = 0.015$), and the presence of AoAC at baseline ($p = 0.001$) were related to AoAC progression [25]. No significant association was found between AoAC progression and the baseline clinical parameters, including gender, obesity, hypertension, and dialysis modality [25]. A multivariate analysis of the data revealed that dialysis duration ($p = 0.003$) and the presence of AoAC at baseline ($p < 0.001$) were independent risk factors for AoAC progression in patients undergoing dialysis [25].

In the NECOSAD study [26], 384 dialysis patients (age 61 ± 15 years, 64% male, 61% hemodialysis) were recruited to assess the associations between the parameters of mineral metabolism and the progression of AoAC [26]. Annual chest X-rays were screened for AoAC, and patients were categorized as having no, moderate, or severe calcification [26]. Progression was defined as an increase in calcification category during follow-up on dialysis. At baseline, 96 (25%) patients had severe, 205 (53%) patients had moderate and 83 (22%) patients had no aortic calcification. For 237 of the 288 patients with no or moderate calcifications at baseline, X-rays were available for follow-up. During follow-up (mean 2.3 years), aortic calcification progressed in 71 patients (30%). In this study, elevated baseline plasma calcium (>9.5 mg/dl) and iPTH (>300 pg/ml) concentrations were associated with AoAC progression (odds ratios of 3.1, 95% CI (1.2–8.2) and 4.4 (1.4–14.1), respectively). Furthermore, progression of aortic calcification was found to be significantly associated with increased risk of all-cause mortality (HR 1.9; 95% CI 1.2–3.1) and cardiovascular mortality (HR 2.7; 95% CI 1.3–5.6) [26].

Finally, the use of the peritoneal route for the administration of potential inhibitors of VC has recently been presented [27], albeit only in an animal model. Pyrophosphate (PPi), an endogenous molecule, appears naturally to cause inhibition of soft tissue calcification, but its concentration is typically reduced in CKD and end-stage renal disease which is one of the reasons for accelerated calcification tendencies in CKD [3]. Although once thought to be a promising therapeutic opportunity, PPi's very short half-life in circulation seemed to curtail earlier interventional studies. The possibility that a slow, continuous entry of PPi into the circulation and prevention of VC might be achieved by daily PD has now been tested in an animal model. Pharmacokinetic studies were first carried out in rats with renal impairment following 5/6 nephrectomy. Efficacy studies were then performed in the apolipoprotein E gene knockout mouse model overlaid with CKD. PPi was delivered by means of a permanent peritoneal catheter in a solution, simulating human PD, but without the timed removal of spent dialysate. von Kossa's staining followed by semiquantitative morphological image processing, with separation of inside (intimal) and outside (presumed medial) lesions, was used to determine aortic root calcification. In comparison to an intravenous bolus, delivery of PPi in a PD solution resulted in a slower, extended delivery over >4 h. Next, the efficacy studies showed that a 6-day/week PD-simulated administration of PPi resulted in a dose-dependent inhibition of aortic calcification in both intimal and medial lesions. A dose-response effect on total aortic calcification was also documented, with a full inhibition seen at the highest dose. Some limited peritoneal catheter-related inflammation was observed, as expected, and included the placebo-treated control groups. This inflammatory response could have masked a lower level PPi-specific adverse effect, but none was observed. It would be now of immense interest to develop this intriguing possible therapeutic intervention to the point where this might be something to be attempted in man.

Conclusions

VC remains a common and severe clinical challenge for all subjects with CKD, and especially so for those patients on dialysis. PD patients are not spared and indeed seem to suffer as much from VC and its complications as do patients on hemodialysis. Better epidemiological cohort studies are now allowing a more mature understanding of the factors which can influence progression, or regression. Several promising new interventions are being trialled or developed, leading to some hope that in the next decade this serious vascular scourge might be able to be conquered. Until it can be, meticulous care to deliver good dialysis adequacy, and good control of CKD-MBD parameters (avoiding calcium-overloading and preventing adynamic bone pathology [4]), seem all that we can currently do.

References

1 Kanbay M, Solak Y, Covic A, Goldsmith D: Sudden cardiac death in patients with chronic kidney disease: prevention is the sine qua non. Kidney Blood Press Res 2011;34:269–276.

2 Kanbay M, Afsar B, Goldsmith D, Covic A: Sudden death in hemodialysis: an update. Blood Purif 2010;30:135–145.

3 Covic A, Kanbay M, Voroneanu L, Turgut F, Serban DN, Serban IL, Goldsmith DJ: Vascular calcification in chronic kidney disease. Clin Sci (Lond) 2010;119:111–121.

4 Covic A, Gusbeth-Tatomir P, Goldsmith DJ: Vascular calcification – a new window on the cardiovascular system: role of agents used to manipulate skeletal integrity. Semin Dial 2007;20:158–169.

5 Haydar AA, Covic A, Colhoun H, Rubens M, Goldsmith DJ: Coronary artery calcification and aortic pulse wave velocity in chronic kidney disease patients. Kidney Int 2004;65:1790–1794.

6 Goldsmith D, Ritz E, Covic A: Vascular calcification: a stiff challenge for the nephrologist: does preventing bone disease cause arterial disease? Kidney Int 2004;66:1315–1333.

7 Shanahan CM, Crouthamel MH, Kapustin A, Giachelli CM: Arterial calcification in chronic kidney disease: key roles for calcium and phosphate. Circ Res 2011;109:697–711.

8 Garrett G, Sardiwal S, Lamb E, Goldsmith DJA: PTH – a particularly tricky hormone – why measure it at all in kidney patients? Clin J Am Soc Nephrol 2012;in press.

9 London GM, Guérin AP, Marchais SJ, Métivier F, Pannier B, Adda H: Arterial media calcification in end-stage renal disease: impact on all-cause and cardiovascular mortality. Nephrol Dial Transplant 2003;18:1731–1740.

10 Rutsch F, Nitschke Y, Terkeltaub R: Genetics in arterial calcification: pieces of a puzzle and cogs in a wheel. Circ Res 2011;109:578–592.

11 Karohl C, Gascón LD, Raggi P: Noninvasive imaging for assessment of calcification in chronic kidney disease. Nat Rev Nephrol 2011;7:567–577.

12 Braun J, Oldendorf M, Moshage W, Heidler R, Zeitler E, Luft FC: Electron beam computed tomography in the evaluation of cardiac calcification in chronic dialysis patients. Am J Kidney Dis 1996;27:394–401.

13 Haydar AA, Hujairi NM, Covic AA, Pereira D, Rubens M, Goldsmith DJ: Coronary artery calcification is related to coronary atherosclerosis in chronic renal disease patients: a study comparing EBCT-generated coronary artery calcium scores and coronary angiography. Nephrol Dial Transplant 2004;19:2307–2312.

14 Chertow GM, Burke SK, Raggi P, Treat to Goal Working Group: Sevelamer attenuates the progression of coronary and aortic calcification in hemodialysis patients. Kidney Int 2002;62:245–252.

15 Russo D, Corrao S, Battaglia Y, Andreucci M, Caiazza A, Carlomagno A, Lamberti M, Pezone N, Pota A, Russo L, Sacco M, Scognamiglio B: Progression of coronary artery calcification and cardiac events in patients with chronic renal disease not receiving dialysis. Kidney Int 2011;80:112–118.

16 Block GA, Spiegel DM, Ehrlich J, Mehta R, Lindbergh J, Dreisbach A, Raggi P: Effects of sevelamer and calcium on coronary artery calcification in patients new to hemodialysis. Kidney Int 2005;68:1815–1824.

17 Matsuoka M, Iseki K, Tamashiro M, Fujimoto N, Higa N, Touma T, Takishita S: Impact of high coronary artery calcification score (CACS) on survival in patients on chronic hemodialysis. Clin Exp Nephrol 2004;8:54–58.
18 Goldsmith DJ, Covic A, Sambrook PA, Ackrill P: Vascular calcification in long-term haemodialysis patients in a single unit: a retrospective analysis. Nephron 1997;77:37–43.
19 Wilson PW, Kauppila LI, O'Donnell CJ, Kiel DP, Hannan M, Polak JM, Cupples LA: Abdominal aortic calcific deposits are an important predictor of vascular morbidity and mortality. Circulation 2001;103:1529–1534.
20 Bellasi A, Ferramosca E, Muntner P, Ratti C, Wildman RP, Block GA, Raggi P: Correlation of simple imaging tests and coronary artery calcium measured by computed tomography in hemodialysis patients. Kidney Int 2006;70:1623–1628.
21 Honkanen E, Kauppila L, Wikström B, Rensma PL, Krzesinski JM, Aasarod K, Verbeke F, Jensen PB, Mattelaer P, Volck B, CORD Study Group: Abdominal aortic calcification in dialysis patients: results of the CORD study. Nephrol Dial Transplant 2008;23:4009–4015.
22 Verbeke F, Van Biesen W, Honkanen E, Wikström B, Jensen PB, Krzesinski JM, Rasmussen M, Vanholder R, Rensma PL, CORD Study Investigators: Prognostic value of aortic stiffness and calcification for cardiovascular events and mortality in dialysis patients: outcome of the calcification outcome in renal disease (CORD) study. Clin J Am Soc Nephrol 2011;6:153–159.
23 Raggi P, Bellasi A, Gamboa C, Ferramosca E, Ratti C, Block GA, Muntner P: All-cause mortality in hemodialysis patients with heart valve calcification. Clin J Am Soc Nephrol 2011;6:1990–1995.
24 Bellasi A, Ferramosca E, Ratti C, Block G, Raggi P: Cardiac valve calcification is a marker of vascular disease in prevalent hemodialysis patients. J Nephrol 2011 Jun 28:0. doi: 10.5301/JN.2011.8446.
25 Kim HG, Song SW, Kim TY, Kim YO: Risk factors for progression of aortic arch calcification in patients on maintenance hemodialysis and peritoneal dialysis. Hemodial Int 2011;15:460–467.
26 Noordzij M, Cranenburg EM, Engelsman LF, Hermans MM, Boeschoten EW, Brandenburg VM, Bos WJ, Kooman JP, Dekker FW, Ketteler M, Schurgers LJ, Krediet RT, Korevaar JC, NECOSAD Study Group: Progression of aortic calcification is associated with disorders of mineral metabolism and mortality in chronic dialysis patients. Nephrol Dial Transplant 2011;26:1662–1669.
27 Riser BL, Barreto FC, Rezg R, Valaitis PW, Cook CS, White JA, Gass JH, Maizel J, Louvet L, Drueke TB, Holmes CJ, Massy ZA: Daily peritoneal administration of sodium pyrophosphate in a dialysis solution prevents the development of vascular calcification in a mouse model of uraemia. Nephrol Dial Transplant 2011;26:3349–3357.

Dr. D.J.A. Goldsmith
Reader in Renal Medicine, King's College London, UK
Guy's Campus, King's Health Partners AHSC
London SE1 9R (UK)
Tel. +44 2071885647, E-Mail david.goldsmith@gstt.nhs.uk

Ronco C, Rosner MH, Crepaldi C (eds): Peritoneal Dialysis – State-of-the-Art 2012.
Contrib Nephrol. Basel, Karger, 2012, vol 178, pp 195–199

Adequacy in Peritoneal Dialysis

Jean-Philippe Ryckelynck · Maxence Ficheux · Cindy Castrale · Patrick Henri · Thierry Lobbedez

Department of Nephrology, Dialysis and Renal Transplantation, University Hospital Center, Caen, France

Abstract

Peritoneal dialysis (PD) adequacy is usually estimated by parameters based on the kinetics of small solutes as total Kt/V_{urea} and total weekly creatinine clearance. However, other aspects (blood pressure, anemia, nutrition, inflammation, mineral metabolism and prevention of cardiovascular events) and, in particular, residual renal function must be taken into account. Although minimal levels are well defined, there are no optimal targets to be achieved. Clinical assessments are more and more relevant. In addition, fluid and sodium removal must be estimated, several studies showing that even in anuric patients adequacy can be obtained. Nutrition and inflammation have to be evaluated and their role seems to be more important than peritoneal membrane status in patient survival. Guidelines and recommendations are available to provide a better follow-up in patients on PD.

Adequacy of peritoneal dialysis (PD) was previously only based on the kinetics (clearances) and removal of small solutes. More recently, it has been established that other parameters should be taken in account: blood pressure control, prevention of cardiovascular complications, dyslipidemia, anemia, control of acidosis, nutritional status, mineral metabolism and quality of life [1]. Moreover, in PD patients, the residual renal function (RRF) is important.

Usually, total (renal and peritoneal) weekly Kt/V_{urea} and total weekly creatinine clearance are evaluated. Daily fluid removal (urinary volume and net peritoneal ultrafiltration) and normalized protein catabolic rate (nPCR) are also important.

Small Solute Clearances

In the CANUSA study, it has been concluded that a low weekly Kt/V_{urea} was associated with increased mortality. The conclusions were that a 0.1 decrease of Kt/V_{urea} is associated with a 5% increase of relative risk of death and a 5 liters/week/1.73 m^2 body surface area decrease in total weekly creatinine clearance also increased the relative risk of death (7%). The technique survival and the incidence of hospitalization were negatively correlated to the total weekly creatinine clearance [2].

The results of the CANUSA study were the basis for the Guidelines from the National Kidney Foundation Dialysis Outcomes Quality Initiative (NKF-DOQI) that recommended a weekly total (renal and peritoneal) solute removal greater than 2.0 in terms of Kt/V_{urea} for CAPD whereas for APD this value should be greater than 2.1 and, in terms of total weekly creatinine clearances, more than 60 liters/week/1.73 m^2 for both CAPD and APD [3].

The ADEMEX study did not show such results. In this study, patients were randomly assigned to receive either a usual volume of PD fluids (four daily 2-liter exchanges) or an increased dose to maintain a total creatinine clearance of greater than 60 liters/week/1.73 m². The total Kt/V_{urea} was 2.27 in the intervention group compared to 1.80 in the control group. The 2-year overall patient survival was similar in both groups (68 and 69%, respectively) [4].

In a study from Hong Kong, 320 incident patients with a renal Kt/V less than 1.0 were recruited. They were randomized into three Kt/V targets: group A, 1.5 to 1.7; group B, 1.7 to 2.0; and group C, more than 2.0 Kt/V. The overall 2-year patient survival was 84.9%. There was no statistical difference in patient survival among the three groups. There was no difference in serum albumin, composite nutritional index scores, and hospitalization rate. However, patients had more clinical problems and severe anemia when Kt/V_{urea} was below 1.7. In these cases, a continuous PD regime seems to be essential whenever possible. If urea symptoms indicating underdialysis are observed, an increased amount of peritoneal dialysate must be prescribed even if Kt/V_{urea} is above the minimal target. A transfer to hemodialysis must be arranged if the clinical situation does not improve [5].

Residual renal function has been shown to be much more predictive of survival than peritoneal clearance. In anuric patients, it is possible to analyze survival according peritoneal Kt/V only. In a retrospective study, over a 10-year period, 150 PD anuric patients were enrolled. The 2- and 5-year survival rates were 88.7 and 66.7%, respectively. Patients with a peritoneal Kt/V below 1.67 had the lowest survival rate. The authors concluded that a minimal Kt/V target of 1.70 and an optimal target of 1.80 in anuric patients are required [6]. However, the correlation between Kt/V and creatinine clearance decreases.

The results of a previous study, The European APD Outcome Study (EAPOS), are particularly interesting: it is a 2-year, prospective, multicenter study of clinical outcomes in anuric patients on APD [7]. At baseline, the residual renal function had to be less than 1 ml/min per 1.73 m². A total of 177 patients were enrolled. The APD prescription was adjusted at the physician's discretion to aim for a creatinine clearance of more than 60 liters/week per 1.73 m² and ultrafiltration (UF) of more than 750 ml/24 h during the first 6 months. At 1 year, 78 and 74% achieved the creatinine clearance and UF targets, respectively. At 2 years, patient survival was 78% and technique survival was 62%. Baseline creatinine clearance and D/P creatinine had no effect on patient or technique survival. This study shows that anuric patients can successfully use APD. Baseline UF, not creatinine clearance and membrane permeability is associated with patient survival. In conclusion, there was no relationship between mall solute clearance and mortality. In the NECOSAD study, in which 102 CAPD patients and 28 APD patients were enrolled, it was concluded that the risk of death in anuric PD patients increased only when weekly Kt/V_{urea} was lower than 1.5 and the creatinine clearance less than 40 liters/week/1.73 m² [8].

Ultrafiltration

These results concerning ultrafiltration, taken from the reanalysis of the CANUSA study, showed that neither net peritoneal ultrafiltration nor total fluid removal was associated with patient survival. Although these results may be explained partly, statistically, by less variability in peritoneal clearance than in GFR, the latter seems to be more important than the former [9].

In the NECOSAD study, a net ultrafiltration below 750 ml/24 h predicted a higher mortality when compared to a higher value. These results confirmed the previous findings from the EAPOS study. However, the patients with an ultrafiltration lower than 1.15 liters/day had a mortality risk of 3.41 but without any statistical significance among five different subgroups. More than a low ultrafiltration, cardiac failure with volume overload could be the main cause of increased mortality [8].

Recently, Paniagua et al. [10] looked at the implications of different dialysis regimens in patients on CAPD, taking into account that fluid removal varies with glucose fluid concentrations. They analyzed ultrafiltration and adequacy indices for 4 different combinations of dialysis fluid. The study concerns 99 patients on CAPD. Each patient performed 4 exchanges in 24 h, including 3 daily exchanges with 1.36% glucose and 1 night exchange with either 1.36% glucose (G1), 2.27% glucose (G2), 3.86% glucose, or icodextrin. Weekly total Kt/V_{urea} and weekly total creatinine clearance were determined.

The mean values of Kt/V_{urea} were significantly lower for the G1 schedule than for the G3 and Ico schedules. The adequacy indices for overnight application of 3.86% glucose and icodextrin were similar. The conclusion of this study is that using dialysis fluids with 1.36 and 2.27% glucose overnight reduces glucose exposure, but those schedules may provide inadequate ultrafiltration and small-solute removal in some patients (UF less than 1 liter/day, Kt/V less than 1.70) [10]. Inflammation and inadequate fluid removal seems to more important than high peritoneal transport rate as risk factors in patients on PD.

Intraperitoneal volume per exchange and intraperitoneal pressure (IPP) have an impact on ultrafiltration. By increasing the IPP after applying an abdominal belt, an increase of Kt/V_{urea} from 1.89 to 2.30 has been observed in 12 patients on CAPD. The authors suggest that the increase in the intra-abdominal pressure produced by wearing an abdominal belt might achieve a better contact of the peritoneal fluid with a larger peritoneal membrane surface area, leading to improved adequacy [11].

Ultrafiltration in relation to membrane permeability and PD fluid osmotic components is detailed by Lameire and Van Biesen [this vol., pp. 47–52].

Peritoneal Dialysis Adequacy and Inflammation

Low RRF, inflammation and an increased peritoneal transport rate (PTR), evaluated by the peritoneal equilibration test, are reported to be associated with increased mortality in PD patients. A total of 117 patients who were started on PD were analyzed retrospectively. Assessment of RRF, inflammation and PTR were evaluated 1 month after the start of PD [12].

The aim of the study was to test the hypothesis that a low RRF at the start of PD might be linked to inflammation, which may be associated with a high PTR, and thus these three factors may be associated with increased mortality in PD patients. The prevalence of an RRF of less than 4 ml/min/1.73 m^2, inflammation with a serum CRP of more than 10 mg/l and high PTR (D/P creatinine ≥0.86) was 46, 31 and 15%, respectively. Of 117 patients, 22% had one, 22% had two, 2% had all three, and 34% had none of these characteristics. Overall patient survival was significantly lower in the patients with low RRF ($p = 0.002$), high serum CRP ($p = 0.004$) and more than two of the three characteristics ($p = 0.0002$). In the group of patients who had none of these characteristics, the 5-year survival was 100% whereas the 5-year survival was only 17.5% in patients with two or more of these characteristics. However, in the high PTR group, patient survival rate was significantly lower only at 1 year of PD but not in subsequent years of PD. These results indicate that low RRF and inflammation are both associated with high overall mortality. Likewise, peritoneal protein clearance, although correlated with volume overload and inflammation, is largely an independent predictor of mortality [13]. Moreover, inflammation interacts with other cardiovascular risk factors in uremia and was shown to increase the risk of death and cardiovascular events [14].

Peritoneal Dialysis Adequacy and Nutrition

Nutrient intake by patients on dialysis can be influenced by many factors [15]. The most important are residual renal function, comorbidities, inflammation, infections, acidosis, initial malnutrition in part due to late referral, age, peritoneal glucose absorption, and inadequacy of PD. There is a strong correlation between nutritional status, inflammation and mortality in an observational study with a 15-year follow-up [16]. Accumulation of uremic toxins with chronic kidney disease progression is associated with anorexia. However, whether increasing dialysis dose leads to better clinical outcomes is still being debated.

First in the CANUSA study, each 1 g/l increase in serum albumin was associated with a 6% decrease in mortality and one unit in the SGA score with a 25% decrease in relative risk of death [2].

Secondary analyses of the ADEMEX trial and of an interventional study conducted in six centers in Hong Kong found no association between higher dialysis dose and improved nutritional status. In another Hong Kong study, patients were divided into tertile groups of daily protein intake (DPI): low (≤0.73 g/kg/day), middle (0.74–0.93 g/kg/day) and high (≥0.94 g/kg/day) tertile groups. Though RRF was significantly lower and CRP higher in the low tertile group in comparison to the high tertile group, there were no significant difference for D/P creatinine, total Kt/V and total creatinine clearance between each group [17]. This study also showed that DPI lower than 0.73 g/kg/day was associated with the worst outcome. Other reports have suggested that the relationship between Kt/V and nPNA is not linear but reaches a plateau at a total Kt/V of approximately 1.8. In a univariate and multivariate Cox regression model on patient survival, serum albumin at baseline and peritoneal protein clearance but neither peritoneal Kt/Vurea nor peritoneal transport status are independent risk factors. In some patients, increasing the dialysis dose could improve nutritional status [15].

Recommendations

The recommendations were reviewed and published as European Best Practice Guidelines (EBPG 2005) and International Society of Peritoneal Dialysis (ISPD 2006) Guidelines.

According to the EBPG [18]
The adequacy targets for dialysis should include both urea removal and fluid removal. The targets should be based on those achieved by PD only.

The minimum peritoneal target for Kt/V_{urea} in anuric patients is a weekly value of 1.7. The presence of residual renal function can compensate when these targets are not achieved.

When the targets are not achieved, patients should be monitored carefully for signs of overhydration, uremic complaints and malnutrition.

Some APD patients who use frequent short exchanges and have a slow transport status can fulfill the above targets, but may have a low peritoneal creatinine clearance. In these patients, an additional target of 45 l/week/1.73 m^2 for peritoneal creatinine clearance should be aimed at in addition to achieving the Kt/V_{urea} target of 1.7.

When malnutrition develops, the adequacy of dialysis prescription should be assessed.

According to the ISPD [19]
Residual renal function, but not peritoneal clearance, is predictive of survival in prospective observational studies and can account for most of the association between total clearance and survival.

Adequacy of dialysis should be interpreted clinically rather than targeting only solute and fluid removal. Clinical assessment should include clinical and laboratory results, peritoneal and renal clearances, hydration status, appetite and nutritional tatus, energy level, hemoglobin concentration, responsiveness to erythropoietin therapy, electrolytes and acid-base balance, calcium phosphate homeostasis, and blood pressure control.

Prospective randomized interventional studies do not provide evidence to support a beneficial effect of increasing dialysis to total Kt/V_{urea} above 2.0, or creatinine clearance above 60 liters/week/1.73 m^2, in patients on CAPD with a total Kt/V_{urea} above 1.70 or creatinine clearance above 50 liters/week/1.73 m^2.

Interventional studies have demonstrated that total Kt/V below 1.70 is associated with poorer primary or secondary outcome.

References

1 Heimburger O: How should we measure peritoneal dialysis adequacy in the clinic; in Ronco C, Crepaldi C, Cruz DN (eds): Peritoneal Dialysis – From Basic Concepts to Clinical Excellence. Contrib Nephrol. Basel, Karger, 2009, vol 163, pp 140–146.
2 Churchill DN, Taylor DW: Adequacy of dialysis and nutrition in continuous peritoneal dialysis: association with clinical outcomes. Canada-USA (CANUSA) Peritoneal Dialysis Study Group. J Am Soc Nephrol 1996;7:198–207.
3 National Kidney Foundation: NKF-DOQI clinical practice guidelines for peritoneal dialysis adequacy. Am J Kidney Dis 1997;30(3 suppl 2): S67–S136.
4 Paniagua R, Amato D, Vonesh E, Correa-Rotter R, Ramos A, Moran J, Mujais S, Mexican Nephrology Collaborative Study Group: Effects of increased peritoneal clearances on mortality rate in peritoneal dialysis: ADEMEX, a prospective, randomized, controlled trial. J Am Soc Nephrol 2002;13:1307–1320.
5 Lo WK, Ho YW, Li CS, Wong KS, Chan TM, Yu AW, Ng FS, Cheng IK: Effect of Kt/V on survival and clinical outcome in CAPD patients in a randomized prospective study. Kidney Int 2003;64:649–656.
6 Lo WK, Lui SL, Chan TM, Li FK, Lam MF, Tse KC, Tang SC, Choy CB, Lai KN: Minimal and optimal peritoneal Kt/V targets: results of an anuric peritoneal dialysis patient's survival analysis. Kidney Int 2005;67:2032–2038.
7 Brown EA, Davies SJ, Rutherford P, Meeus F, Borras M, Riegel W, Divino Filho JC, Vonesh E, van Bree M, EAPOS Group: Survival of functionally anuric patients on automated peritoneal dialysis: The European APD Outcome Study. J Am Soc Nephrol 2003;14:2948–2957.
8 Jansen MA, Termorshuizen F, Korevaar JC, Dekker FW, Boeschoten E, Krediet RT, for the NECOSAD Study Group: Predictors of survival in anuric peritoneal dialysis patients. Kidney Int 2005;68:1199–1205.
9 Bargmann JM, Thorpe KE, Churchill DN, CANUSA Peritoneal Dialysis Study Group: Relative contribution of residual renal function and peritoneal clearance to adequacy of dialysis: a reanalysis of the CANUSA study. J Am Soc Nephrol 2001;12:2158–2162.
10 Paniagua R, Debowska M, Ventura M, Avila-Diaz M, Prado-Uribe C, Mora C, Garcia-Lopez E, Lindholm B, Waniewski J: Ultrafiltration and dialysis adequacy with various daily schedules of dialysis fluids. Perit Dial int 2012, in press.
11 Alhwiesh A, Fahd K: The influence of increased peritoneal membrane surface area on dialysis adequacy. Saudi J Kidney Dis Transpl 2011;22:1717–1722.
12 Chung SH, Heimbürger O, Stenvinkel P, Qureshi AR, Lindholm B: Association between residual renal function, inflammation and patient survival in new peritoneal dialysis patients. Nephrol Dial Transplant 2003;18:590–597.
13 Dong J, Xu Y, Li Y, Yang Z: Does association with volume status and inflammation account for the increased death risk from high peritoneal protein clearance in peritoneal dialysis? Blood Purif 2010;30:127–134.
14 Stenvinkel P, Barany P: Can cardiovascular risk in dialysis patients be decreased? Nat Rev Nephrol 2012;8:72–74.
15 Han SH, Han DS: Nutrition in patients on peritoneal dialysis. Nat Rev Nephrol 2012;8:163–175.
16 Avram MM, Fein PA, Rafiq MA, Schloth T, Chattopadhyay J, Mittman N: Malnutrition and inflammation as predictors of mortality in peritoneal dialysis patients. Kidney Int 2006;70:S4–S7.
17 Dong J, Li Y, Xu Y, Xu R: Daily protein intake and survival in patients on peritoneal dialysis. Nephrol Dial Transplant 2011;26:3715–3721.
18 European Best Practice Guidelines for Peritoneal Dialysis (EBPG): Adequacy of peritoneal dialysis. Nephrol Dial Transplant 2005;20(suppl 9):ix24–ix27.
19 Lo WK, Bargman JM, Burkart J, Krediet RT, Pollock C, Kawanishi H, Blake PG, ISPD Adequacy of Peritoneal Dialysis Working Group: Guideline on targets for solute and fluid removal in adult patients on chronic peritoneal dialysis. Perit Dial Int 2006;26:520–522.

Prof. J.-P. Ryckelynck
Nephrology, Dialysis and Transplantation, CHU Clemenceau
Avenue G. Clemenceau
FR–14033 Caen Cedex (France)
Tel. +33 2 31 27 25 76, E-Mail ryckelynck-jp@chu-caen.fr

Ronco C, Rosner MH, Crepaldi C (eds): Peritoneal Dialysis – State-of-the-Art 2012.
Contrib Nephrol. Basel, Karger, 2012, vol 178, pp 200–204

Setting Up Research in Peritoneal Dialysis

Janusz Witowski

Department of Pathophysiology, Poznan University of Medical Sciences, Poznan, Poland

Abstract

Over the past 30 years, peritoneal dialysis (PD) not only developed into a valuable treatment modality, but also stimulated basic science research. Here, we summarize some of such PD-inspired studies that addressed more general aspects of immunology and pathology and helped us to appreciate the complexity of peritoneal biology.

The establishment of clinical PD stimulated research on many related topics. Over the years, different themes were pursued with different fervor. Early studies dealt mainly with the technical problems, such as peritoneal access, fluid composition, and delivery systems. Ultimately, they helped to make PD a safer and more reliable technique. With elementary issues resolved, the research efforts focused on basic sciences (see Jörres and Witowski [1] for a brief history of PD research). In recent years, our understanding of peritoneal biology significantly increased and now we are trying to reconcile the data from in vitro studies, animal experiments, and clinical investigations to create a coherent picture of what really happens in the peritoneum during long-term PD. Here, we will remind you of three stories of research that originated in PD, but produced results going beyond PD itself.

Peritoneal Cytokine

The early days of peritoneal dialysis (PD) were plagued by frequent episodes of infection. Not surprisingly, therefore, the problem of peritonitis drew the attention of both clinicians and basic science researchers. Whilst the former were interested in the means of preventing and treating infections, the latter saw in PD a unique opportunity to study the pathophysiology of inflammation. Although the peritoneal cavity of experimental animals has long been used as a convenient site to investigate the host defence, the availability of PD effluent made it possible to look into the peritoneal homeostasis in humans. The effluent contains both the resident cells and the cells recruited to the peritoneum during inflammation. It also contains a plethora of inflammatory mediators, including those responsible for the cell fluxes. Thus, by examining the effluents drained before, during, and after peritonitis, it became possible to gain an insight into the mechanisms controlling each individual phase of the peritoneal inflammatory response.

This approach was fully exploited in the investigations that helped to define the role of interleukin-6 (IL-6) in immunity. In 1990, Goldman et al. [2] were the first to observe that the initiation of peritonitis in PD patients was accompanied by a massive increase (100- to 10,000-fold) in the concentration of IL-6 in the effluent. At that time, the source of this cytokine and the mechanism by which its levels increased so dramatically could not be identified. However, subsequent measurements revealed that the levels of IL-6 in effluent were much higher than could be explained by its simple diffusion from the circulation. This observation pointed to local IL-6 production. Initially, the source of IL-6 was thought to be peritoneal macrophages. Their careful phenotyping has revealed that they become increasingly immature with the duration of PD and secrete increased quantities of IL-6 [3]. It has soon become apparent, however, that there is an even more potent source of IL-6 in the peritoneum.

The development of cell culture techniques made it possible to cultivate peritoneal mesothelial cells in vitro and expose them to conditions similar to those occurring in the dialyzed peritoneum. Such experiments quickly revealed an enormous potential of human peritoneal mesothelial cells to generate huge amounts of IL-6 in response to pro-inflammatory stimuli [4]. Although it was an important step forward in untangling the peritoneal cytokine network, the role of IL-6 in this system was still unclear. The mystery began to unravel when a model of acute peritonitis in normal and IL-6-deficient mice was established [5]. In this model the animals are challenged intraperitoneally with a standardized dose of cell-free supernatant of *Staphylococcus epidermidis*, a major cause of PD-associated peritonitis. Subsequent events reproduce the pattern of peritonitis in humans and begin with a rapid influx of neutrophils. It occurs in response to specific chemokines (of the CXC family) generated largely by mesothelial cells. Neutrophils are progressively cleared by apoptosis, the production of CXC chemokines gradually decreases and the migration of neutrophils is suppressed. At the same time, mesothelial cells initiate the production of CC chemokines, which activate and recruit monocytes and lymphocytes. These spectacular switches, from the production of one class of chemokines to another and from the neutrophil influx to mononuclear cell infiltration, are central to the resolution of inflammation. In a series of elegant experiments, the Cardiff group has demonstrated that IL-6 is a key mediator of this regulation and acts in combination with its soluble receptor (sIL-6R).

During peritonitis sIL-6R is delivered by neutrophils that shed it from their surfaces after proteolytic cleavage of membrane-bound IL-6 receptors [5]. Unlike other soluble cytokine receptors, sIL-6R displays agonistic rather than antagonistic properties. So when IL-6 binds to sIL-6R, the resulting complex can stimulate, through so-called trans-signaling, those cells that lack their own IL-6 receptor [6]. Accordingly, mesothelial cells, which are deprived of IL-6R, remain unresponsive to IL-6 unless sIL-6R is present. When stimulated by an IL-6-sIL-6R complex, they react by suppressing the secretion of CXC chemokines (which promotes neutrophil removal), and by upregulating the production of CC chemokines (which promotes the recruitment of mononuclear leukocytes).

These seminal observations spurred further research on IL-6 trans-signaling. It has soon been demonstrated that IL-6-regulated processes of intraperitoneal neutrophil trafficking and apoptosis are mediated via a transcription factor STAT3 and further controlled by interferon-γ [7]. Moreover, IL-6 trans-signaling was found to be instrumental in recruiting T cells into the inflamed peritoneum. Thus, it became clear that by mediating the transition from a neutrophil to mononuclear cell population, IL-6 regulated a switch from innate to acquired immunity [6].

While this transition leads to the ultimate resolution of inflammation, it may become dysregulated by repeated episodes of infection and/or uremia and the peritoneum may enter a state of chronic inflammation. This may, in turn, impinge on peritoneal membrane function. The dialytic function of the peritoneum varies greatly among patients already at the start of PD and changes further with time. This variability has been linked to several factors, including local IL-6 production [8]. Accumulating data from the Global Fluid Study strongly suggest that higher dialysate levels of IL-6 predict higher solute transport rates. These data have robust support in the analysis of the IL-6 gene polymorphisms, which revealed that the variants linked with higher IL-6 production were also associated with increased solute permeability [9].

Peritoneal Cell

The development of structural changes in the peritoneum during long-term PD has been well documented. The most consistently observed alterations are the submesothelial thickening, fibrosis, neoangiogenesis and vasculopathy, all of which increase significantly with time on PD [10]. This peritoneal remodeling may be seen as a consequence of disturbed wound healing response to repeated injuries inflicted by continuous irritation by PD fluids. Investigations into the morphology of the dialyzed peritoneum have confirmed that during PD mesothelial cells undergo continues injury and regeneration. Repeated PD fluid exchanges may lead to the occasional detachment of some cells from the peritoneal surface. These cells can be found in the drained effluent in low numbers, but they still can be isolated, propagated in vitro, and analyzed. Such analyses of the effluent-derived mesothelial cells were pioneered by the Madrid group, and revealed the trail of the process that was not previously recognized to occur in the peritoneal membrane [11].

Mesothelial cells isolated from different PD patients were found to vary markedly in their phenotypic appearance. It ranged from a cobblestone morphology typical of epithelial cells to the spindle-like appearance typical of fibroblasts, with mixed populations in between. Although mesothelial cells are of mesodermal origin, they typically display characteristics of epithelial cells with a polygonal appearance, clear apical-basal polarity, and the expression of cytokeratin filaments. They may, however, undergo so-called epithelial-to-mesenchymal transition (EMT) and adopt a fibroblast-like phenotype. During the process they activate the transcription factors *snail* and *slug*, which then decrease the expression of cytokeratins and epithelial adhesion protein E-cadherin, and upregulate the expression of fibroblast-specific protein 1, vimentin, and α-smooth muscle actin (α-SMA). By analyzing these biomarkers in effluent-derived cells, it could be demonstrated that, indeed, in some patients mesothelial cells had been going through EMT [12]. During EMT cells become motile so that they can loosen and then leave the tight epithelial monolayers, and migrate into the underlying stroma. Indeed, in peritoneal biopsies from PD patients, trans-differentiated mesothelial cells were detected in the interstitium at various distances form the peritoneal surface. Later, Margetts et al. [13] documented the whole process of EMT in rats by sequential dual labeling for epithelial and fibroblast markers.

The regulation of EMT is not fully understood. It appears to be controlled by several growth factors, of which transforming growth factor-β_1 (TGF-β_1) emerged as the most potent EMT inducer. TGF-β_1 has been shown to induce EMT of peritoneal mesothelial cells both in culture and in vivo in experimental rodents [11]. Its effect is mediated largely (but not exclusively) through a transcription factor Smad 3 [13].

An immediate interest in peritoneal EMT was spurred by its clinical context when it transpired that trans-differentiated cells were detected in the effluents drained from some patients but not from others. Characterization of the secretory cell phenotype showed that trans-differentiated cells produced significantly more mediators of fibrosis and angiogenesis compared to cells with the classic epithelial appearance [14]. Moreover, the incidence of EMT appeared to increase with time on PD [12]. These findings suggested that mesothelial cells exhibiting a mesenchymal phenotype might contribute to the development of structural alterations typical of long-term PD.

What still remains unclear, however, is the mechanism by which PD initiates EMT. The association with the duration of therapy suggests that EMT may be related to the cumulative exposure to PD fluids. In this respect, it has been demonstrated that the incubation of mesothelial cells in high glucose led to the up-regulation of TGF-β1 [15]. The increased expression of TGF-β_1 in association with EMT was also observed in animals receiving intraperitoneal injections of methylglyoxal, a glucose degradation product (GDP) [16]. More recently, Bajo et al. [14] have documented a clear relationship between biocompatibility of PD fluids and the induction of peritoneal EMT. They have shown that the incidence of EMT in mesothelial cells is higher in patients treated with conventional PD fluids with high GDP levels compared with patients receiving newer low-GDP solutions.

An interesting aspect of peritoneal EMT was addressed by Pletinck et al. [17]. They have investigated how dietary intake of salt impacts on the peritoneal morphology. They were inspired by earlier observations suggesting that increased salt intake may lead to tissue fibrosis and increased TGF-β_1 expression independently of changes in blood pressure or volume status. During the experiment the rats were allowed to drink either pure water or a 2% salt solution. The morphological analysis of the peritoneal membrane revealed thickening, fibrosis, and mesothelial EMT, as well as an increased expression of IL-6 and TGF-β_1. These effects were not associated with increased blood pressure and were evident already after 2 weeks of increased salt consumption. This finding deserves further exploration in view of the suggestions that excess sodium plays an adverse role in the pathogenesis of organ damage in renal failure.

Peritoneal Foreign Body

Over the past years, a great deal of effort was devoted to biocompatibility issues in PD. This usually meant the assessment of various PD fluids, while other aspects of the PD system seemed to be somewhat neglected. Recent studies revived an interest in the peritoneal catheter. Flessner et al. [18] have compared the response of the peritoneum to the same PD solution instilled in rodents either through an implanted silicone catheter or via daily needle injections. After a few weeks, they found a significantly thickened and more vascularized peritoneum in animals with a catheter. These changes were accompanied by an increase in the expression of pro-angiogenic and pro-fibrotic growth factors, and by an increased transport of small solutes and albumin. The authors hypothesized that the presence of a catheter caused a foreign body reaction and resulted in local inflammation. They went on to examine this effect more precisely by placing small catheter fragments intraperitoneally rather than implanting a whole catheter tunneled to the outside [19]. This approach minimized the trauma, eliminated the formation of a biofilm, and reduced the risk of infection. Already after 1 week, a distinct layer of adherent cells could be identified on the catheter surface. The analysis of its cellular makeup revealed the presence of macrophages, T cells, dendritic cells, as well as mesothelial and fibroblast-like cells. Interestingly, many cells stained distinctly for a myofibroblast marker, α-SMA, which could signify the formation of a fibrotic capsule around the catheter. Such fibrous encapsulation may compromise the catheter patency and lead to its malfunction. The origin of cells expressing α-SMA is not certain. They might be trans-differentiated mesothelial cells and/or macrophages. Mooney et al. [20] have demonstrated that macrophages display a great potential for cellular plasticity and are capable of trans-differentiating from a myeloid to mesenchymal phenotype.

In addition to changes on the catheter itself, Flessner et al. [19] have observed clear alterations in the neighboring parietal peritoneum, which exhibited an increased submesothelial thickness, vascular density, and altered permeability for macromolecules. These data show the strength of the peritoneal foreign body response and its potential impact on the peritoneal transport properties.

On the other hand, the same reaction may be turned into a benefit. The experimental studies indicate that the peritoneal cavity may provide a sterile location, in which myofibroblast-rich tissue is generated under controlled conditions. In this respect, the peritoneal cavity may serve as a bioreactor for tissue engineering [20].

Conclusion

The above stories serve to remind us about the significance of basic science research. They show how in-depth analysis of a single molecule, a cell type, or a foreign material found in the peritoneal cavity may increase our understanding of basic pathophysiological processes. The knowledge thus gained will certainly affect future clinical developments in PD.

References

1 Jörres A, Witowski J: Lessons from basic research for PD treatment. Perit Dial Int 2005;25(suppl 3):S35–S38.

2 Goldman M, Vandenabeele P, Moulart J, Amraoui Z, Abramowicz D, Nortier J, Vanherweghem JL, Fiers W: Intraperitoneal secretion of interleukin-6 during continuous ambulatory peritoneal dialysis. Nephron 1990;56:277–280.

3 McGregor SJ, Topley N, Jörres A, Speekenbrink AB, Gordon A, Gahl GM, Junor BJ, Briggs JD, Brock JH: Longitudinal evaluation of peritoneal macrophage function and activation during CAPD: maturity, cytokine synthesis and arachidonic acid metabolism. Kidney Int 1996;49:525–533.

4 Witowski J, Jörres A, Coles GA, Williams JD, Topley N: Superinduction of IL-6 synthesis in human peritoneal mesothelial cells is related to the induction and stabilization of IL-6 mRNA. Kidney Int 1996;50:1212–1223.

5 Hurst SM, Wilkinson TS, McLoughlin RM, Jones S, Horiuchi S, Yamamoto N, Rose-John S, Fuller GM, Topley N, Jones SA: Il-6 and its soluble receptor orchestrate a temporal switch in the pattern of leukocyte recruitment seen during acute inflammation. Immunity 2001;14:705–714.

6 Jones SA: Directing transition from innate to acquired immunity: defining a role for IL-6. J Immunol 2005;175:3463–3468.

7 McLoughlin RM, Witowski J, Robson RL, Wilkinson TS, Hurst SM, Williams AS, Williams JD, Rose-John S, Jones SA, Topley N: Interplay between IFN-gamma and IL-6 signaling governs neutrophil trafficking and apoptosis during acute inflammation. J Clin Invest 2003;112:598–607.

8 Davies SJ, Mushahar L, Yu Z, Lambie M: Determinants of peritoneal membrane function over time. Semin Nephrol 2011;31:172–182.

9 Gillerot G, Goffin E, Michel C, Evenepoel P, Biesen WV, Tintillier M, Stenvinkel P, Heimburger O, Lindholm B, Nordfors L, Robert A, Devuyst O: Genetic and clinical factors influence the baseline permeability of the peritoneal membrane. Kidney Int 2005;67:2477–2487.

10 Williams JD, Craig KJ, Topley N, Von Ruhland C, Fallon M, Newman GR, Mackenzie RK, Williams GT: Morphologic changes in the peritoneal membrane of patients with renal disease. J Am Soc Nephrol 2002;13:470–479.

11 Aroeira LS, Aguilera A, Sanchez-Tomero JA, Bajo MA, del Peso G, Jimenez-Heffernan JA, Selgas R, Lopez-Cabrera M: Epithelial to mesenchymal transition and peritoneal membrane failure in peritoneal dialysis patients: pathologic significance and potential therapeutic interventions. J Am Soc Nephrol 2007;18:2004–2013.

12 Yanez-Mo M, Lara-Pezzi E, Selgas R, Ramirez-Huesca M, Dominguez-Jimenez C, Jimenez-Heffernan JA, Aguilera A, Sanchez-Tomero JA, Bajo MA, Alvarez V, Castro MA, del Peso G, Cirujeda A, Gamallo C, Sanchez-Madrid F, Lopez-Cabrera M: Peritoneal dialysis and epithelial-to-mesenchymal transition of mesothelial cells. N Engl J Med 2003;348:403–413.

13 Devuyst O, Margetts PJ, Topley N: The pathophysiology of the peritoneal membrane. J Am Soc Nephrol 2010;21:1077–1085.

14 Bajo MA, Perez-Lozano ML, Albar-Vizcaino P, del Peso G, Castro MJ, Gonzalez-Mateo G, Fernandez-Perpen A, Aguilera A, Sanchez-Villanueva R, Sanchez-Tomero JA, Lopez-Cabrera M, Peter ME, Passlick-Deetjen J, Selgas R: Low-GDP peritoneal dialysis fluid ('balance') has less impact in vitro and ex vivo on epithelial-to-mesenchymal transition (EMT) of mesothelial cells than a standard fluid. Nephrol Dial Transplant 2011;26:282–291.

15 Wong TY, Phillips AO, Witowski J, Topley N: Glucose-mediated induction of TGF-beta 1 and MCP-1 in mesothelial cells in vitro is osmolality and polyol pathway dependent. Kidney Int 2003;63:1404–1416.

16 Hirahara I, Ishibashi Y, Kaname S, Kusano E, Fujita T: Methylglyoxal induces peritoneal thickening by mesenchymal-like mesothelial cells in rats. Nephrol Dial Transplant 2009;24:437–447.

17 Pletinck A, Consoli C, Van Landschoot M, Steppan S, Topley N, Passlick-Deetjen J, Vanholder R, Van Biesen W: Salt intake induces epithelial-to-mesenchymal transition of the peritoneal membrane in rats. Nephrol Dial Transplant 2010;25:1688–1696.

18 Flessner MF, Credit K, Henderson K, Vanpelt HM, Potter R, He Z, Henegar J, Robert B: Peritoneal changes after exposure to sterile solutions by catheter. J Am Soc Nephrol 2007;18:2294–2302.

19 Peters T, Potter R, Li X, He Z, Hoskins G, Flessner MF: Mouse model of foreign body reaction that alters the submesothelium and transperitoneal transport. Am J Physiol Renal Physiol 2011;300:F283–F289.

20 Mooney JE, Rolfe BE, Osborne GW, Sester DP, van RN, Campbell GR, Hume DA, Campbell JH: Cellular plasticity of inflammatory myeloid cells in the peritoneal foreign body response. Am J Pathol 2010;176:369–380.

Prof. Janusz Witowski
Department of Pathophysiology, Poznan University of Medical Sciences, Collegium Anatomicum
Święcickiego 6
PL–60–781 Poznań (Poland)
Tel. +48 61 8546575, E-Mail jwitow@ump.edu.pl

Ronco C, Rosner MH, Crepaldi C (eds): Peritoneal Dialysis – State-of-the-Art 2012.
Contrib Nephrol. Basel, Karger, 2012, vol 178, pp 205–215

Continuous Flow Peritoneal Dialysis: Update 2012

Richard Amerling[a] · James F. Winchester[a] · Claudio Ronco[b]

[a]Division of Nephrology and Hypertension, Beth Israel Medical Center, New York, N.Y., USA;
[b]Nephrology Division, San Bortolo Hospital, Vicenza, Italy

Abstract

Continuous flow peritoneal dialysis (CFPD) is a technique of renal replacement therapy (RRT) dating back to the 1950s. Its essential features are a fixed intraperitoneal volume and rapid, continuous movement of dialysis solution into and out of the peritoneal cavity. Inlet and outlet catheters and a means of generating a large volume of sterile dialysate are required. External regeneration of dialysate via conventional hemodialysis equipment or sorbent technology mitigates the need for large volumes of sterile fluid and makes the technique feasible. Clearance depends on peritoneal mass transfer coefficient, rate of dialysate flow and efficiency of external regeneration. Studies to date all demonstrate small solute clearances 3–8 times greater than conventional automated peritoneal dialysis (APD). Catheter design is crucial to the clinical success of the technique and will be discussed. Potential applications include daily home dialysis, treatment of acute renal failure in the ICU, ultrafiltration of ascites, and the wearable artificial kidney.

Standard continuous ambulatory and automated peritoneal dialysis (CAPD, APD) have experienced slow growth, and even declining market share in recent years [1]. This is at least partially due to the failure of these techniques to adequately dialyze larger, anephric patients with high body mass index (BMI) and larger body surface area (BSA) [2]. Peritoneal solute clearance is not limited by membrane surface area or blood flow in most patients. The technique of extended dwell and cycling of exchanges is inefficient [3]. As solute transfer progresses during a typical exchange, the transfer rate begins to fall off quickly as the transperitoneal concentration gradient dissipates. Solute transfer rate towards the end of a typical 6-hour dwell is practically nil. This is partially remedied by increasing the frequency of exchanges, as in acute PD. With more frequent exchanges, the in and outflow time begins to seriously impact the total effective dialysis time of fluid in contact with the membrane. This limits any gain in efficiency. The conceptual solution to this problem is continuous flow peritoneal dialysis (CFPD). A constant, large intraperitoneal volume of fluid is continuously replenished, either by synchronized ingress and egress of sterile dialysate (single-pass CFPD), or by recirculating a single large exchange through an external regenerating apparatus. This latter can be either a conventional hemodialysis system, or a sorbent-based circuit. Dialysate is constantly in contact with the membrane, and intraperitoneal solute concentration is kept low. This maximizes the transperitoneal solute concentration gradient, which drives solute transport maximally for the entire duration of the treatment [4].

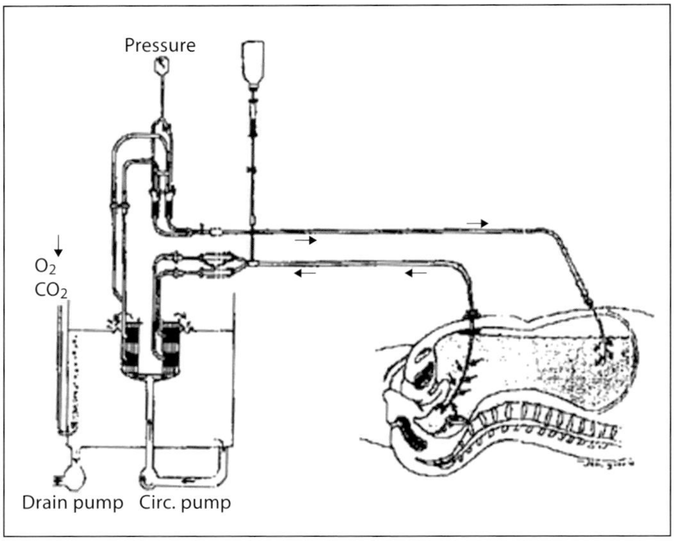

Fig. 1. System for CFPD used by Shinaberger; modified.

In 1965, Shinaberger et al. [5] reported a series of patients treated with CFPD. He used two peritoneal catheters inserted acutely at opposite ends of the peritoneal cavity, and instilled 3 liters of sterile intraperitoneal dialysate refreshed by an external Kiil dialyzer in 100 liters of dialysate (fig. 1). Dialysate flow rates ranged from 120–300 ml/min. Clearances of urea varied from 46 to as high as 125 ml/min!

Variations on this method were reported by other groups over the next two decades and met with mixed success [6–12]. Most employed dual lumen catheters and either sterile dialysate in single pass mode, or externally regenerated dialysate. Urea clearances were in the region of 30–50 ml/min. More recently, our [13] and others' [14–16] experience confirm the enhanced solute clearance abilities of CFPD.

Kinetics and Ultrafiltration in Continuous Flow Peritoneal Dialysis

Mathematical models of solute fluxes in CFPD have been developed [17]. They vary for single pass CFPD and external regeneration techniques. Total body urea clearance depends on the peritoneal mass transfer area coefficient (MTACurea), peritoneal dialysate flow rate (Qp), and dialysance in the external circuit (D). This latter depends on external dialysate flow and membrane surface area. Clearly, the MTACurea will be rate limiting, and total urea clearance will approach this number. When modeling the Shinaberger data, Gotch [17] calculated $MTAC_{urea}$ in the 60–70 range. A high-efficiency external circuit is necessary to maximize the concentration gradient and enhance the driving force for solute movement.

The need to match internal and external ultrafiltration rates in CFPD has been an ongoing technical challenge. If the internal rate exceeds the external rate, the intraperitoneal volume will swell; the converse will result in emptying the abdominal cavity. Thus, an important element of a successful home CFPD machine will be a mechanism to simply and automatically match internal and external ultrafiltration. Possible solutions include volume sensing via bioimpedance, abdominal girth strain gauge sensors, and using intraperitoneal pressure as a surrogate for volume [Ash, pers. commun.]. One advantage is that if glucose is retained as an osmotic agent, less will be required to maintain ultrafiltration. Gotch [17] predicts constant ultrafiltration of 0.2–0.45 liters/h with 1–1.5% dextrose

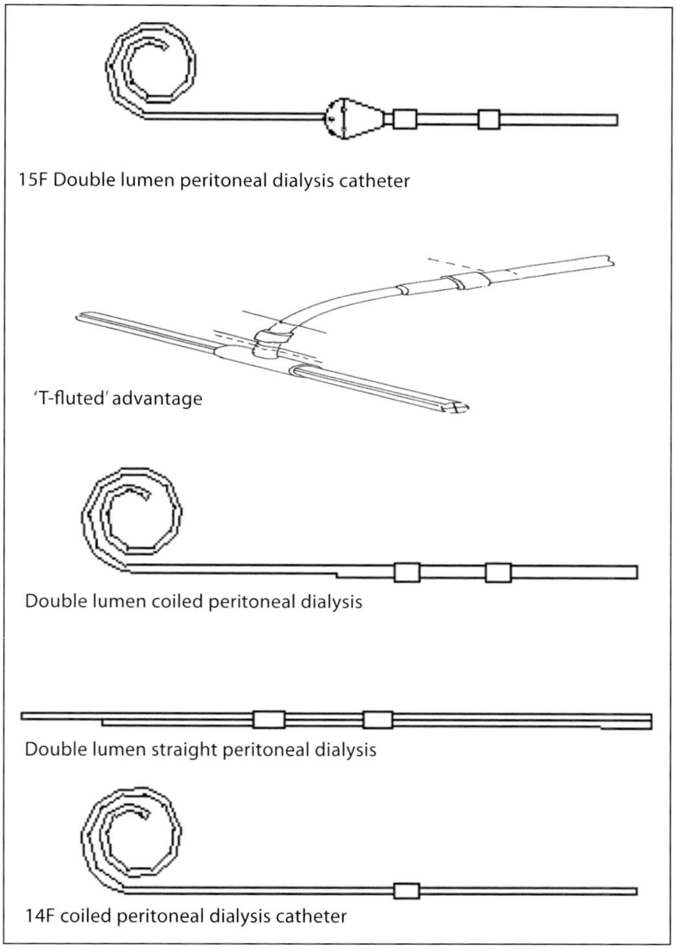

Fig. 2. Catheter configurations for CFPD.

solution. This has been confirmed in vivo by Freida [pers. commun.], who achieved a mean of 587 ml of ultrafiltration over 4 hours of single pass CFPD using 1.36% (anhydrous)dextrose. Glucose absorption is still considerable with CFPD and an alternative osmotic agent would be welcome. Based on our experience in patients with ascites, albumin would be an ideal agent [18].

Catheter Design for CFPD (fig. 2)

For CFPD to be successful, adequate mixing of intraperitoneal dialysate is crucial. Port to port 'streaming' limits this, and with it, both solute clearance and ultrafiltration [19]. It is of interest that historically, Shinaberger et al. [5], who used two catheters placed as far apart as possible, achieved the best clearances. The subsequent studies, which used different dual lumen catheters, rarely achieved urea clearances above 35 ml/min. Of course, this is still three times better than conventional PD. But we should strive to maximize clearances to reduce treatment times and optimal catheter design is critical. McKee et al. [20] compared urea clearances using a dual lumen vs. two catheters in a micropig model of CFPD with DFR of 50–100 ml/min and found no differences. It is likely, however, that higher flows will induce a degree of internal recirculation, or streaming.

We [13] and Mineshima et al. [21] have tried a simple side-by-side dual lumen catheter for CFPD. The 'streaming' with this catheter is tremendous: over 50% in our study. Streaming in our patients with two intrapelvic catheters was around 40%. In our patient with two catheters in 'one up, one down' configuration (see below), streaming was 11%.

Ash and co-workers have designed a catheter with a t-shape configuration in order to maximally separate the tips of the two lumens [22]. We have designed a novel catheter for CFPD equipped with a thin-walled silicone diffuser used to gently infuse the inflow dialysate into the peritoneum [23]. The holes on the round tapered diffuser are positioned to allow dialysate to exit perpendicularly 360° from the diffuser, thereby reducing trauma to the peritoneal walls and allowing the dialysate to mix in the peritoneum. The fluid is then drained through the second lumen whose tip is positioned in the lower pelvis. The different catheters are schematically depicted below.

The new catheter with diffuser is also equipped with a special removable hub that allows for easy creation of the subcutaneous tunnel without increasing the size of the exit site. The results thus far are impressive, with high flows, minimal intra-abdominal pressure, and negligible recirculation.

We recently inserted this catheter, at the bedside, into a patient with end stage renal disease, severe heart failure due to prolonged use of a high flow arteriovenous fistula, massive ascites and edema, and refractory hypotension that made hemodialysis impossible. Using CFPD we dialyzed and removed almost 10 liters of ascitic fluid over two 4-hour sessions. We also banded his AVF externally which improved blood pressure. The sessions were well tolerated and he improved fairly dramatically. Urea reduction over 4 h was trivial, however. We attribute this to the need to first reduce urea levels within the massive ascites before being able to significantly affect serum levels. After this initial success, we used the catheter for standard PD, also successfully. Unfortunately, the patient expired from cardiac failure after a month.

Applications

Daily Home Dialysis

As a high clearance peritoneal technique, CFPD would be a logical choice for home dialysis. As of yet, there have been no reports of patients maintained at home on CFPD. Clearly, the issues of catheter design, ultrafiltration management, and machine design still need to be worked out. Nevertheless, a user-friendly CFPD machine would offer significant advantages over home hemodialysis. First, it is inherently safer than hemodialysis. There is no risk of accidental disconnection leading to hemorrhage, no possibility of air embolism, and sepsis is very unlikely. The peritoneal membrane certainly can become infected, but bacteremia is rare in PD peritonitis. A urea clearance of 40 ml/min for 8 h in a 70-kg patient would generate a Kt/V of 0.5. Five nights of CFPD would produce a weekly Kt/V of 2.5, comfortably above the current DOQI recommendations. Besides higher clearances, CFPD has clear advantages over standard CAPD or APD: Use of bicarbonate buffer; minimal peritoneal exposure to glucose degradation products and advanced glycation end products; minimal protein loss, and a completely dry abdomen during the day [24].

Treatment of Acute Kidney Injury

With enhanced solute clearance, CFPD becomes an attractive alternative for the ICU treatment of ARF. In patients in which anticoagulation is problematic, patients who do not tolerate hemodialysis because of hemodynamic instability, patients with ARF associated with acute pancreatitis, CFPD could be useful. We reported a hemodialysis patient with venous catheter associated *Pseudomonas* sepsis who underwent CFPD in the ICU over 2 days when blood access was unavailable [25]. He already had two PD catheters in place that were being used

Table 1. ICU CFPD data

	BUN, mg/dl	Creatinine, mg/dl	CO_2, mmol/l	K, mmol/l	Ca, mg/dl	Phosphate, mg/dl	Mg, mg/dl
Treatment 1							
Before	50	5.2	23	5	8.6	7.1	2.2
After	36	4.2	22	4.4	8.2	4.7	1.9
Treatment 2							
Before	54	7.1	19	4.6	8.0	5.8	1.9
After	39	4.8	18	4.7	8.2	4.5	1.9
Kinetics		Kt/V (Daugirdas)		Ku, ml/min			
Treatment 1		0.46		25			
Treatment 2		0.39		20			

for ascites ultrafiltration (see below). Two treatments of 12 h each were performed using the Fresenius 2008H in CRRT mode, 2 liters of 1.5% (hydrous) dextrose intraperitoneal solution recirculated at 250 ml/min through an F40 dialyzer, bathed in a 2.5 mEq/l Ca, 4.0 mEq/l K external dialysate at 300 ml/min. Kt/V for these sessions averaged 0.43, which corresponded to a urea clearance of only about 23 ml/min (table 1). The dialyzer had become clogged with fibrin after an unknown time, which limited clearance. This patient developed Pseudomonas peritonitis, seeded from the blood, and had the PD catheters removed. He eventually returned to hemodialysis with another venous catheter.

We have had two experiences treating acute kidney injury (AKI) with CFPD [26]. Both patients developed AKI in hospital and were in the ICU, though one was stable enough to be transported to the inpatient dialysis unit for treatment. Both had considerable ascites, which facilitated catheter insertion and ultrafiltration. Both had pigtail catheters inserted percutaneously in opposing lower abdominal quadrants by ICU physicians. We used the Fresenius 2008H in CRRT mode and an F-80 polysulfone hollow fiber artificial kidney.

Patient 1 was a 66-year-old woman with AKI in the setting of a thyroid storm, multidrug resistant sepsis, anasarca, ascites, severe hypoalbuminemia, and marked hemodynamic instability. She was unable to tolerate an ultrafiltration of 100 ml/h via slow hemodialysis. She underwent two CFPD treatments with a Qp of 200 ml/min, Qd 100–300 ml/min and UFR of 50–200 ml/h. In the first treatment 3.6 liters were removed in 24 h. The BUN decreased from 54 to 22 mg/dl for a urea reduction ratio of 59%. Applying the Daugirdas equation yielded a Kt/V of 1.11 and a urea clearance (V = 40 liters) of 31 ml/min. The procedures were well tolerated, but she developed peritonitis and the catheters were removed. She expired about a month later, with no further attempts at renal replacement.

Patient 2, a 65-year-old man with cirrhosis developed AKI, likely from drug-induced allergic interstitial nephritis. He presented with oliguria, severe ascites and peripheral edema, and was refractory to diuretics. He underwent 3 consecutive days of CFPD for 5–8 h/day via percutaneous pigtail catheters placed in the ICU. Qp was 250–300 ml/min, Qd 500 ml/min, and the UFR was 400–500 ml/h. Over 10 kg of fluid was removed over 3 days by ultrafiltration of his ascites. He was hemodynamically stable throughout. Urea clearance averaged 50 ml/min (table 2) and BUN and creatinine declined with each treatment (fig. 3). The catheters were removed after 3 days. His renal function

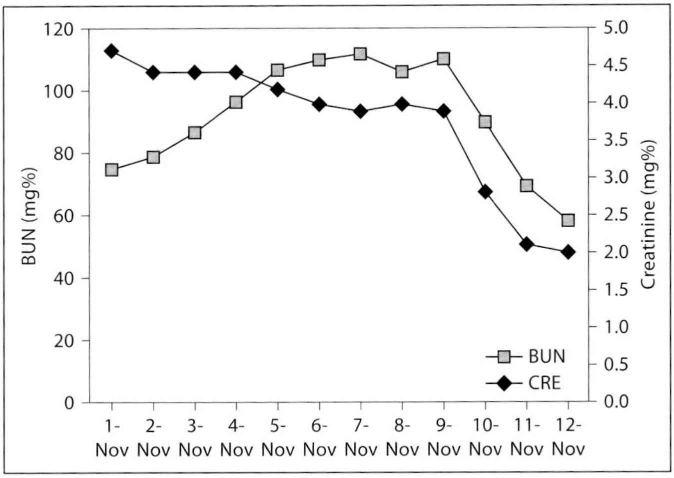

Fig. 3. Evolution of BUN and creatinine in patient 2 (AKI) with 3 consecutive days of treatment with CFPD.

Table 2. Summary of 3 CFPD treatments on patient 2

Date	UF volume, liters	URR, %	kt/V	V, ml	Rx time, min	Ku, ml/min
Nov. 9	2	18	0.26	72,000	354	52.88
Nov. 10	3.7	23	0.35	70,000	485	50.52
Nov. 11	4.4	18	0.29	68,000	400	49.30

Kt/V calculated from pre-/post-BUN by the Daugirdas equation. Average urea clearance was 50 ml/min.

recovered and he was transferred to another institution for liver transplantation.

CFPD has been used successfully in pediatric anasarca and AKI. Sagy reported the use of CFPD in 6 pediatric cases of ARDS with anasarca [27]. They used percutaneously inserted Tenckhoff catheters and 2.5% dextrose dialysate in single pass CFPD. All patients had significant improvement in their respiratory status, though 2 of the 6 died.

More recently, Raaijmakers et al. [28] reported using CFPD in a single-pass mode in 6 pediatric patients with AKI. Patients were treated with both CFPD and conventional PD for 8–16 h. CFPD was performed with two catheters inserted at the bedside.

After initial filling, dialysate flow rate (100 ml/1.73 m^2/min) was maintained with an adapted continuous venovenous hemofiltration machine. Ultrafiltration flow rate was set at 2.5 ml/1.73 m^2/min. Mean ultrafiltration was 0.20 ml/1.73 m^2/min with conventional PD vs. 1.8 ml/1.73 m^2/min with CFPD. Mean clearances of urea and creatinine were 5.0 and 7.6 ml/1.73 m^2/min with conventional PD vs. 15.0 and 28.8 ml/1.73 m^2/min with CFPD, respectively. No complications occurred.

Treatment of Dialysis Ascites

Dialysis ascites is a not infrequent complication of chronic hemodialysis. It may be associated with cirrhosis, heart failure, or previous peritoneal

Table 3. Results, patient 1 (CFPD of ascites)

	0 min	30 min	60 min	90 min	120 min	URR, %	Kt/V	Ku, ml/min
BUN, mg%	52.3	53	50	49.7	46.9	12.50	0.18	48
Creatinine, mg%	7.5	7.6	7.8	7.9	7.8			

Table 4. Treatment data for patient 2 (CFPD of ascites)

Filter	Pre-weight	Post-weight	Weight loss, kg	Pre-BUN	Post-BUN	URR, %	kt/V	Ku, ml/min	Qp, ml/min	Qd, ml/min
AV400	101	93	8	56	47	16.1	0.3	73.5	260	300
F70	104.1	98.4	5.5	65	61	6.1	0.14	34.3	300	300
F70	101.9	95.6	6.3	75	53	29.3	0.49	120	300	300
F70	99.6	93.5	6.1	66	59	10.6	0.2	49	300	500
AV400	96.3	89.8	6.5	54	46	14.8	0.27	66.2	300	500
Average	100.58	94.06	6.48	63.2	53.2	15.38	0.28	68.6		

dialysis. Treatment is problematic and usually consists of repeated paracentesis. This results in ongoing protein loss and malnutrition. We treated three hemodialysis patients with refractory ascites with CFPD [29]. Two patients had two Cruz PD catheters placed, with the coiled section in the pelvis. The third patient had a Cruz catheter placed in the usual position, and a standard Tenckhoff catheter inserted with the coiled portion in the upper abdomen (see below, patient 2). Treatments were from 2 to 4 h, with ultrafiltration of approximately 1 liter/h. Ascitic fluid was heparinized with 2,000 units of heparin and pumped at 200–300 ml/min through a hemofilter, typically the Fresenius F70. External dialysate flow rate was 300–500 ml/min. Dialysate calcium was 2.5 mEq/l, and the K was from 2–4 mEq/l. Blood and ascitic fluid chemistries were sampled and the patient was weighed before and after each session. Solute clearances were derived from these measurements using the Daugirdas equation. The patients underwent a total of 9 treatments. Data are presented in tables 3–6.

Patient 1 was a 67-year-old man with diabetes, coronary artery disease, peripheral vascular disease and dialysis ascites. He was receiving thrice-weekly hemodialysis treatments using a Permcath, due to multi-access failure. He had idiopathic dialysis ascites for which he would have paracentesis every 4–6 weeks.

The 12.5% urea reduction is equivalent to a Kt/V of 0.18. With V of approximately 32 liters, the urea clearance is 48 ml/min for this treatment.

BUN was measured every 30 min in patient 1 (fig. 4). There was no change over the first 30 min. This is because the external dialyzer must first reduce the ascitic fluid urea level before any significant transperitoneal urea transport can be established. The time required will vary with the volume of ascites and the efficiency of the extracorporeal circuit. Based on serial measurements of ascitic fluid urea nitrogen in another patient, this requires at least 60 min (fig. 5).

This is significant because in a pure CFPD, with sterile, urea-free dialysate being used rather than ascites, a higher rate of urea removal will begin immediately. Urea reduction and clearance numbers will be correspondingly higher. For example, if we recalculate the urea clearance for patient 1 using 90 min rather than 120 min of dialysis, the clearance jumps from 48 to 64 ml/min.

Table 5. Changes in ascites composition in patient 2 after 4 h of CFPD/UF of ascites

Date	Pre-ascites TP	Post-TP	Pre-UN	Post-UN	Pre-creatinine	Post-creatinine	UF volume
Nov. 23	3.4	7.3	53	16	7.8	2	3,968
Jan. 8	2.8	6.9	77	21	8.3	1.8	4,019
Jan. 21	3.3	11.2	74	19	9.1	2.2	4,897
Average	3.17	8.47	67.50	17.25	8.30	1.83	4,160

Table 6. Small solute reduction in patient 2

Treatment no.	URR, %	Creatinine RR, %	Phosphate RR, %	K RR, %	Dialysate K, mmol/l
1	16	7		8	4
2	6	6		6	4
3	29	32	26	28	2
4	11	14	9	4	2
5	15	16	14	12	3
Average	15.4	15	16.33	11.6	

Patient 1 had only one session of CFPD for ascites removal. He was then hospitalized with Permcath sepsis as described above.

Patient 2 was a 60-year-old man with ESRD from diabetes, and congestive heart failure secondary to valvular heart disease. He had peritoneal catheters implanted in a one-up, one-down configuration (fig. 6). He underwent five 4-hour sessions of CFPD over a 2-month period. Treatments were performed in the hospital in-patient dialysis unit, on an ambulatory basis. Previously, he had been admitted every few weeks in congestive heart failure for emergency hemodialysis and paracentesis.

Below (tables 5, 6) are pre-/post-ascites chemistries and reduction ratios (RR) for other small solutes. The ascitic protein becomes concentrated by ultrafiltration of water. This undoubtedly creates a driving force for transperitoneal ultrafiltration.

Patient 2 developed resistant *Staphylococcus aureus* peritonitis following an episode of venous catheter sepsis. The catheters were removed and he continued on hemodialysis, with regular admissions for paracentesis.

Patient 3 was a 76-year-old man with ESRD from diabetes mellitus and cirrhosis. He had refractory ascites, and required weekly paracentesis. There was pericatheter leakage of ascites for a week postoperatively due to rapid ascites reaccumulation. This was resolved by draining the abdomen every 6 h for 2 days. This patient underwent three CFPD treatments. Unfortunately, his first treatment was performed after a considerable amount of ascites had been drained, and there were frequent alarms due to low flow in the peritoneal circuit. There was also some discomfort to the patient, and he became reluctant to have further treatments. He preferred to have fluid drained during hemodialysis. He became cachectic and agreed to two more CFPD treatments. Results are shown below (table 7).

Patient 3 had a bout of peritonitis that resolved with antibiotics. He failed to thrive due to advanced liver failure and elected to discontinue dialysis.

Wearable Artificial Kidney

We are developing a wearable device using CFPD concepts [30]. This provides a significant

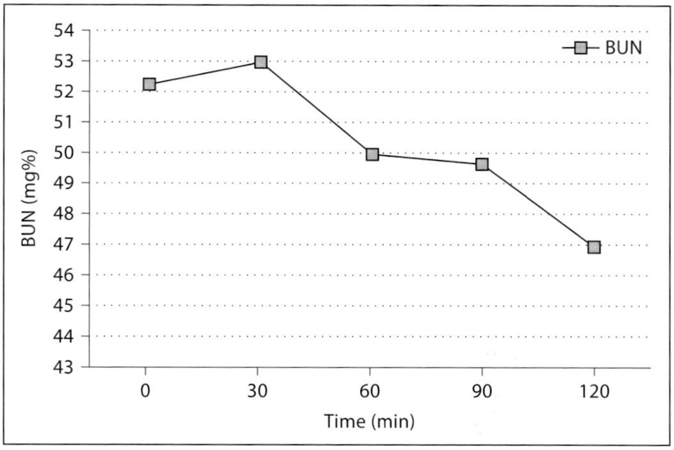

Fig. 4. BUN reduction during 2 h CFPD of ascites in patient 1.

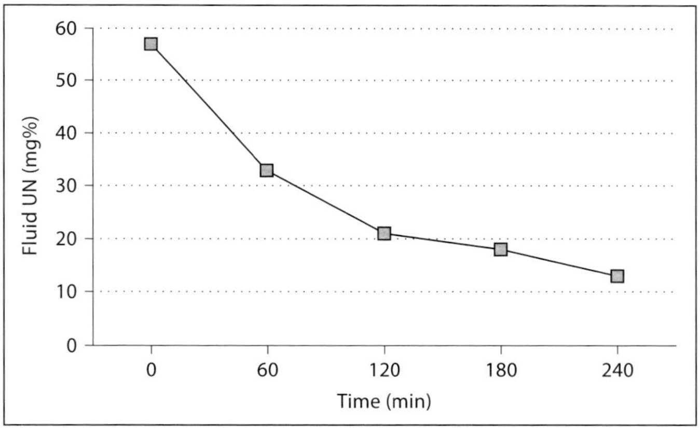

Fig. 5. Decline in ascites UN over 4 h in patient 2.

advantage over blood-based wearable systems in the lack of need for prolonged anticoagulation, among others. The system consists of: (1) a double lumen peritoneal catheter, (2) a dialysate outflow line, (3) a miniaturized rotary pump, (4) a circuit for dialysate regeneration featuring a waterproof container with 4 cartridges in parallel with a mixture of activated carbon and polystyrenic resins, (5) a filter for deaeration and microbiological safety, (6) a dialysate inflow line, and (7) a handheld computer as a remote control. The system is designed as a simple mechanical aid to perform CAPD. A typical schedule could be summarized as follows:

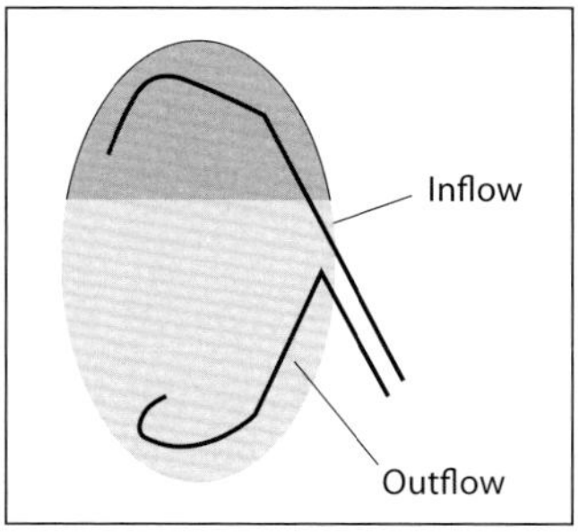

Fig. 6. Catheter configuration in patient 2 (CFPD ascites).

Table 7. Results for 3 CFPD of ascites in patient 3: bottom row is the mean

Pre-TX WT	Post-TX WT	Delta WT	UF volume	Pre-BUN	Post-BUN	URR, %	kt/V	Ku, ml/min	Filter
81.5	76.6	4.9	3,700	41	38	7	0.15	30.6	F70
83.5	81.5	2	3,850	59	46	22	0.35	71.5	F70
82.4	74.5	7.9	4,600	73	67	8	0.2	40	F70
82.5	77.5	4.9	4,050	57.7	50.3	12.5	0.2	47.4	

the peritoneal cavity is loaded in the morning with 2 liters of fresh PD solution. After approximately 2 h, when 50% dialysate/plasma equilibration has occurred, recirculation is activated for 10 h at a rate of 20 ml/min (range between 15 and 30). After this period, recirculation stops and a complete equilibration is obtained in the remaining indwelling solution. Glucose could be optionally added to the peritoneal cavity to achieve ultrafiltration if needed through a line connected to a small reservoir placed on the belt. The patient via handheld computer can activate this function. After 2 h, the fluid is drained and a 2-liter icodextrin exchange is performed overnight to achieve further ultrafiltration. Assuming a daily clearance of 12 liters obtained by the minicycler, as demonstrated by the experimental findings, an additional clearance of 4–5 liters can therefore be provided by the equilibrated solution drained in the evening and by the overnight exchange. Such efficiency should provide a weekly creatinine clearance 100 liters/week and may represent an important treatment for larger patients unable to meet the adequacy targets.

Discussion

Assuming the access and ultrafiltration problems are solved technically, the combination of high clearance and less risk should make CFPD highly competitive as a choice for home dialysis. Online manufacture of external dialysate from purified water will minimize the expense of sterile prepared solutions in bags. Glucose concentrations will be created and maintained by the external dialysate; levels at or under 1% should be adequate for ultrafiltration in most patients. Bicarbonate will be the buffer, also generated externally, resulting in a more physiologic environment for the peritoneal membrane. Daytime exchanges will be unnecessary, and 5–6 treatments per week of 5–8 h should provide adequate Kt/V in most patients.

CFPD should be considered in patients with AKI, especially when blood access is difficult. Two PD catheters can readily be implanted at the bedside, either surgically or laparoscopically. It should also be considered in children, where single pass mode is efficient and economical.

CFPD is effective in dialysis ascites. Given the propensity for secondary infection of the peritoneal catheter from blood-borne bacteria, we recommend confining this to patients with an A-V fistulae or using it as the primary modality. The progressive concentration of protein in the ascitic fluid as water is removed causes transperitoneal ultrafiltration. This is helpful in edematous patients, but nonedematous patients may become volume depleted and require intravenous saline for support.

CFPD is a rational basis for a wearable artificial kidney and is currently in development.

References

1 Blake PG, Bloembergen WE, Fenton SS: Changes in the demographics and prescription of peritoneal dialysis during the last decade. Am J Kidney Dis 1998;32(suppl 4):S44–S51.
2 McDonald SP, Collins JF, Johnson DW: Obesity is associated with worse peritoneal dialysis outcomes in the Australia and New Zealand patient populations. J Am Soc Nephrol 2003;14:2894–901.
3 Nolph KD, Twardowski ZJ: The peritoneal dialysis system; in Nolph KD (ed.): Peritoneal Dialysis, ed 3. Amsterdam, Kluwer Academic Publishers, 1989, pp 13–27.
4 Amerling R, Ronco C, Levin NW: Continuous-flow peritoneal dialysis. Perit Dial Int 2000; 20(suppl 2):S172–S177.
5 Shinaberger JH, Shear L, Barry KG: Peritoneal-extracorporeal recirculation dialysis. A technique for improving efficiency of peritoneal dialysis. Investigative Urology 1965;2:555–565.
6 Lange K, Treser G, Mangalat J: Automatic continuous high flow rate peritoneal dialysis. Arch Klin Med 1968;214:201–206.
7 Stephen RL, Atkin-Thor E, Kolff WJ: Recirculating peritoneal dialysis with subcutaneous catheter. Trans Am Soc Artif Int Organs 1976;22:575–585.
8 Raja RM, Kramer MS, Rosenbaum JL: Recirculation peritoneal dialysis with sorbent Redy cartridge. Nephron 1976;16:134–142.
9 Gordon A, Lewin AJ, Maxwell MH, Morales ND: Augmentation of efficiency by continuous flow sorbent regeneration peritoneal dialysis. Trans Am Soc Aftif Int Organs 1976;22:599–604.
10 Warden GD, Maxwell G, Stephen RL: The use of reciprocation peritoneal dialysis with a subcutaneous peritoneal catheter in end-stage renal failure in diabetes mellitus. J Surg Res 1978;24:495–500.
11 Kablitz C, Stephen RL, Jacoblsen SC, et al: Reciprocating peritoneal dialysis. Dial Transplant 1978;7:211–214.
12 Kraus MA, Shasha SM, Nemas M, Better OS, Khoushy A: Ultrafiltration peritoneal dialysis and recirculating peritoneal dialysis with a portable kidney. Dial Trans 1983;12:385–388.
13 Amerling R, DeSimone L, Inciong-Reyes R, Pangilinan A, Folden T, Ronco C, Gotch FA, Levin N: Clinical experience with continuous flow and flow-through peritoneal dialysis. Semin Dial 2001;14:388–390.
14 Mineshima M, Watanuki M, Yamagat K, et al: Development of continuous recirculation peritoneal dialysis using a double lumen catheter. ASAIO J 1992;38:M377–381.
15 Cruz C, Melendez A, Gotch FA, Folden T, Crawford TL, Diaz-Buxo JA: Single-pass continuous flow peritoneal dialysis using two catheters. Semin Dial 2001;14:391–394.
16 Ash SR, Janle EM: Continuous flow-through peritoneal dialysis (CFPD): comparison of efficiency to IPD, TPD and CAPD in an animal model. Perit Dial Int 1997;17:365–372.
17 Gotch FA: Kinetic modeling of continuous flow peritoneal dialysis. Semin Dial 2001;14:378–383.
18 Amerling R: Treatment of dialysis ascites by continuous flow peritoneal diafiltration, two catheters and the Fresenius 2008H. Perit Dial Int 2002;22(suppl 1):S33.
19 Diaz-Buxo JA: Streaming, mixing, and recirculation: role of the peritoneal access in continuous flow peritoneal dialysis (clinical considerations). Adv Perit Dial 2002;18:87–90.
20 McKee JS, Marchand JR, DeLeo M, Rudell S: Solute clearance during continuous flow PD (CFPD): one vs. two catheters. Perit Dial Int 2001;21(suppl 1):S35.
21 Mineshima M, Suzuki S, Sato Y, et al: Solute removal characteristics of continuous recirculation peritoneal dialysis in experimental and clinical studies. ASAIO J 2000;46:95–98.
22 Ronco C, Gloukhoff A, Dell'Aquila R, Levin NW: Catheter design for continuous flow peritoneal dialysis. Blood Purif 2002;20:40–44.
23 Ronco C, Levin NW, D'Acquila R, Sergeyeva O: New dual lumen catheter with diffuser for continuous flow peritoneal dialysis. J Am Soc Nephrol 2002;13:1A.
24 Passlick-Deetjen J, Lage C, Jorres A: Continuous flow peritoneal dialysis: solution formulation and biocompatibility. Semin Dial 2001;14:384–387.
25 Amerling R, Savransky E: Continuous flow peritoneal dialysis (CFPD) in the ICU: case report. Blood Purif 2002;20:320.
26 Amerling R, Merouani A: Continuous-flow peritoneal dialysis as acute therapy; in Ronco C, Bellomo R, Kellum JA (eds): Critical Care Nephrology, ed 2. New York, Elsevier, 2009, pp 1509–1515.
27 Sagy M, Silver P: Continuous flow peritoneal dialysis as a method to treat severe anasarca in children with acute respiratory distress syndrome. Crit Care Med 1999;27:2532–2536.
28 Raaijmakers R, Schröder CH, Gajjar P, Argent A, Nourse P: Continuous flow peritoneal dialysis: first experience in children with acute renal failure. Clin J Am Soc Nephrol 2011;6:311–318.
29 Amerling R, Glezerman I, Savransky E, Dubrow A: Enhanced small solute clearance during continuous flow peritoneal dialysis (CFPD) using two catheters. J Am Soc Nephrol 2002;13:1A.
30 Ronco C, Fecondini L: The Vicenza wearable artificial kidney for peritoneal dialysis (ViWAK PD). Blood Purif 2007;25:383–388.

Prof. Richard Amerling
Beth Israel Medical Center
350 East 17th Street
New York, NY 10003 (USA)
Tel. +1 212 420 4070, E-Mail ramerlin@chpnet.org

Ronco C, Rosner MH, Crepaldi C (eds): Peritoneal Dialysis – State-of-the-Art 2012.
Contrib Nephrol. Basel, Karger, 2012, vol 178, pp 216–220

Combination Therapy: Five Days PD and One Day HD – What Are the Benefits?

John Burkart

Wake Forest University Medical Center, Winston Salem, N.C., and Health Systems Management, Tifton, Ga., USA

Abstract

Other than renal transplantation, the two major treatment options for patients with stage V kidney disease are hemodialysis and peritoneal dialysis. Both therapies have advantages and disadvantages while there are obvious physical differences in the way they are delivered. In clinical practice, one typically uses one therapy at a time in patients. However, there are medical and patient lifestyle reasons why you may want to use both on a weekly basis. Early clinical experience with this approach has been encouraging. With emerging data suggesting that more frequent hemodialysis or slower ultrafiltration rates may be beneficial for the patient there are now even more compelling reasons to consider this approach. This paper reviews the published literature on combined modality therapy and suggests reasons why we may want to utilize combination therapy more often.

In health, the kidneys remove retained solutes and excess fluids while maintaining electrolyte balance 24 h a day, 7 days a week. Patients with stage V chronic kidney disease on dialysis typically receive replacement renal therapy that no way approximates solute clearance rates that one experiences in health. For instance, a typical standardized Kt/V_{urea} for three times a week center hemodialysis (CHD) patients is 2.1 while the minimal Kt/V_{urea} for a typical peritoneal dialysis (PD) patient is at least 1.7/week. Both are markedly different than the weekly Kt/V_{urea} of about 25.2 for patients with normal kidney function (say a urea clearance of 100 ml/min) and a volume of distribution for urea of 40 liters, a value at least 10 times as high! Similarly, when it comes to volume homeostasis, in health, excessive fluid intake is often eliminated within hours and weight varies little from day to day. Whereas we recognize that it is not uncommon to see a CHD patient who gains 5–7 kg between treatments or a PD patient who is volume overloaded. Despite these obvious differences in solute and fluid removal between health and patients on dialysis, dialysis patients often do very well. But, do they all do well and of those that 'do well' could they do even better? Despite over 33 years of experience with renal replacement therapies, our patients still experience a high mortality rate, most of it cardiovascular related. Is this due to failure of our current therapies or a failure in how the renal replacement community delivers these therapies?

Both PD and hemodialysis (HD) therapies have their individual advantages and disadvantages, some of which overlap and some of which are divergent. HD allows for intermittent bouts of highly efficient solute removal, while PD allows for slow continuous ultrafiltration but has less vigorous rates of solute removal. We typically utilize one modality at a time in a patient. We occasionally use both modalities as a patient 'transitions' from one therapy to another, but in these cases, usually for only a very short time. However, there really are no rules or medical contraindications for chronically using both modalities in an individual patient. In fact there may be some advantages. Our major hesitancy to using combined therapy usually has to do with – Will we get paid to do that? Don't you now have two accesses that can both have complications? And, Will the patient really do that? In fact, the answer to those questions seems to be YES/Yes, but-/Sometimes.

Experience with Combined Dialysis

Dr. Kawanishi published the first report on 12 patients treated with combination therapy in 1999 stating that it was one of the simplest ways to maintain adequacy of continuous ambulatory peritoneal dialysis (CAPD) [1]. This report was followed by a review of quality of life reporting on 6 Japanese patients [2] and a retrospective observational trial of Japanese patients treated with this approach over a 5-year period [3]. The first non-Japanese experience was an observational cohort study and a multicenter survey on 31 patients who were placed on combined therapies for various medical problems [4]. Those authors stated that in general the patient's signs or symptoms that the combined modality was used for improved with the intervention. These were followed by multiple cohort observational studies mainly from Japan that have further defined the therapy, describing how to calculate dialysis dose (Kt/V_{urea}), and the effect of the therapy on clinical outcomes such as LVH [5–10]. Along the way, other terms were used to describe this approach – including bimodal [11] therapy (8 incident patients) and complimentary therapy [12]. In a recent survey of dialysis patients and dialysis centers in Japan, approximately 20% were on combined (complimentary) therapy, most on PD 5 days a week and HD once a week [13].

Reported Indications for Combined Modality Approach

Suggested indications for considering use of combined modalities include but are not limited to the medical conditions listed below. These have not been proven in prospective randomized clinical trials. However, in selected reports, individual patients or cohorts of patients have reported these benefits.

Suggested Indications When One Should Consider Use of Combination Therapy

For patients currently on PD:

1 Patients who need an increase in their PD dose that would result in a prescription that is too difficult to do or incompatible with the patient's lifestyle.
2 Patients who are unable to maintain euvolemia due to UF failure or reluctance by the center to use hypertonic glucose solutions.
3 Medical reasons which limit the ability to do PD:
decreased PD capacity, hernia, hydrothorax.
4 Inability to do daily PD therapy.
5 Minimizing glucose expose and potentially preventing peritoneal membrane damage.

For patients on HD:

1 Prevention of complications of intermittent HD (minimize loss of RKF, prevent hypotension and cardiac stunning).
2 Cardiovascular instability due to valvular heart disease or CHF.
3 Patients needing daily ultrafiltration who do not want to switch to PD alone because of the desire not to use cycler therapy or perform multiple daytime PD exchanges.

For all patients:

1 Supplemental treatment (adding the second modality) to patients on single therapy (PD or HD) who had done well but are now failing to thrive and have residual syndrome.

Reported Benefits of Combined Modality Approach

In early studies, reports suggested that use of this approach made it easier to achieve minimal adequacy targets without having a PD prescription that was too burdensome for the patient [1]. Subsequent reports suggested that in selected patients who had manifestations of uremia not treated well by a 'full' dose of PD alone, that adding supplemental weekly CHD treatments generally resulted in a self-reported improvement in that sign or symptom for that patient [2, 4]. More recent observational studies have examined other issues.

In an observational cohort study (n = 6) Fukui et al. [5] evaluated QOL and found an overall improvement in scores (124.2 ± 26.1 vs. 141.7 ± 20.1; $p = 0.0025$). In another cohort study of nondiabetic patients who had been on PD at least 2 years and were less than 50 years old, Kawanishi et al. [6] reported that there was a better technique survival ($p < 0.02$) for patients on combination therapy (n = 32) compared to those on PD alone (n = 48). They also reported an improvement in anorexia, edema and restless legs while also showing an improvement in blood pressure and a lowering of serum β_2-microglobulin levels [6, 7]. This improvement in serum β_2-microglobulin levels was also seen at 1 year of follow-up in a retrospective observational cohort study of 53 patients with declining residual kidney function who were placed on combination therapy because of overhydration and or underdialysis [8]. These authors also demonstrated a reduction in number of antihypertensive medications used. There are other potential cardiovascular benefits to combined therapy. McIntyre et al. [11] reported a reduction in use of antihypertensive medications and an improvement in left ventricular mass index (LVMI) as did Tanaka et al. [9]. Finally, one report suggested that the monthly costs for combination therapy in Japan (5 days of PD and 1 day of CHD/week) was the least expensive therapy (CAPD USD 3,346, HD USD 2,833, APD USD 4,649 and combined therapy USD 2,769) [7].

Although not well investigated, it is possible that the daily ability to remove excess fluid (the continuous slow ultrafiltration associated with PD) may prevent the need to have large UF volumes during a short HD session and therefore avoid potential hypotensive episodes and resultant cardiac stunning [14] with its associated increased relative risk of death. A regimen of once or twice a week standard HD with 4–6 days of PD/week should avoid these needs for excessive ultrafiltration rates during a HD treatment because of the subsequent daily fluid removal by PD while maintaining optimal solute removal. At present there are no data to confirm this.

In Japan there tends to be a reluctance to use hypertonic glucose solutions, in part due to the fear that in the long term this will lead to peritoneal membrane damage [15] and encapsulating peritoneal sclerosis (EPS). As a result, one approach to maintain euvolemia and minimize glucose exposure is to do one or two HD treatments/week during which one can ultrafiltrate any accumulated fluid without exposing patient and peritoneal membrane to excessive amounts of glucose or glucose degradation products (GDPs). Data on whether or not this does in fact 'protect' the peritoneal membrane remains controversial.

Possible Complications

When using both therapies one must have two accesses – A PD catheter and a HD access. The concern is that there will be twice as many access related complications. The observational cohort studies did not examine these potential complications very well. In general, peritonitis rates were similar when on combined therapy to those reported for PD alone. Unfortunately, there are little data on HD-related access complication rates. In our experience, when the patient had an access complication related to one therapy (fistula clotting, revision, or need to replace PD catheter due to unresolving peritonitis), it was relatively easier to take care of that complication because one could just use the other access and do the other therapy until the access complication resolved. There was no need for a temporary access. Furthermore, in general, most patients who did combined therapy were already on PD. The PD catheter is generally a problem free access. If patients were to just transition to HD, unless the reason for transition was an episode of peritonitis that would not resolve and catheter removal was needed, patients would typically have a functioning PD catheter that was removed. When transitioning to HD you would add a new HD access. In these cases, you just add the HD catheter and keep the PD catheter.

Possible Regimens

Many possible regimens exist for combination therapy. The most common is one using 5 or 6 days/week of PD and one HD treatment/week. Occasionally one may have to use 2 HD treatments/week and 4 or 5 days/week of PD. There are many possible variations and which one was used would depend on if one is trying to treat an incident patient or a patient with long standing ESRD and minimal residual kidney function. It would depend on the patient and the clinical sign or symptom one is trying to improve as to what frequency of HD or PD one would choose. However, another situation where you may want to consider a combination therapy is in the long-term patient who is on a single therapy and is meeting current minimal adequacy targets and minimal ultrafiltration rates yet is still failing to thrive and just not doing well.

Recent prospective randomized trials [16, 17] and multiple observational reports have suggested that there is an advantage to frequent hemodialysis therapies (most reports were on patients dialyzing for 6 sessions/week). Despite these reported benefits, just over 1% of the dialysis population in the United States utilizes this form of HD. The reasons for this are multifactorial but one of them is just the burden it would place on the patient who may or may not have a partner or suitable home to do daily home dialysis. An option for these patients to consider would be the addition of PD to the three times a week center HD therapy. Patients could do 1 or 2 PD dwells on non-HD days or a daily overnight PD dwell. Solutions with a prolonged UF profile such as Icodextrin would be ideal in this case. By doing 3/week HD and additional PD on off days, one could have daily UF and solute removal that would be greater than what one typically achieves in short daily HD and approaching that of the shorter nocturnal regimens.

Conclusions

The combination of PD and HD therapies in a single patient is doable and in fact complementary in many ways. One can optimize the benefits of each therapy while minimizing their potential downsides. Multiple observational cohort studies have shown that it is feasible to do this and there seems to be some potential benefits for patients. Certainly one can augment solute removal over that often possible with one therapy alone and one could likely better maintain euvolemia on a day-to-day basis. More data are needed to confirm the validity of this approach as a recommended therapy for all. However, when caring for the individual patient, in certain instances, it appears as if this would be a safe and perhaps beneficial approach that needs to continue to be considered.

Disclosure Statement

J.B. is an ad hoc consultant for Baxter healthcare and serves on the medical advisory board for NxStage Renal.

References

1 Kawanishi H, Moriishi M, Katsutani S, Sakikubo E, Tsuchiya S: Hemodialysis together with peritoneal dialysis is one of the simpilest ways to maintain adequacy in continuous ambulatory peritoneal dialysis. Adv Perit Dial 1999;15:1270131.

2 Hashimoto Y, Matsubara T: Combined PD and HD therapy improves QOL in ESRD patients. Adv Perit Dial 2000;16:108–112.

3 Kawanishi H, Moriishi M, Tsuchiya S: Five years' experience of combination therapy: PD and HD. Adv Perit Dial 2002;18:62–67.

4 Agarwal M, Clinard P, Burkart J: Combined peritoneal dialysis and hemodialysis: Our experience compared to others. Perit Dial Int 2003;23:157–161.

5 Fukui H, Hara S, Hashimoto Y, et al: Review of combination peritoneal dialysis and hemodialysis as a modality treatment for end stage renal diseases. Ther Apheresis Dial 2004;86:56–61.

6 Kawanishi H, Moriishi M: Clinical effects of combined therapy with peritoneal dialuysis and hemodialysis. Perit Dial Int 2007;27(S2):S126–S129.

7 Kawanishi H, Hashimoto Y, Nakamoto H, Nakayama M, Tranaeus A: Combination therapy with peritoneal dialysis and hemodialysis. Perit Dial Int 2006;26:150–154.

8 Matsuo N, Yokoyama K, Maruyama Y, Ueda Y, Yoshida H, Tanno Y, Yamamoto R, Terawaki H, Ikeda M, Hanaoka K, Yamamoto H, Ogura M, Watanabe S, Kimura Y, Hosoya T: Clinical impact of a combined therapy of peritoneal dialysis and hemodialysis. Clin Nephrol 2010;74:209–216.

9 Tanaka M, Mise N, Nakajima H, Uchida L, Ishimoto Y, Kotera N, Tanaka S, Kurita N, Sugimoto T: Effects of combination therapy with peritoneal dialysis and hemodialysis on LVH. Perit Dial Int 2011;31:598–600.

10 Hoshi H, Nakamoto H, Kanno Y, Takane H, Ikeda N, Sugahara S, Okada H, Suzuki H: Long-term follow-up of patients treated with a combination of continuous ambulatory peritoneal dialysis and hemodialysis. Adv Perit Dial 2006;22:136–140.

11 McIntyre CW: Bi-modal dialysis (BMD): an integral approach to renal replacement therapy. Perit Dial Int 2004;24:547–553.

12 Kawanishi H, McIntyre C: Complementary use of peritoneal and hemodialysis. Therapeutic synergies in the treatment of end stage renal failure patients. Kidney Int Suppl 2008;108:S63–S67.

13 Survey JSDT 2011.

14 McIntyre CW, Burton JO, Selby NJ, et al: Hemodialysis induced effects on myocardial blood flow. Clin J Am Soc Nephrol 2008;3:19–26.

15 Davies SJ, Phillips L, Naish PF, Russell GI: Peritoneal glucose exposure and changes in peritoneal membrane solute transport with time on dialysis. J Am Soc Nephrol 2001;12:1046–1051.

16 Cullerton BF, Walsh M, Klarenbach SW, et al: Effect or frequent nocturnal hemodialysis vs conventional hemodialysis on left ventricular mass and quality of life. A randomized controlled trial. JAMA 2007;298:1291–1299.

17 FHN Trials Group: In-center hemodialysis six times a week versus three times a week. N Engl J Med 2010;363:2287–2300.

John Burkart, MD
Professor of Medicine/Nephrology, Wake Forest University Medical Center
Medical Center Blvd.
Winston Salem, NC 27157–1053 (USA)
Tel. +1 336 716 3963, E-Mail jburkart@wfubmc.edu

Ronco C, Rosner MH, Crepaldi C (eds): Peritoneal Dialysis – State-of-the-Art 2012.
Contrib Nephrol. Basel, Karger, 2012, vol 178, pp 221–227

Peritoneal Dialysis Access: What's the Best Approach?

Miguel C. Riella[a] · Domingos C. Chula[b]

[a]Department of Medicine, Catholic University of Parana, and [b]Pro-Renal Foundation Brazil, Curitiba, Brazil

Abstract

There are many procedures for placement of an intra-abdominal peritoneal catheter for peritoneal dialysis. Each one has its own advantages and disadvantages. Although the blind technique with a trocar was the initial procedure utilized, over the years interventional nephrologists and surgeons have evolved to more modern techniques that allow more direct visualization of the peritoneal cavity, minimizing complications catheter-related. Novel techniques such as peritoneoscopy and laparoscopy appear to be associated with a reduced number of exit site infections, lower incidence of peritonitis, decreased risk of leakage and improved catheter survival. Since some studies have not seen all these benefits associated with these procedures, one recognizes the importance of the experience obtained with each procedure in every center and the impossibility of generalization.

'The best approach is the one in which the team has the most experience and acceptable results'.

Despite the overall prevalence of hemodialysis (HD) around the world, peritoneal dialysis (PD) is an effective and attractive home modality of renal replacement therapy associated with independence and good quality of life [1–3].

Similar to vascular access for HD, peritoneal access is also the patient's 'life line' since successful PD depends on adequate and sustainable access to the peritoneal cavity [4, 5].

Immediate mechanical complications after catheter insertion may have a negative effect on patient's acceptance of this modality. Management of access is a key factor for the improvement of PD technique survival. It requires the establishment of a dedicated team that should ideally consist of nephrologists, surgeons and nurses. Nowadays, laparoscopists or interventional radiologists may also be part of the team. The preference of one technique over another must take into account the incidence of complications (pericatheter leakage, dislodgment, exit site and tunnel infection) and long-term catheter survival associated with each technique, cost, ease and timely insertion of the catheter, and factors contributing to mortality risk (general anesthesia) [6, 7].

The experience of the team is more important than the type of catheter and the implantation technique used [8].

Peritoneal Dialysis Access Techniques

Techniques for PD catheter insertion include placement by percutaneous guide-wire (performed blindly or with fluoroscopic guidance) [9], open surgical dissection [10],

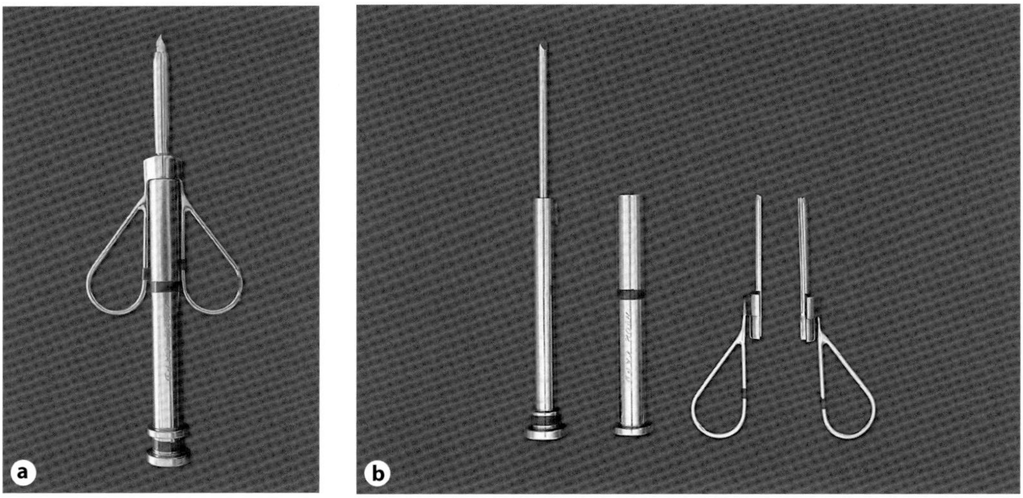

Fig. 1. Tenckhoff trocar for blind placement of peritoneal catheter.

peritoneoscopic and laparoscopic implantation [11–16]. A modified fluoroscopic technique by adding ultrasound-assistance has also been proposed [17].

Percutaneous Insertion

This could be accomplished in two ways: blind insertion using Tenckhoff's trocar (fig. 1) or under fluoroscopy using the Seldinger technique. One should be aware that these techniques are associated with a higher risk of placement failure and bowel perforation in patients with a previous history of major abdominal surgery, gross obesity or suspected intra-abdominal adhesions. However, in selected cases, bedside placement by the nephrologist has outcomes at least comparable with the surgical technique [8, 18].

Blind Percutaneous Insertion with Tenckhoff's Trocar

For the past three decades we have routinely used this technique in our unit due to several reasons: our team is familiar with the procedure and has had good results; there is no dependence on radiology suite availability for fluoroscopic guidance and it is the lowest cost procedure since there is no specific reimbursement for peritoneoscopy or laparoscopic PD catheter insertion.

We have prospectively evaluated over 24 months the outcome of PD catheter insertion in 121 patients under three conditions: blind percutaneously – group P (n = 53), percutaneously under fluoroscopy – group F (n = 26) and surgical implant – group C (n = 42).

Infectious and noninfectious complications were not different among the groups and catheter survival at the end of follow-up was 70% for group P, 85% for group F and 70% for group C (p = 0.95) (fig. 2, 3).

However, one should be aware that positioning the catheter deep cuff in the subcutaneous tissue external to the muscle fascia might be associated more often with catheter mal-position, hernia and leaks [19].

One should be aware, however, that despite being a convenient procedure that can be performed anywhere in the hospital, of low cost, bowel perforation is an occasional complication and no visualization of the peritoneal space is provided. The deep cuff normally is left outside the abdominal musculature unless specific care is taken to bury the cuff into the rectus muscle.

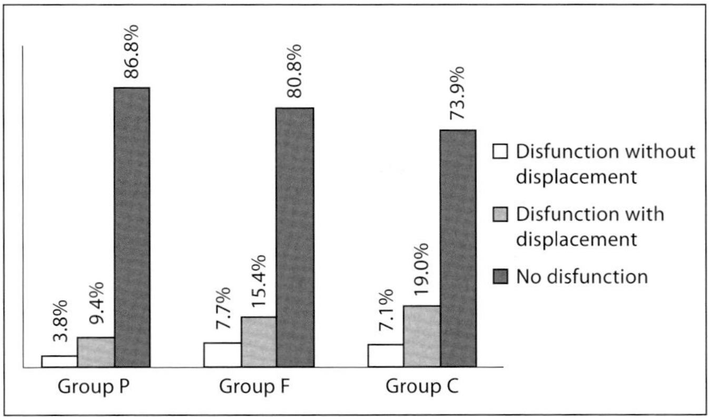

Fig. 2. Displacement or catheter obstruction according to technique employed. Group P = Blind percutaneous insertion; group F = fluoroscopy guided insertion; group C = surgical insertion.

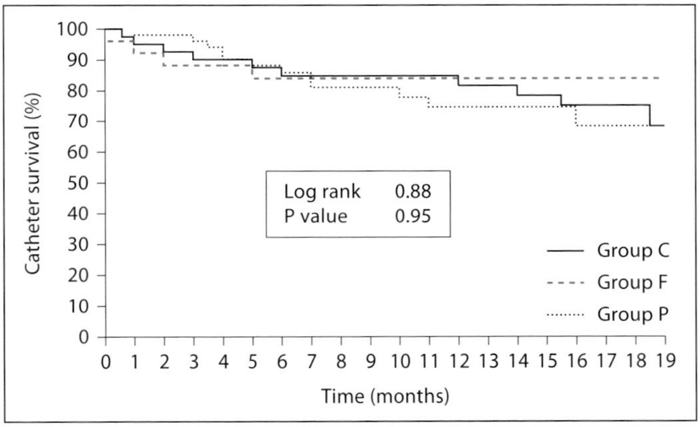

Fig. 3. Catheter survival. Group P = Blind percutaneous insertion; group F = fluoroscopy guided insertion; group C = surgical insertion.

Seldinger Technique under Fluoroscopy

Placement of PD catheters under this technique has been described before [9]. In general, the procedure is carried out under strict aseptic conditions, with parenteral sedation and local anesthesia. Using a 16-gauge lumbar puncture needle, 2 liters of dialysis solution is infused into the peritoneal space by puncture at the midline 1–2 cm below the umbilicus, approximately 1 h prior to procedure [18]. A 3-cm paramedian incision is made, followed by blunt dissection of the subcutaneous tissue until the fascia of the rectus muscle is reached. The peritoneum is punctured using a 16-gauge needle. A Cook peel-away sheath and introducer is inserted over a guide-wire [18]. The guide is introduced only after the previously administered dialysis solution appeared in the needle. The introducer is removed leaving the guide-wire and the peel-away sheath in situ. The catheter is advanced through the peel-away sheath over the guide-wire and directed caudally toward the left iliac fossa. The guide-wire is then removed and the peel-away sheath is split. The inner cuff of the catheter is secured by suture on the fascia of the rectus muscle. An 8- to 12-cm subcutaneous tunnel is fashioned by using a hook-shaped stylet. The end of the catheter is attached to the stylet and the tip of the hook is pushed through the subcutaneous tissue in a latero-caudal direction to the incision. The proximal end of the catheter is pulled through the exit site and positioned so that the inner cuff is located at the peritoneal entry at the fascia of the rectus muscle and the second cuff is more than 3 cm from the exit site. The original incision is then closed and the catheter is flushed with 2 liters of heparinized dialysis solution to confirm catheter patency and to check for intra-abdominal bleeding [18].

Ultrasound/Fluoroscopy-Assisted Placement
A modified fluoroscopic technique by adding ultrasound-assistance has been proposed and described by Maya [17]: after initial dissection of the subcutaneous tissue anterior to the anterior rectus sheath, a needle is inserted into the abdominal cavity under the guidance of ultrasound. The position of the epigastric artery is also examined using ultrasonography to avoid the risk of arterial injury.

Three milliliters of contrast are injected into the peritoneal cavity under fluoroscopy to assure location. A wire is introduced through the needle, and the needle is exchanged for a 4-Fr catheter. The cope mandrel wire is exchanged for a stiff glide-wire and the 4-Fr catheter is exchanged for a 6-Fr catheter sheath (Pinnacle R/O II, 10 cm; Boston Scientific, Medi-Tech). Two hundred cc of normal saline are infused through the catheter sheath into the peritoneal cavity. The 6-Fr catheter sheath is exchanged for a series of dilators (8-, 12-, and 14-Fr). Finally an 18-Fr peel-away sheath is left in place. A double-cuff, swan neck, peritoneal catheter (Quinton, Swan-Neck, Peritoneal Catheter, 62.2 cm; Tyco Healthcare Group, Mass., USA) is introduced over the stiff glide-wire into the peritoneal cavity. The coil portion is placed in the pelvic area. The inner cuff is advanced into the muscle prior to removal of the peel away sheath. Holding the inner cuff into the rectus muscle with a set of forceps, an assistant removes the peel-away sheath leaving the cuff buried into the muscle. The peritoneal catheter is tunneled to an exit site located distal, lateral, and below the initial incision and the outer cuff is buried in the subcutaneous tissue. Patency of the PD catheter is tested with 300 ml of normal saline, infusion time is faster than retrieval and usually takes 8–10 min to complete this task. Finally, 20 ml of contrast is injected through the peritoneal catheter to assess placement. The catheter is flushed and locked with heparin. A locking adapter piece (Titanium Adapter; Baxter Healthcare Corporation, Deerfield, Ill., USA) is attached to the end of the catheter and connected to a transfer set.

It has been pointed out that while fluoroscopy can confirm catheter position and configuration, it cannot anticipate problems with adhesions or redundant omentum. Using fluoroscopic imaging to merely verify catheter location does not significantly improve outcomes over conventional open catheter placement [23]. Furthermore, fluoroscopically guided revisionary procedures for catheter malposition and flow obstruction are associated with high failure rates, principally because there is no opportunity to correct the underlying pathology that led to the dysfunction [25, 26].

Open Surgery
A minilaparotomy is the most widely used technique for implantation of the catheter. In this technique layers of tissue are separated under direct vision. An experienced and skilled operator, either a physician or a surgeon, in a dedicated room, under sterile conditions, is required. To choose the localization of catheter placement, the left side is recommended because it avoids the caecum. Currently, the most usual procedure is a paramedian incision on the left side, with a trans-rectus dissection of the muscle [6].

As described by Ash [20], a 3- to 5-cm 'primary' skin incision and a 2- to 3-cm incision through the rectus muscle are made. The parietal peritoneum is identified, incised, and lifted to create an air space between parietal and visceral peritoneum. The catheter and internal stylet are advanced by feel into the peritoneum, until the deep cuff is within the rectus muscle (for Tenckhoff-type catheters). For the Missouri and Toronto-Western catheters, the ball is advanced into the abdomen and the parietal peritoneum sewn between the ball and Dacron disc. Dissective placement is generally performed under light general anesthesia, but can be done with local anesthesia if desired [20].

Peritoneoscopy

As described by Ash [20], who uses a laparoscopic catheter insertion technique marketed under the proprietary name of Y-TEC peritoneoscopic implantation system (Medigroup, Oswego, Ill., USA), the peritoneoscope has a 2.2-mm diameter and is 15 cm long. Under local anesthesia, a trocar is inserted into the peritoneal cavity and the abdomen is insufflated with room air. The laparoscope, equipped with an overlying plastic sleeve, is used to identify a clear space in the peritoneal cavity. After choosing the proper location of the peritoneal catheter, it follows the same course when the scope is removed [20].

A cannula, internal trocar, and surrounding Quill guide are inserted into the abdomen, the intraperitoneal position confirmed using the scope, and then about 1 liter of air is manually injected to create a pneumoperitoneum [20]. The cannula is advanced between the visceral and parietal peritoneum under vision, the scope and cannula are removed, the Quill is expanded with dilators, and the peritoneal catheter advanced through the Quill. The deep cuff enters the musculature by expanding the Quill, with the Cuff Implanter tool advancing the cuff so that the outer portion is just below the external rectus sheath. A second spiral guide encloses the catheter with the intraperitoneal limbs folded forward. This spiral guide is advanced through the Quill guide, and when the Quill guide and spiral guide are retracted, the limbs open against the parietal peritoneum. The deep cuff is automatically positioned within the rectus muscle. Peritoneoscopic placement of Tenckhoff is generally done with local anesthesia (as opposed to laparoscopic placement).

Tunneling the catheter is similar for each method of insertion. The exit site is determined by laying the catheter over the skin in a gentle downward bend (for straight subcutaneous segment catheters) or in an arcuate course (for Swan Neck catheters). The exit site is chosen at a point 2 cm external to the subcutaneous cuff (if present). A 'secondary' incision is made by inserting a No. 11 scalpel blade to the hub. A Tunnelor Tool or similar device is advanced through the subcutaneous fat from the secondary incision to the primary incision. The tip of the catheter is attached to the Tunnelor, and the tip brought through the secondary incision. Hemostats are lightly applied to the catheter tubing (outside the superficial cuff) and the tips of the hemostats are drawn into the tunnel. When the tips of the hemostats reach the desired position of the subcutaneous cuff, the tips are spread and the hemostat removed. The catheter is pulled through the exit site and the subcutaneous cuff is drawn into the tunnel, to rest 2 cm from the exit site [20].

Some authors point out the peritoneoscopic placement is associated with the lowest rate of catheter complications and a catheter half-life of more than 3 years [20].

Laparoscopy

As stated by Crabtree [22], laparoscopy provides a minimally invasive approach with complete visualization of the peritoneal cavity during the catheter implantation procedure. Laparoscopically enabled techniques of rectus sheath catheter tunneling, omentopexy, adhesiolysis, epiploectomy, and colopexy minimize the risk of catheter migration, pericatheter leak and hernia, omental entrapment, and flow obstruction.

On the other hand, others have pointed out that laparoscopic techniques use larger trocars in diameter compared to the peritoneoscope and the procedure usually requires general anesthesia, the use of CO_2 to inflate the abdomen, potentially more irritating to the peritoneum than air, requires two punctures to the peritoneum (one for the scope and the other for the catheter) and placement of the deep cuff on the rectus requires additional maneuvers [20].

A number of studies have been published on laparoscopic catheter implantation [21, 22], including randomized controlled trials [13, 23–25]. The technique has been associated with a reduced number of exit site infections, a lower incidence of peritonitis, a decreased risk of leakage and an improved catheter survival, although the latter could not be confirmed in one study [23]. In addition, the laparoscopic technique enables the simultaneous correction of adhesions and hernias. The possibility of dealing with adhesions, allowing more patients that ordinarily might not be considered PD candidates because of prior surgery or peritonitis is an important feature of this procedure. One single-center study reported no beneficial effect of the laparoscopic technique [25]. This underlines the importance of the experience obtained in every center, and the impossibility of generalization [8].

Which Is the Best Technique?

As well pointed out by Asif, the preference of one technique over another must take into account the incidence of complications (pericatheter leakage, exit site and tunnel infection) and long-term catheter survival associated with each technique, cost, ease and timely insertion of the catheter, and factors contributing to mortality risk (general anesthesia) [6].

Blind placement procedures are convenient, can be performed anywhere in a hospital, and have the advantage of being low cost [20]. Bowel perforation is an occasional complication (about 1 in 100 placements) and no visualization of the peritoneal space is provided to avoid impinging the catheter tip on adhesions or visceral surfaces. The standard procedure leaves the deep cuff outside of the abdominal musculature, not within the rectus sheath, unless specific further steps are taken, such as grasping the cuff with hemostats and driving the cuff into the rectus muscle [20].

There are advantages and disadvantages of each technique of catheter placement, and the overall success of the catheter is highly dependent upon the method of placement [20].

Open surgical technique allows placement of the deep cuff within the abdominal musculature but pericatheter leaks are frequent if the catheter is used immediately after placement. This technique also provides no visualization of adhesions or best area free of adhesions for placement of the catheter.

Peritoneoscopic placement allows visualization of the peritoneal space, avoinding some of the pitfalls associated with blind or surgical technique such as placing the catheter against adhesions or under the omentum. Nephrologists using this technique have compared it with surgical and blind techniques and have documented better results in terms of incidence of catheter complications such as infection, outflow failure and catheter survival [6, 24, 26].

Laparoscopy allows better visualization of the peritoneal cavity than peritoneoscopy.

References

1 Vonesh EF, Snyder JJ, Foley RN, Collins AJ: The differential impact of risk factors on mortality in hemodialysis and peritoneal dialysis. Kidney Int 2004;66:2389–2401.
2 Merkus MP, Jager KJ, Dekker FW, Boeschoten EW, Stevens P, Krediet RT: Quality of life in patients on chronic dialysis: self-assessment 3 months after the start of treatment. The Necosad Study Group. Am J Kidney Dis 1997;29(4):584–592.
3 Rubin HR, Fink NE, Plantinga LC, Sadler JH, Kliger AS, Powe NR: Patient ratings of dialysis care with peritoneal dialysis vs. hemodialysis. JAMA 2004;291:697–703.
4 Saran R, Pisoni RL, Weitzel WF: Epidemiology of vascular access for hemodialysis and related practice patterns. Contrib Nephrol. Basel, Karger, 2004, vol 142, pp 14–28.
5 Riella MC: Challenges in interventional nephrology. Contrib Nephrol. Basel, Karger, 2005, vol 149, pp 131–137.
6 Asif A: Peritoneal dialysis access-related procedures by nephrologists. Semin Dial 2004;17:398–406.
7 Campos RP, Chula DC, Riella MC: Complications of the peritoneal access and their management. Contrib Nephrol. Basel, Karger, 2009, vol 163, pp 183–197.
8 Dombros N, Dratwa M, Feriani M, et al: European best practice guidelines for peritoneal dialysis. 3. Peritoneal access. Nephrol Dial Transplant 2005;20(suppl 9):ix8–ix12.
9 Zappacosta AR, Perras ST, Closkey GM: Seldinger technique for Tenckhoff catheter placement. ASAIO Trans 1991;37:13–15.
10 Washburn KK, Currier H, Salter KJ, Brandt ML: Surgical technique for peritoneal dialysis catheter placement in the pediatric patient: a North American survey. Adv Perit Dial 2004;20:218–221.
11 Copley JB, Lindberg JS, Tapia NP, Back SN, Snyder PA: Peritoneoscopic placement of Swan neck peritoneal dialysis catheters. Perit Dial Int 1994;14:295–296.

12 Kelly J, McNamara K, May S: Peritoneoscopic peritoneal dialysis catheter insertion. Nephrology (Carlton) 2003;8:315–317.
13 Tsimoyiannis EC, Siakas P, Glantzounis G, Toli C, Sferopoulos G, Pappas M, et al: Laparoscopic placement of the Tenckhoff catheter for peritoneal dialysis. Surg Laparosc Endosc Percutan Tech 2000;10:218–221.
14 Ogunc G: Videolaparoscopy with omentopexy: a new technique to allow placement of a catheter for continuous ambulatory peritoneal dialysis. Surg Today 2001;31:942–944.
15 Zaman F, Pervez A, Atray NK, Murphy S, Work J, Abreo KD: Fluoroscopy-assisted placement of peritoneal dialysis catheters by nephrologists. Semin Dial 2005;18:247–251.
16 Degesys GE, Miller GA, Ford KK, Dunnick NR: Tenckhoff peritoneal dialysis catheters: the use of fluoroscopy in management. Radiology 1985;154:819–820.
17 Maya ID: Ultrasound/fluoroscopy-assisted placement of peritoneal dialysis catheters. Semin Dial 2007;20:611–615.
18 Ozener C, Bihorac A, Akoglu E: Technical survival of CAPD catheters: comparison between percutaneous and conventional surgical placement techniques. Nephrol Dial Transplant 2001;16:1893–1899.
19 Crabtree JH: Fluoroscopic placement of peritoneal dialysis catheters: a harvest of the low-hanging fruits. Perit Dial Int 2008;28:134–137.
20 Ash SR: Chronic peritoneal dialysis catheters: overview of design, placement, and removal procedures. Semin Dial 2003;16:323–334.
21 Ash SR: Bedside peritoneoscopic peritoneal catheter placement of Tenckhoff and newer peritoneal catheters. Adv Perit Dial 1998;14:75–79.
22 Crabtree JH, Fishman A, Huen IT: Videolaparoscopic peritoneal dialysis catheter implant and rescue procedures under local anesthesia with nitrous oxide pneumoperitoneum. Adv Perit Dial 1998;14:83–86.
23 Wright MJ, Bel'eed K, Johnson BF, Eadington DW, Sellars L, Farr MJ: Randomized prospective comparison of laparoscopic and open peritoneal dialysis catheter insertion. Perit Dial Int 1999;19:372–375.
24 Gadallah MF, Pervez A, el-Shahawy MA, et al: Peritoneoscopic versus surgical placement of peritoneal dialysis catheters: a prospective randomized study on outcome. Am J Kidney Dis 1999;33:118–122.
25 Eklund B, Groop PH, Halme L, Honkanen E, Kala AR: Peritoneal dialysis access: a comparison of peritoneoscopic and surgical insertion techniques. Scand J Urol Nephrol 1998;32:405–408.
26 Pastan S, Gassensmith C, Manatunga AK, Copley JB, Smith EJ, Hamburger RJ: Prospective comparison of peritoneoscopic and surgical implantation of CAPD catheters. ASAIO Trans 1991;37:M154–M156.

Miguel C. Riella, MD, PhD, FACP
Av. Iguassu 2689
Curitiba, Parana, 80240–030 (Brazil)
Tel. +55 41 3342 5849, E-Mail mcriella@pro-renal.org.br

Ronco C, Rosner MH, Crepaldi C (eds): Peritoneal Dialysis – State-of-the-Art 2012.
Contrib Nephrol. Basel, Karger, 2012, vol 178, pp 228–231

Time between Peritoneal Dialysis Catheter Insertion and Use

Elwaleed Elhassan[a] · Isaac Teitelbaum[b]

[a]Department of Medicine, University of Khartoum School of Medicine, Khartoum, Sudan; [b]Division of Renal Diseases and Hypertension, University of Colorado, Aurora, Colo., USA

Abstract

Successful performance of peritoneal dialysis (PD) is predicated upon the presence of a properly functioning catheter. Several techniques are available for placing PD catheters among which peritoneoscopic and laparoscopic techniques are gaining broader acceptance. Once placed, PD catheters may be used immediately with low dialysate volumes and a dry day. Alternatively, utilizing what is now referred to as the Moncrief- Popovich technique, they may be embedded subcutaneously for later use. Embedding PD catheters following implantation is an attractive option with multiple potential advantages. Such advantages may encourage wider use of the Moncrief-Popovich technique in PD units Observational studies indicate that the duration of catheter embedment between implantation and externalization does not appear to affect catheter survival. Larger studies are still awaited to further explore the optimum duration of embedment.

A well-functioning catheter is the cornerstone for the successful performance of PD. PD catheter insertion may be performed by nephrologists, surgeons, or interventional radiologists. Catheter insertion is gaining popularity among nephrologists and it has been shown that PD utilization increases when catheter insertion is performed by nephrologists [1–3].

Placement of the catheter to secure access to the peritoneal cavity can be accomplished by any of a variety of techniques (surgical, blind or Seldinger, laparoscopic/peritoneoscopic, or fluoroscopic) [4]. Choosing between these techniques must take into account the incidence of complications (e.g. pericatheter leakage and exit site or tunnel infections), the extent of long-term catheter survival associated with each technique, cost, ease, timely insertion of the catheter, and factors that contribute to mortality risk (e.g. general anesthesia). Surgical implantation is the most common method for placement of a chronic PD catheter. With the recent improvements in technique, peritoneoscopic or laparoscopic-assisted implantations are now being widely implemented and their use is expanding. The major advantage of this approach is that it is minimally invasive while still allowing for direct visualization of the intraperitoneal structures [4, 5]. The peritoneoscopic technique has been shown in randomized controlled clinical trials to result in decreases in the incidence of early peritonitis, exit site infections, and pericatheter leaks, as well as longer catheter survival [6, 7].

Once a catheter is inserted, a decision is made regarding whether to use it immediately or to embed it under the skin for later use. Since tissue dissection with peritoneoscopy or laparoscopy is minimal, the postoperative course is brief and the catheter can be used immediately if needed. Under these circumstances it is generally recommended that, for the first several days of PD, one should use low dialysate volumes at night with a dry (empty) abdomen during the day. By minimizing intra-abdominal pressure, particularly in the upright position, this decreases the probability of pericatheter leakage. There is no consensus in the literature on the optimal time interval that should elapse between peritoneal catheter insertion and commencement of dialysis when urgent initiation of dialysis is not necessary; thus, practices vary between different centers. Nevertheless, a period of 2–3 postoperative weeks for complete wound healing is recommended before implementing continuous ambulatory PD [8, 9].

Embedding the Peritoneal Catheter

An alternative to nonembedded catheter insertion with the potential for immediate catheter use is the method first described by Moncrief and Popovich in 1993 [10]. This method, commonly referred to as the Moncrief-Popovich (MP) technique, involves subcutaneous burial of the distal part of the catheter at the time of implantation. Externalization of the distal part of the catheter under local anesthesia is performed subsequently, after a variable period of time, when initiation of dialysis is deemed necessary [11]. The rationale for introducing this technique was the potential reduction in exit site and peritoneal infections due to both the initial absence of an exit site which serves as an entry port for bacteria, and the elimination of biofilm. Despite these assumptions, the MP technique has not been consistently shown to decrease the incidence of PD-related infections [12, 13]. However, this technique does offer several potential advantages: it is more cost effective, as follow up clinic visits and catheter flushing are unnecessary; it applies to PD the concept of early access that is analogous to the arteriovenous fistula in hemodialysis [14], and subcutaneous burial of the distal portion of the catheter may be more cosmetically acceptable to certain patients. Moreover, it essentially eliminates early pericatheter leakage by virtue of tissue in-growth around the cuffs and immobilization of the catheter.

Does Embedding the Catheter Worsen Outcomes?

At least theoretically, prolonged embedding of the peritoneal dialysis catheter may increase the likelihood of catheter failure because of mechanical or structural problems and it may increase the risk for infectious complications. Moreover, prolonged presence of the catheter in the peritoneal cavity may itself be injurious to the intact peritoneum. In a rodent model of PD, Flessner et al. [15] demonstrated that the presence of the PD catheter in the peritoneal cavity results in increased production of inflammatory cytokines leading to structural and functional changes in the peritoneal membrane. They speculated that the PD catheter serves as a platform for the activation of mesothelial cells that are shed from the basement membrane and for their subsequent transition from an epithelial to a fibroblastic phenotype with increased cytokine production within the peritoneal cavity.

A large retrospective Canadian study has examined the relationship between embedment duration and catheter outcomes in patients undergoing PD catheters placement by the MP technique. Those investigators found that, compared with either a shorter (11–47 days) or longer (134–2,041 days) embedment period, an intermediate embedment duration of 48–133 days resulted in the best catheter survival and the lowest primary catheter failure rate [16]. In contrast, another recently published study of 180 catheters placed using the MP technique demonstrated no association between duration of catheter embedment and risk of obstruction [17]. This was a retrospective study intended to investigate the rate of catheter-related complications and survival according to the method of catheter implantation. When compared to

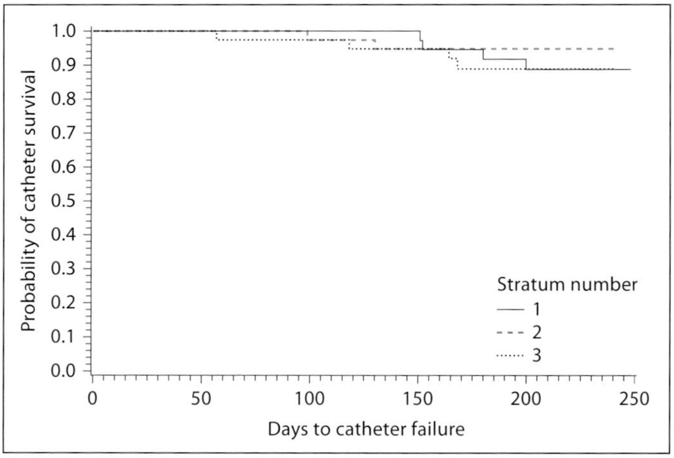

Fig. 1. Catheter survival until mechanical failure, hernia, leak, or infectious complications, by the embedment time group. Catheters were embedded for 2–34 days in group 1, 34–53 days in group 2, and 53–788 days in group 3. Group 1 vs. group 2, p = 0.51; group 1 vs. group 3, p = 0.33; group 2 vs. group 3, p = 0.75. Reprinted from Elhassan et al. [18], with permission.

catheter placement by mini-laparotomy with immediate catheter externalization, placement by mini-laparotomy in conjunction with the MP technique was associated with significantly lower rates of early exit-site infection (6.7 vs. 14.2%; $p = 0.021$), pericatheter leakage (2.2 vs. 11.4%; $p < 0.0001$), and catheter obstruction (7.2 vs. 14.2%; $p = 0.034$) in spite of prolonged embedment time (median 55 days, range 0–991 days).

We, too, have retrospectively analyzed the outcomes of 122 PD catheters inserted by the MP technique at our center between 2000 and 2008. Our primary outcome was catheter survival defined by the absence of pericatheter hernia or leakage, mechanical catheter problems, and catheter-related infections [18]. Secondary outcomes were the likelihood of catheter patency (defined by the absence of a fibrin plug or omental wrap) and the likelihood of complications within 90 days after externalization. We also analyzed the distribution pattern of the standard peritoneal equilibration test (PET) to determine whether there was a relationship between the duration of catheter embedment and peritoneal membrane transport status. The effect of embedment duration on catheter survival was modeled both categorically, by dividing the total number of catheters into tertiles of embedment duration (tertile I: 2–34 days; tertile II: 34–53 days; tertile III: 53–788 days), and as a continuous variable.

After controlling for sex, race, age, and diabetes status, embedment duration did not have a significant effect on catheter survival as a continuous predictor or as a categorical variable (fig. 1; $p \geq 0.33$ for all comparisons). Furthermore, our study showed no correlation between embedment duration and membrane transport status as determined by the standard PET test. Regarding secondary outcomes, our study was most notable for a very high overall catheter utilization rate (99.2%). Initial utilization was 109 of 122 catheters (89.3%). Primary mechanical complications were observed in 13 of 122 catheters (10.7%) – 10 with a fibrin plug or kink and 3 with an omental wrap. However, 12 of those 13 catheters were subsequently used after simple laparoscopic manipulation. Overall, therefore, 99.2% of buried catheters were successfully used for PD.

A randomized controlled trial is currently underway in Australia to determine the optimal time for initiation of PD after insertion of a Tenckhoff catheter [19]. The patients will be randomized to one of three treatment groups: group 1 will start PD 1 week after catheter insertion, group 2 at 2 weeks and group 3 at 4 weeks. The primary end point is the complication rate (leaks and infection) after initiation of PD. Unfortunately, there is no embedment duration longer than four weeks being examined, thereby limiting the potential significance of this study.

Conclusion

Successful application of PD entails the presence of a well-functioning catheter. Among the different insertion techniques, peritoneoscopy and laparoscopy are gaining more interest and wider utilization. Evidence supports their superiority in terms of reduced adverse catheter outcomes compared to the open surgical technique. PD catheters can be used immediately after insertion if needed, but embedding them offers some specific advantages. The duration of catheter embedment before externalization does not seem to affect catheter survival, although randomized controlled studies are awaited to consolidate such results.

References

1 Kang SH, Do JY, Cho KH, Park JW, Yoon KW: Blind peritoneal catheter placement with a Tenckhoff trocar by nephrologists: a single-center experience. Nephrology (Carlton). 2012;17:141–147.

2 Gadallah MF, Ramdeen G, Torres-Rivera C, Ibrahim ME, Myrick S, Andrews G, Quin A, Fang C, Crossman A: Changing the trend: a prospective study on factors contributing to the growth rate of peritoneal dialysis programs. Adv Perit Dial 2001;17:122–126.

3 Asif A, Pflederer TA, Vieira CF, Diego J, Roth D, Agarwal A: Catheter insertion by nephrologists and its impact on peritoneal dialysis utilization. Semin Dial 2005;18:157–160.

4 Asif A: Peritoneal dialysis access-related procedures by nephrologists. Semin Dial 2004;17:398–406.

5 Maio R, Figueiredo N, Costa P: Laparoscopic placement of Tenckhoff catheters for peritoneal dialysis: a safe, effective, and reproducible procedure. Perit Dial Int 2008;28:170–173.

6 Pastan S, Gassensmith C, Manatunga AK, Copley JB, Smith EJ, Hamburger RJ: Prospective comparison of peritoneoscopic and surgicalimplantation of CAPD catheters. Trans Am Soc Artif Organ 1991;37:M154–M156.

7 Gadallah MF, Pervez A, El-Shahawy MA, Sorrells D, Zibari G, McDonald J, Work J: Peritoneoscopic versus surgical placement of peritoneal dialysis catheters: a prospective randomized study on outcome. Am J Kidney Dis 1999;33:118–122.

8 Ash SR: Chronic peritoneal dialysis catheters: procedures for placement, maintenance and removal. Semin Nephrol 2002;22:221–236.

9 CARI Guidelines: Timing of commencement of dialysis after peritoneal dialysis catheter insertion. 2004. http://www.cari.org.au/dialysis_ptp_publ2004.php.

10 Moncrief JW, Popovich RP, Broadrick LJ, et al: The Moncrief–Popovich catheter. A new peritoneal access technique for patients on peritoneal dialysis. ASAIO J 1993;39:62–65.

11 Page DE, Turpin C: A simple and inexpensive method of subcutaneous implantation of catheter distal segment using a Tenckhoff curled catheter. Perit Dial Int 2000;20:85–87

12 Danielsson A, Blohme L, Tranaeus A, et al: A prospective randomized study of the effect of a subcutaneously 'buried' peritoneal dialysis catheter technique versus standard technique on the incidence of peritonitis and exit-site infection. Perit Dial Int 2002;22:211–219.

13 Wu CC, Su PF, Chiang SS: A prospective study to compare subcutaneously buried peritoneal dialysis catheter technique with conventional technique. Blood Purif 2007;25:229–232.

14 Dasgupta MK: Moncrief-Popovich catheter and implantation technique: the AV fistula of peritoneal dialysis. Adv Ren Replace Ther 2002;9:116–124.

15 Flessner MF, Credit K, Henderson K, Vanpelt HM, Potter R, He Z, Henegar J, Robert B: Peritoneal changes after exposure to sterile solutions by catheter. J Am Soc Nephrol 2007;18:2294–2302.

16 Brown PA, McCormick BB, Knoll G, Su Y, Doucette S, Fergusson D, Lavoie S: Complications and catheter survival with prolonged embedding of peritoneal dialysis catheters. Nephrol Dial Transplant 2008;23:2299–2303.

17 Brum S, Rodrigues A, Rocha S, Carvalho MJ, Nogueira C, Magalhães C, et al: Moncrief-Popovich technique is an advantageous method of peritoneal dialysis catheter implantation. Nephrol Dial Transplant 2010;25:3070–3075.

18 Elhassan E, McNair B, Quinn M, Teitelbaum I: Prolonged duration of peritoneal dialysis catheter embedment does not decrease catheter success rates. Perit Dial Int 2011;31:558–564.

19 Ranganathan D, Baer R, Fassett RG, Williams N, Han T, Watson M, Healy H: Randomised controlled trial to determine the appropriate time to initiate peritoneal dialysis after insertion of catheter to minimise complications (Timely PD study). BMC Nephrol 2010;11:11.

Dr. Isaac Teitelbaum
Division of Renal Diseases and Hypertension, University of Colorado, Denver
12605 E. 16th Avenue, F774
Aurora, CO 80045 (USA)
Tel. +1 720 848 7601, E-Mail isaac.teitelbaum@ucdenver.edu

Ronco C, Rosner MH, Crepaldi C (eds): Peritoneal Dialysis – State-of-the-Art 2012.
Contrib Nephrol. Basel, Karger, 2012, vol 178, pp 232–237

Peritoneal Dialysis Membrane Evaluation in Clinical Practice

Raymond T. Krediet[a] · Dirk G. Struijk[b]

[a]Division of Nephrology, Department of Medicine, Academic Medical Centre University of Amsterdam and
[b]Dianet Foundation, Amsterdam, The Netherlands

Abstract
A review is given on the various methods to assess the quality of the peritoneum as a dialysis membrane. The quality of the peritoneum in patients who are treated with chronic peritoneal dialysis (PD) has mainly focused on solute transport. Only recently have biomarkers in effluent been considered as useful, but are not generally applied. Peritoneal function tests should not be performed only when clinical problems are present, but rather on a regular basis, for instance every 6–12 months. Only in this way can the natural cause become apparent.

Peritoneal Equilibration Test

The peritoneal equilibration test (PET) was described in 1987 and is still the most used method [1]. It is based on a dialysis dwell of four hours, using a 2-liter exchange with a 2.27%/2.5% glucose-based dialysis solution; the preceding exchange is with a 1.36%/1.5% glucose solution. Dialysate samples are taken at 2 and 4 h; a blood sample is also obtained. Laboratory investigations include creatinine and glucose, and the results are expressed as the dialysate/plasma (D/P) ratio of creatinine, the dialysate glucose concentration at a certain time point/the initial dialysate glucose concentration (D_t/D_o), and the drained volume. Due to simplicity of the calculations of D/P creatinine and D_t/D_o glucose, the PET has become popular.

Based on the PET, patients have been divided into four transport categories. These are high and low average (mean of the population ±1 SD) and high and low (between 1 and 2 SD). These terms are confusing because the transport of LMW solutes such as urea is mainly dependent on the drained volume. Therefore high transporters can have low values for Kt/V_{urea} because of a small drained volume [2, 3]. Therefore, the term 'high' could better be changed to 'fast'; similarly 'low' should be renamed 'slow'. The so-called 'fast PET' is a modification of the PET in which dialysate samples are taken after only 4 h [4]. This does not influence the results.

Personal Dialysis Capacity Test

The personal dialysis capacity (PDC) test has been developed by Haraldsson [5]. It is performed by the patients themselves with five exchanges per 24 h; the preceding long exchange is also used. The five exchanges differ in terms of dwell time and glucose concentration. Laboratory investigations in two blood samples and every dialysate sample include urea, creatinine, glucose and albumin.

Table 1. Comparison between the PET and the PDC test

	PET	PDC test
Number of exchanges	1	5
Glucose concentration, %	2.27	variable
Dwell time, h	4	2, 3, 4, 5, 10
Number of dialysate samples	1 or 2	6
Serum and dialysate albumin	no	yes
Volume marker	no	no
Calculations	simple	kinetic modelling

Using kinetic modeling with a computer program based on the three-pore model [6], three parameters are determined: the area parameter (A_o/Δ_x), the absorption (JV_{AR}) and the large pore flow rate (JV_L). A_o/Δ_x is the unrestricted pore area available for exchange over the diffusion distance. This is related to MTACs or D/P ratios of LMW solutes. JV_{AR} is a combination of lymphatic absorption and transcapillary backfiltration. JV_L is based on the transport of albumin or total protein. A comparison between the PET and PDC is given in table 1.

It has been claimed that the unrestricted pore area is a better indicatior of peritoneal function than D/P creatinine [7]. However, this was based on a comparison with intraperitoneally administered iohexol, the disappearance of which is by both diffusion and lymphatic uptake. Normal values for the PDC test were determined in a multicenter study in 336 patients [8]. Not unexpectedly, the area parameter showed a positive relationship with peritoneal creatinine clearance and a negative relationship with UF.

The large pore flux was related to area. This parameter was also associated with hypoalbuminemia and mortality in a single-center study [9]. A link between JV_L and C-reactive protein has been described [10]. Such a relation was not present for the other PDC parameters, nor for D/P creatinine. Based on these findings superiority of the PDC over the PET has been claimed. However, a more recent study in a large number of patients could not confirm these results [11].

The question may arise whether the PET should be replaced by the PDC test. Besides its benefits, the PDC test has a number of disadvantages: five exchanges are needed, which carries the risk of more inaccuracies; second, the number of laboratory investigations is much larger than in the PET; third, kinetic modeling requires the need of assumptions, which may not always be correct, and, fourth, no sodium kinetics are included. However, the PET in its original form provides only limited information. This underlines the need for modifications.

Standardized Peritoneal Permeability Analysis

Standardized peritoneal permeability analysis (SPA) provides the most extensive information on peritoneal transport. It is based on a 4-hour dwell, initially with a 1.36%/1.5% glucose-based solution [12]. Later, the tonicity of the solution was changed to 3.86%/4.25% [13]. Dextran 70 1 g/l is added to the test solution as a volume marker. The instillation of the test solution is preceded by a rinsing exchange with a 1.36%/1.5% glucose dialysis solution. Dialysate samples are obtained at various time points during the dwell; blood samples are taken at the beginning and the end of the test dwell. The peritoneal cavity is drained after 4 h. This is followed by another rinsing procedure to determine the residual volume, which is necessary for the determination of fluid kinetics. The following solutes are measured in the dialysate and the blood samples: urea, creatinine, urate, glucose, sodium (Na^+), potassium (K^+), total dextran, and various plasma proteins. Using the results of these investigations, the following parameters are calculated: MTAC of urea, creatinine and urate, peritoneal glucose absorption, D/P sodium, peritoneal clearances of the above mentioned proteins. Transcapillary UF is calculated from the dilution of Dextran 70 and the effective lymphatic absorption rate from its

Table 2. Advantages and limitations of the various peritoneal function test without a volume marker

Test[1]	Advantages	Limitations
Original PET	widely used gold standard for small solute transport	limited information on ultrafiltration no Na^+ sieving no FWT no OC
Modified PET	definition for UFF Na^+ sieving D/P creatinine similar to original PET	no FWT no OC
PDC test	large pore flow using albumin peritoneal absorption area parameter	no Na^+ sieving no FWT no OC
Mini-PET	FWT	D/P creatinine difficult to compare with PET values no OC
Modified PET with temporary drainage	definition of UFF Na^+ sieving FWT D/P creatinine similar to original PET	no OC

FWT = Free water transport; OC = osmotic conductance.
[1] The value of the test is increased when an effluent CA125 determination is added.

disappearance. Net UF is the difference between the two. The sieving of sodium (D/P sodium) gives an indication of free water transport. The intra-individual coefficients of variation for the MTAC of LMW solutes are less than 10%, and those for fluid kinetics less than 20%.

Although it is evident that the SPA provides the most detailed information on peritoneal transport that can be obtained in individual patients, the test is too complicated for routine clinical practice.

Refinements of the PET

The variations that will be discussed are the modified PET, the mini-PET and the modified PET with temporary drainage. Their advantages and limitations are given in table 2. An algorithm is given in figure 1.

Modified PET

The differences between the modified and the original PET are the use of a 3.86%/4.25% glucose solution and an additional dialysate sample at 1 h for the determination of sodium. The modified PET has been advocated by the committee on UF management of the International Society for Peritoneal Dialysis [14]. The test provides more accurate information on net UF, because the drained volume is larger than in the original PET. The D/P sodium at 1 h gives information on free water transport. UF failure is defined by the 3 × 4 rule: net UF is less than 400 ml after a dwell of 4 h with a 3.86%/4.25% dialysis solution [14, 15]. Increasing the dialysate glucose concentration to 3.86%/4.25% does not affect D/P creatinine. The modified PET is feasible in routine clinical practice [16] and can be used in the follow-up of patients [17].

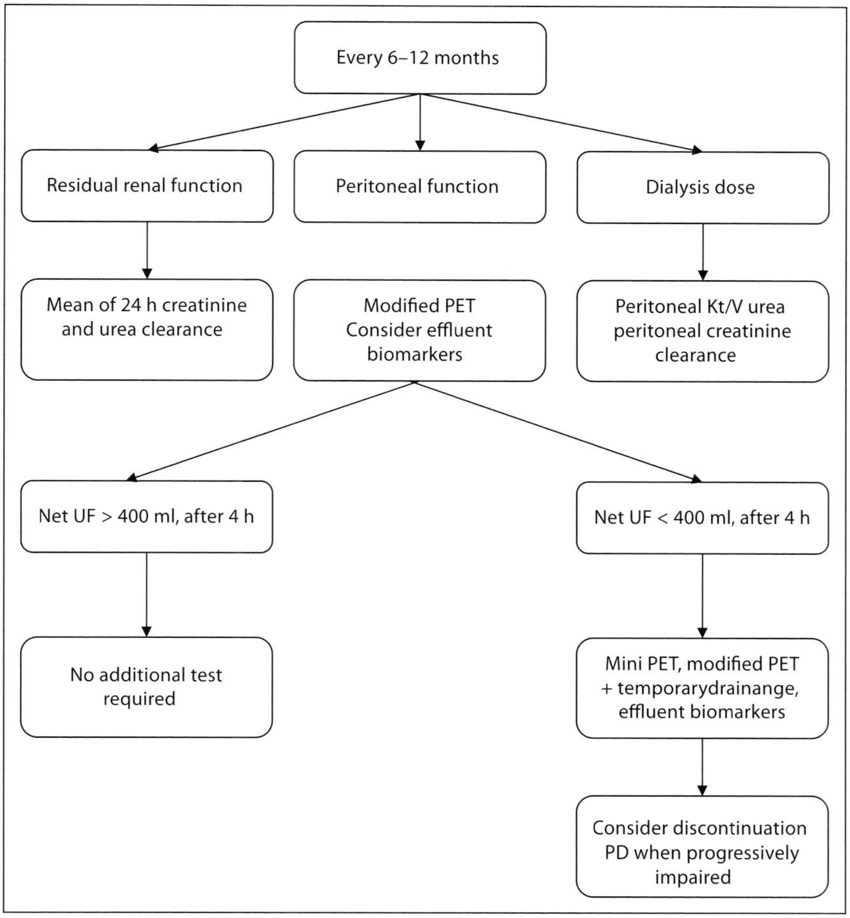

Fig. 1. A suggested algorithm for follow-up of patients on PD.

Mini-PET

The mini-PET is performed with a 3.86%/4.25% glucose-based solution, but the dwell time is only 1 h [18]. It allows the calculation of small pore fluid transport and free water transport. The assumptions are as follows: the diffusion through small pores can be neglected compared with convective transport because of the high UF rates during the first hour, small pores offer no hindrance to the transport of sodium and there is little contribution of lymphatic absorption to fluid transport during the first hour. In such cases, the removal of sodium after 1 h (amount drained minus amount instilled) divided by the plasma sodium concentration yields the small pore fluid transport. Free water transport can be calculated easily as the difference between net UF after 1 h and small pore fluid transport in the same period. The contribution of free water transport to total UF averaged 46%, but had a very wide range among patients.

The above technique has also been used in the SPA at various time points during four hour dwells [19]. It appears that free water transport is linearly related to the decrease in the osmotic pressure gradient.

The original paper on the mini-PET reported a good relationship with the modified PET on the division of patients in transport categories. However, it has been shown that MTAC values are higher during the first hour of a four hours dwell than in the period thereafter [16]. This makes it unlikely that the mini-PET can replace the modified PET completely.

Modified PET with Temporary Drainage
The modified PET and the mini-PET can be combined when the peritoneal cavity is drained after one hour to determine the volume at that time by weighing. After taking a dialysate sample, the drained volume is reinfused and left for another 3 h. Using this approach, no differences were found for net UF and small solute transport compared to those in a modified PET [19]. The contribution of free water transport after 1 h averaged 44% of net UF.

Effluent Biomarkers

Peritoneal tissues and cells are likely to shed some of their products in the fluid that surrounds them. Determination of these in effluent may provide information on the status of the peritoneum. Local production estimation must take possible contribution of diffusion from the serum into account. Most information is present on effluent cancer antigen 125 (CA125), which can be considered a marker of mesothelial cell mass [20]. It has an intraindividual coefficient of variation of 15% and shows a decrease during follow-up [21]. IL-6 concentrations in effluent are higher than in serum. This cytokine has a coefficient of variation of 28%. No clear effect of duration of PD has been found. Recently, it was established that the combination of effluent CA125 appearance rate <33 U/min and IL-6 >350 pg/min had a specificity of 89% for the development of encapsulating peritoneal sclerosis [22]. These data will have to be confirmed.

Conclusion

The best way to measure peritoneal transport in the absence of a volume maker is by using a 4-hour dwell with a 3.86%/4.25% glucose-based dialysis solution with a temporary drainage after 1 h for determination of the intraperitoneal volume and sampling, followed by reinfusion. Laboratory investigations should include sodium, creatinine, glucose and, probably, albumin. This test provides useful information on D/P creatinine, D_t/D_0 glucose, peritoneal albumin clearance, net UF and free water transport, and is therefore the best choice for use in routine clinical practice. Determination of biomarkers in effluent is likely to increase the possibility to detect peritoneal membrane abnormalities.

References

1 Twardowski ZJ, Nolph KD, Khanna R, et al: Peritoneal equilibration test. Perit Dial Int 1987;7:138–147.
2 Wang T, Heimburger O, Waniewski J, et al: Increased peritoneal permeability is associated with decreased fluid and small-solute removal and higher mortality in CAPD patients. Nephrol Dial Transplant 1998;13:1242–1249.
3 Churchill DN, Thorpe KE, Nolph KD, et al: Increased peritoneal membrane transport is associated with decreased patient and technique survival for continuous peritoneal dialysis patients. J Am Soc Nephrol 1999;9:1285–1292.
4 Twardowski ZJ: The fast peritoneal equilibration test. Semin Dial 1990;3:141–142.
5 Haraldsson B: Assessing the peritoneal dialysis capacities of individual patients. Kidney Int 1995;47:1187–1198.
6 Rippe B, Haraldsson B: Transport of macromolecules across microvascular walls. The two-pore theory. Physiol Rev 1994;74:163–219.
7 Johansson E, Johansson A-C, Andreasson B-I, et al: Unrestricted pose area (A_0/Δ_x) is a better indicator of peritoneal membrane function than the PET. Kidney Int 2000;58:1773–1779.
8 Van Biesen W, Carlsson O, Bergia R, et al: Personal dialysis capacity PDC™) test: a multicenter clinical study. Nephrol Dial Transplant 2003;18:788–796.

9 Heaf JG, Sarac S, Afzal S: A high peritoneal large pore fluid flux causes hypoalbuminaemia and is a risk factor for death in peritoneal dialysis patients. Nephrol Dial Transplant 2005;20:2194–2201.
10 Van Biesen W, Van Der Tol, A, Veys N, et al: the personal dialysis capacity test is superior to the peritoneal equilibration test to discriminate inflammation as the cause of fast transport status in peritoneal dialysis patients. Clin J Am Soc Nephrol 2006;1:269–274.
11 Balafa O, Halbesma N, Struijk DG, et al: Peritoneal albumin and protein losses do not predict outcome in peritoneal dialysis. Clin J Am Soc Nephrol 2011;6:561–566.
12 Pannekeet MM, Imholz ALT, Struijk DG, et al: The standard peritoneal permeability analysis: a tool for the assessment of peritoneal permeability characteristics in CAPD patients. Kidney Int 1995;48:866–875.
13 Smit W, Van Dijk P, Schouten N, et al: Peritoneal function and assessment of reference values using a 3.86% glucose solution. Perit Dial Int 2003;23:440–449.
14 Mujais S, Nolph K, Gokal R, et al: Evaluation and management of ultrafiltration problems in peritoneal dialysis. Perit Dial Int 2000; 20(suppl 4):S5–S21.
15 Krediet RT, Lindholm B, Rippe B: Pathophysiology of peritoneal membrane failure. Perit Dial Int 2000;20(suppl 4):S22–S42.
16 Rodrigues AS, Silva S, Bravo F, et al: Peritoneal membrane evaluation in routine clinical practice. Blood Purif 2007;25:447–504.
17 Rodrigues AE, Martins M, Korevaar JC, et al: Evaluation of peritoneal transport and membrane status peritoneal dialysis: focus on incidents fast transporters. Am J Nephrol 2007;27:84–91.
18 La Milia V, Di Filippo S, Crepaldi M, et al: Mini-peritoneal equilibration test: a simple and fast method to assess free water and small solute transport across the peritoneal membrane. Kidney Int 2005;68:840–846.
19 Cnossen TT, Lijten INM, Konings JCA, et al: Peritoneal transport and ultrafiltration quantification of free water transport during the peritoneal equilibration test. Perit Dial Int 2009;29:523–527.
20 Krediet RT: Dialysate cancer antigen 125 concentration as marker of peritoneal membrane status in patients treated with chronic peritoneal dialysis. Perit Dial Int 2001;21:132–136.
21 Lopes-Barreto D, Coester AM, Noordzij M, et al: Variability of effluent cancer antigen 125 and interleukin-6 determination in peritoneal dialysis patients. Nephrol Dial Transplant 2011;26:3739–3744.
22 Sampimon DE, Korte MR, Lopes Barreto D, et al: Early diagnostic markers for encapsulating peritoneal sclerosis: a case-control study. Perit Dial Int 2010;30:163–169.

Prof. Raymond T. Krediet, MD, PhD
Academic Medical Center, Division of Nephrology, Department of Medicine
Meibergdreef 9
NL–1105 AZ Amsterdam (The Netherlands)
Tel. +31 20 566 5990, E-Mail r.t.krediet@amc.uva.nl

Ronco C, Rosner MH, Cresaldi C (eds): Peritoneal Dialysis – State-of-the-Art 2012.
Contrib Nephrol. Basel, Karger, 2012, vol 178, pp 238–245

Bioelectrical Impedance Analysis in the Assessment of Hydration Status in Peritoneal Dialysis Patients

Mikko Haapio[a,c] · Paolo Lentini[a,b] · Andrew A. House[a,d] · Massimo de Cal[a] · Dinna N. Cruz[a] · Dehua Gong[a] · Maria Pia Rodighiero[a] · Roberto Dell'Aquila[a,b] · Claudio Ronco[a]

[a]San Bortolo Hospital, Department of Nephrology, International Renal Research Institute (IRRIV), Vicenza, and [b]San Bassiano Hospital, Department of Nephrology, Bassano del Grappa, Italy; [c]Helsinki University Central Hospital, Division of Nephrology, Helsinki, Finland; [d]London Health Sciences Centre, Division of Nephrology, London, Ont., Canada

Abstract

Objective: Assessment of fluid status in chronic peritoneal dialysis (PD) patients is complex. Clinical evaluation based solely on body weight, blood pressure, volume of ultrafiltration (UF) and peripheral edema is insufficient. A non-invasive test, bioelectrical impedance analysis (BIA) might be of potential benefit. **Aim:** To test whether BIA correlates with other ancillary markers of extracellular fluid volume, namely B-type natriuretic peptide (BNP), residual renal function (RRF) and UF, and whether BIA provides complementary information in categorizing PD patients vis-à-vis hydration status. **Methods:** A cross-sectional study of 61 out-patients on chronic PD. Single-frequency BIA measurements of resistance/height were divided into tertiles (lowest: <253 Ω/m; middle: ≥253 Ω/m and <316 Ω/m; highest: ≥316 Ω/m). **Results:** Compared to patients in the highest tertile of BIA (least fluid), patients in the lowest tertile (most fluid) had highest BNP, RRF and UF (93.5 vs. 55.0 pg/ml, p = 0.029; 850 vs. 300 ml/day, p = 0.05; and 1.75 vs. 1.21 l/day, p = 0.023, respectively). **Conclusions:** BIA tertiles categorized PD patients who differed in BNP, RRF and UF in a stepwise pattern, suggesting BIA may better inform hydration status, and serve as an additional clinical tool in management of chronic PD patients.

Prevention of extracellular fluid volume overload is a primary target of dialysis therapy; there is an increasing body of evidence that fluid status is an important determinant of clinical outcome in peritoneal dialysis (PD) patients [1]. Despite efforts to maintain optimal fluid balance, volume overload is relatively frequent in patients on PD especially after residual renal function declines [2, 3]. Correct estimation of the so-called 'dry weight' represents a major practical issue in the clinical assessment of chronic dialysis patients. Underestimation of dry weight can lead to hypovolemia, hypotension and cramping, whereas overestimation can lead to hypertension, and pulmonary and peripheral edema [4]. Fluid overload of PD patients has been associated with development of pathological cardiovascular findings, including left ventricular hypertrophy, elevated diastolic blood pressure and end-diastolic volume on echocardiogram [5, 6], with increased cardiovascular and overall mortality [1].

Clinical variables in estimation of dry weight (e.g. body weight, blood pressure, peripheral edema) are inaccurate, nonspecific and subjective, and thus there is a need for reliable, noninvasive tests to guide our targeting of dry weight. B-type natriuretic peptides (BNPs) have emerged as markers of cardiac stretch in patients with volume overload, and high levels of these hormones strongly correlate with poor prognosis in both chronic hemodialysis (HD) and PD patients [7–9]. In HD patients, elevated plasma BNP concentration may serve as a useful tool to detect overhydration [10, 11]. Levels of BNPs in patients on PD are reported to be lower than in HD patients, but the correlation with left ventricular dysfunction and abnormal cardiac structure is clear in both dialysis modalities [12–15].

Bioelectrical impedance analysis (BIA) technique is a simple way to measure body fluid composition noninvasively, rapidly and inexpensively [16]. The technique employs measurement of impedance, which is inversely related to tissue fluid content [17]. BIA analysis further calculates impedance into resistance and reactance, and produces such estimates of body composition parameters as total body water (TBW), intracellular fluid volume (ICV) and extracellular fluid volume (ECV) [18].

In earlier studies BIA has shown some usefulness in assessment of fluid status in PD patients [19–23], but the data remain limited. In the current study we wished to further explore whether categorization of hydration status based on BIA would correlate with plasma BNP, residual renal function (RRF, i.e. amount of diuresis) and ultrafiltration (UF), and whether BIA could serve as a useful means to evaluate volume status of chronic PD patients.

Patients and Methods

We performed a cross-sectional analysis of 61 stable out-patients that had been on chronic PD for at least 3 months, on their routine appointment at the PD clinic at St. Bortolo Hospital, Vicenza, Italy. We received informed consent from all participating patients, and approval for the study from the hospital's Ethics Review Board. Patients with incomplete data at any predestined point of data collection were excluded, as were patients with a history of limb amputation which hinders interpretation of BIA results. Enrolled patients collected 24-hour dialysate fluid and urine on the day prior to PD clinic visit, and a standard peritoneal equilibration test (PET) [24] was performed during the visit. Seated blood pressure was obtained with multiple measurements using a mercury sphygmomanometer. Subject characteristics are listed in table 1.

Plasma and dialysate concentrations of urea, creatinine and glucose were determined as per standard methodology. Blood sampling for BNP was performed after 20–30 min of resting in a semi-recumbent position, and all samples were drawn into chilled EDTA vacuum blood-collection tubes, placed immediately on ice, and centrifuged within 30 min at 4°C. The plasma was stored at –80°C until assayed (for a maximum of 6 months). BNP Triage MeterPro® (Biosite® Inc. Diagnostics, San Diego, Calif., USA) point-of-care immunoassay method was used for measuring plasma BNP.

Single-frequency BIA measurements were obtained using a plethysmograph emitting 800 μÅ and 50 kHz alternating sinusoidal current (EFG Electrofluidgraph, Akern s.r.l., Pontassieve, Florence, Italy), chosen for its previous validation in patients with renal failure [19, 20]. After at least 20 min in a supine position, with arms and legs abducted at a 30° angle from the trunk, and cleaning the skin to ensure good contact, electrodes were attached to the right wrist and ankle in a standardized fashion, according to instructions of the BIA device manufacturer. All BIA measurements were conducted by the same operator, who was blinded to other measurements of fluid status. Current was passed between the electrodes followed by measurements of resistance (R, total body water) and reactance (X, intracellular water). BIA measurements were standardized by height (H) of subjects, thus producing R/H and X/H (both in Ohm/m or Ω/m). These values were then used to calculate the phase angle (PA, reactance/resistance), perform a vector plot (R/H against X/H), and calculate ECV as a proportion of estimated TBW, using the software Bodygram® (Akern s.r.l., Pontassieve, Florence, Italy). The results of BIA measurements were divided into tertiles using 253

Table 1. Characteristics of patients according to PD modality

	CAPD (n = 43)	APD (n = 18)	p value
Age, years	65 (51–72)	61 (49–77)	0.99
Gender, % male	51	56	0.49
Duration of dialysis, months	40 (34–62)	53 (45–78)	0.007
BMI	27 (25–32)	25 (23–28)	0.027
Systolic BP, mm Hg	140 (130–158)	138 (128–153)	0.60
Diastolic BP, mm Hg	80 (73–90)	80 (80–100)	0.69
BNP, pg/ml	78 (50–241)	52 (28–81)	0.024
Residual renal function, ml/day	800 (275–1,550)	300 (0–1,163)	0.13
Ultrafiltration, liters/day	1.60 (1.20–1.95)	1.38 (1.06–2.05)	0.55
Kt/V	2.1 (1.8–2.3)	2.1 (1.9–2.3)	0.78
PET category, n for H/HA/LA/L*	10/19/11/1	18/0/0/0	–

Values (except for gender and PET category) are expressed as median (interquartile range, IQR).
CAPD = Continuous ambulatory peritoneal dialysis; APD = automated peritoneal dialysis; BMI = body mass index; BP = blood pressure; BNP = B-type natriuretic peptide; Kt/V = urea clearance; PET = peritoneal equilibration test (transporter types: H = high; HA = high average; LA = low average; L = low).
* n = 41 (PET test not completed in 2 patients).

and 316 Ω/m as cutoff values for R/H, to define three patient groups (lowest tertile [most fluid]: <253 Ω/m, n = 20; middle tertile: ≥253 and <316 Ω/m, n = 21; highest tertile [least fluid]: ≥316 Ω/m, n = 20). Table 2 describes characteristics of these patient groups.

All analyses were performed using the statistical package PASW Statistics 18 (SPSS Inc., Chicago, Ill., USA). As many variables were not normally distributed, nonparametric comparisons were performed using Mann-Whitney U test and Kruskal-Wallis test for independent samples. Values are expressed as median (IQR) unless otherwise stated. $p < 0.05$ was required for statistical significance.

Results

Bioelectrical Impedance Analysis

The analysis of BIA measurements according to R/H tertiles revealed significant differences between the groups. Compared to the patients in the highest tertile (least fluid), the patients in the lowest tertile (most fluid) had highest BNP (93.5 vs. 55.0 pg/ml, p = 0.029), RRF (850 vs. 300 ml/day, p = 0.05) and UF (1.75 vs. 1.21 l/day, p = 0.023). BIA tertiles appeared to distinguish BNP, RRF and UF in a largely dose-dependent fashion as illustrated in figure 1.

B-Type Natriuretic Peptide

We explored the relationship between BNP and both RRF and UF by comparing BNP between dichotomized groups of subjects. We found BNP not to be statistically different between groups according to RRF using the median value of 600 ml/day as a cutoff, with minimal RRF having a mean (SE) BNP of 301 (115) pg/ml and those with higher RRF having BNP of 166 (45) pg/ml (p = 0.27). Likewise, using the median amount of daily UF to categorize subjects did not reveal any differences in BNP, with the group below 1.50 liters/day having mean (SE) BNP of 251 (100) pg/ml and the group above having BNP of 212 (68) pg/ml (p = 0.75).

Modality

Comparing continuous ambulatory peritoneal dialysis (CAPD) patients (n = 43) to automated peritoneal dialysis (APD) patients (n = 18),

Table 2. Patients divided according to tertiles of bioelectrical impedance analysis (BIA) test results

	BIA tertiles			p value*
	'normal fluid' ≥253 and <316 Ω/m (n = 21)	'most fluid' <253 Ω/m (n = 20)	'least fluid' ≥316 Ω/m (n = 20)	
Age, years	66 (52–78)	62 (52–67)	66 (48–74)	0.38
Gender, % male	67	15	75	<0.001
Duration of dialysis, months	53 (40–69)	36 (31–61)	43 (37–69)	0.42
BMI	28 (24–32)	27 (24–33)	35 (23–27)	0.021
Systolic BP, mm Hg	135 (130–155)	150 (128–160)	140 (126–144)	0.23
Diastolic BP, mm Hg	80 (72–100)	88 (80–100)	80 (71–85)	0.013
BNP, pg/ml	61 (35–189)	94 (59–389)	55 (31–104)	0.029
Residual renal function, ml/day	850 (100–1,650)	850 (375–1,413)	300 (0–775)	0.05
Ultrafiltration, liters/day	1.62 (1.22–2.07)	1.75 (1.32–2.07)	1.21 (0.94–1.67)	0.023

Values (except for gender) are expressed as median (interquartile range, IQR).
* p value expressing comparison between groups 'most fluid' and 'least fluid'.
BIA = Bioelectrical impedance analysis; BMI = body mass index; BP = blood pressure; BNP = B-type natriuretic peptide.

neither the median amount of RRF nor UF was significantly different (800 vs. 300 ml, p = 0.13, and 1.60 vs. 1.38 l, p = 0.55, respectively). Also the weekly Kt/V was approximately the same between these groups (2.08 vs. 2.14, p = 0.78). The level of BNP, however, was significantly higher in CAPD patients (77.5 vs. 51.5 pg/ml, p = 0.024).

Discussion

The management of optimal fluid status is a challenging task for clinicians treating chronic dialysis patients. RRF is best preserved when daily ultrafiltration target is modest, using biocompatible PD fluids that contain a small but still sufficient concentration of glucose [2]. Whilst preserving RRF, adequate dialysis dose and toxin clearance need to be ensured. Furthermore, use of dietary salt should be minimized and daily fluid intake kept stable [25]. At the same time, fluid homeostasis is affected by hypertension and antihypertensive and diuretic regimens [26, 27]. Adding to this complexity are the insensitive clinical tools used to try to assess appropriate extracellular fluid volume status. The results of our study indicated that BIA may play an important complementary role in defining categories of hydration in PD patients.

Loss of salt and water homeostasis is an invariable feature of progressive chronic renal disease [28]. Hydration status is dependent mostly on the balance of fluid intake, and fluid removal by dialysis and urine output. All intake and output are targeted to be balanced in order to reach an ideal 'dry weight', with normotension and trivial peripheral edema. The relationship between correct 'dry weight' targeting and preservation of RRF is crucial [29]. Reanalysis of the CANUSA data revealed that RRF is one of the most powerful predictors of outcome in PD patients [30]. Unfortunately, for most PD patients RRF declines gradually and ceases within 3–5 years after the start of PD, though this rate is slower than that experienced with conventional intermittent HD [30–32]. Based on these observations, several authors have advocated keeping patients 'wet' for the protection of RRF, but this runs the risk of potentially contributing to volume overload with peripheral edema, hypertension, pulmonary congestion and left ventricular hypertrophy [33]. Up to 40% of chronic PD patients have been reported to develop one or more episodes of circulatory congestion during prospective follow-up of 3 years [34]. Maintenance of RRF appeared to be protective because it allowed patients to better manage fluid balance. Taking care of strict dietary salt restriction could be the first step to maintaining 'equilibrium' between RRF and normovolemia [30].

ADEMEX study clearly showed that hypervolemia of CAPD patients is an important and independent predictor of overall survival and cardiovascular death [35]. Chronic fluid overload causes hypertension and eventually development of left ventricular hypertrophy, followed by poor prognosis [34]. Wang [34] reported over 90% of prevalent PD patients to present with left ventricular hypertrophy. However, if clinical research and practice are to evolve recognizing the importance of fluid volume in PD patient outcomes, then improving our bedside assessments is an overarching goal that requires further study. The 'gold standard' method for measuring total body water (deuterium oxide dilution) is a cumbersome and labor-intensive technique [36]. Several other techniques are currently under development (e.g. densitometry, neutron activation analysis, and measurement of total body potassium), and many of these have provided accurate and precise data, but are still to date too costly, time-consuming and impractical for routine clinical use [37]. Therefore, there is an urgent need for simple-to-use, reproducible and reliable means to estimate fluid volume status, particularly in patients who do not present with clinically overt volume overload.

In our study, we explored the usefulness of BIA in evaluation of fluid status in chronic PD patients, and found it to correlate with other markers of fluid volume in a stepwise pattern. Based on BIA measurements, the patients who were most 'wet' (lowest BIA tertile), had higher BNP, RRF and UF than the normovolemic or least wet patients (highest BIA tertile). Acknowledging that the level of BNP is elevated in states of circulatory hypervolemia and cardiac distension, our results suggest that BIA is capable of detecting

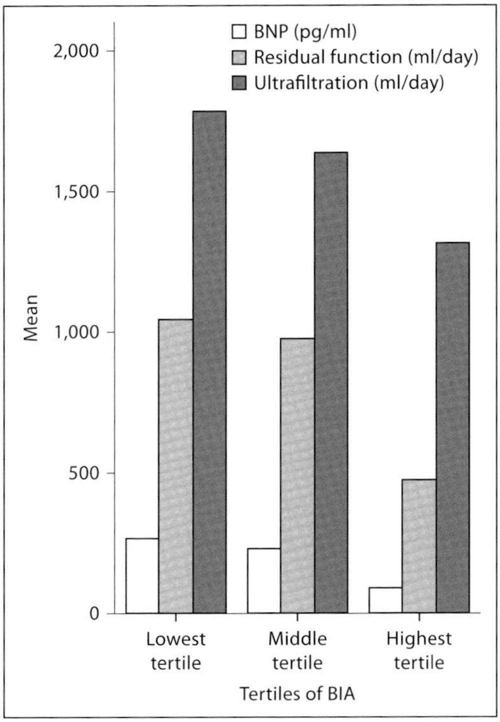

Fig. 1. Mean level of BNP, RRF and UF according to BIA results divided into tertiles.

hypervolemia also in PD patients. This is in line with earlier observations, where BIA has worked best in distinguishing hypervolemia, rather than normo- or hypovolemia [5, 18–20, 38]. Considering the serious consequences of hypervolemia on cardiac morbidity and mortality, this characteristic of BIA highlights its potential importance in the clinical armamentarium.

Importantly, in our study the patients for whom BIA indicated hypervolemia had also higher amount of RRF and UF. The explanation for this is somewhat speculative. It would be tempting to suggest that the patients with better preserved RRF drink more freely and thus have an increased amount of hydration, and likewise the daily UF required to maintain a neutral balance would necessarily be higher. The same reasoning could also explain why the patients who had only very limited RRF had higher R/H by BIA and lower levels of BNP, both variables reflecting normo- or hypovolemia. In other words, lack of RRF led to self-imposed dietary fluid restriction and hence a less hydrated state. An alternative explanation is that patients who were chronically underhydrated were more prone to hypotension and tissue hypoperfusion, and had a resultant loss of RRF. Only a prospective trial using BIA to target a particular category could tease out some of the causal relationships between our cross-sectional observations.

Another interesting aspect of our study was the comparison pertaining to the subgroups of CAPD and APD patients. Specifically, the subjects using CAPD had significantly higher levels of BNP compared to patients receiving APD. This is in concordance with some earlier results [1]. The matter is, however, very complex and subject to tremendous degrees of bias based on patient selection. In a large study by Paniagua et al. [1] with 753 prevalent dialysis patients, CAPD patients (n = 230) had higher TBW and ECV, and systolic and diastolic blood pressures compared to APD patients (n = 135), thus suggesting CAPD patients to have had more fluid overload. Opposed to these results, Bavbek et al. [39] found APD patients to have higher BNP levels in their study of 62 PD patients. Their APD patients (n = 30), however, although with somewhat lower blood pressure compared to CAPD patients, presented with significantly higher left ventricular mass index, which is often caused by chronic fluid overload.

The limitations of our study merit discussion. First of all, these results represent a single-center experience, with a relatively small number of patients. Although our results establish correlation between fluid overload by BIA technique and elevated BNP, these results are cross-sectional and do not establish any causality. A long-term prospective study with greater statistical power would be required to determine if targeting dry weight based on BIA is a clinically useful strategy to achieve euvolemia in PD patients, and if BNP or NT-pro BNP are valid and independent markers for hypervolemia in this population. Furthermore, some questions remain with respect to the use of BIA in dialysis patients in general [40]. Firstly, although single-frequency BIA has great potential to probe the complex combinations of body composition abnormalities, the technique has limitations. BIA assumes that the body behaves as a uniform electrical conductor, which it not entirely correct in reality as limbs provide a disproportionate contribution to impedance with their smaller cross-sectional area compared to trunk – a characteristic to which BIA is relatively insensitive [41, 42]. Secondly, position and posture of the subject are particularly important, and measurements should be performed after a standard period of recumbency [43]. Thirdly, single-frequency BIA is insensitive to free peritoneal fluid [44–46]. To correct for these technical limitations we took all possible precautions to perform measurements correctly, and only after drainage of PD fluid.

Conclusions

In our study, we explored the relationship of BIA measurements with BNP, RRF and UF in chronic PD patients, and found hypervolemia by BIA correlate to and distinguish patients with higher levels of BNP, RRF and UF in a stepwise pattern. This suggests that BIA may better inform hydration status, and serve as an additional clinical tool in management of chronic PD patients.

Acknowledgments

The authors wish to thank the nurses and patients of the peritoneal dialysis program at the St. Bortolo Hospital, Vicenza, Italy.

Disclosure Statement

Statement of financial support: BNP kits and BNP Triage MeterPro® device were provided by Biosite® Inc. Diagnostics, San Diego, Calif., USA, without charge and influence on the content of the manuscript. No kits were freely on market at the time of the study.

References

1 Paniagua R, Ventura MD, Avila-Díaz M, et al: NT-proBNP, fluid volume overload and dialysis modality are independent predictors of mortality in ESRD patients. Nephrol Dial Transplant 2010;25:551–557.

2 van den Wall Bake AW, Kooman JP, Lange JM, et al: Adequacy of peritoneal dialysis and the importance of preserving residual renal function. Nephrol Dial Transplant 2006;21(suppl 2):ii34–ii37.

3 Cheng LT, Chen W, Tang W, et al: Residual renal function and volume control in peritoneal dialysis patients. Nephron Clin Pract 2006;104:c47–c54.

4 Asghar RB, Green S, Engel B, et al: Relationship of demographic, dietary, and clinical factors to the hydration status of patients on peritoneal dialysis. Perit Dial Int 2004;24:231–239.

5 Konings CJ, Kooman JP, Schonck M, et al: Assessment of fluid status in peritoneal dialysis patients. Perit Dial Int 2002;22:683–692

6 Wang X, Axelsson J, Lindholm B, et al: Volume status and blood pressure in continuous ambulatory peritoneal dialysis patients. Blood Purif 2005;23:373–378.

7 Svensson M, Gorst-Rasmussen A, Schmidt EB, et al: NT-pro-BNP is an independent predictor of mortality in patients with end-stage renal disease. Clin Nephrol 2009;71:380–386.

8 Wang AY, Lam CW, Yu CM, et al: N-terminal pro-brain natriuretic peptide: an independent risk predictor of cardiovascular congestion, mortality, and adverse cardiovascular outcomes in chronic peritoneal dialysis patients. J Am Soc Nephrol 2007;18:321–330.

9 Rutten HJ, Korevaar JC, Boeschoten EW, et al, NECOSAD Study Group: B-type natriuretic peptide and amino-terminal atrial natriuretic peptide predict survival in peritoneal dialysis. Perit Dial Int 2006;26:598–602.

10 Sheen V, Bhalla V, Tulua-Tata A, et al: The use of B-type natriuretic peptide to assess volume status in patients with end-stage renal disease. Am Heart J 2007;153:244.e1–e5.

11 Roueff S, Martin E, Chauffert ML, et al: Brain natriuretic peptide variations are linked to volume status in hemodialysis patients. Clin Nephrol 2008;70:508–513.

12 Lee JA, Kim DH, Yoo SJ, et al: Association between serum n-terminal pro-brain natriuretic peptide concentration and left ventricular dysfunction and extracellular water in continuous ambulatory peritoneal dialysis patients. Perit Dial Int 2006;26:360–365.

13 Gangji AS, Helal BA, Churchill DN, et al: Association between N-terminal propeptide B-type natriuretic peptide and markers of hypervolemia. Perit Dial Int 2008;28:308–311.

14 David S, Kümpers P, Seidler V, et al: Diagnostic value of N-terminal pro-B-type natriuretic peptide (NT-proBNP) for left ventricular dysfunction in patients with chronic kidney disease stage 5 on haemodialysis. Nephrol Dial Transplant 2008;23:1370–1377.

15 Woodard GE, Rosado JA: Recent advances in natriuretic peptide research. J Cell Mol Med 2007;11:1263–1271.

16 Matthie J, Zarowitz B, De Lorenzo A, et al: Analytic assessment of the various bioimpedance methods used to estimate body water. J Appl Physiol 1998;84:1801–1816.

17 Bosy-Westphal A, Danielzik S, Dörhöfer RP, et al: Patterns of bioelectrical impedance vector distribution by body mass index and age: implications for body-composition analysis. Am J Clin Nutr 2005;82:60–68.

18 Konings CJ, Kooman JP, Schonck M, et al: Influence of fluid status on techniques used to assess body composition in peritoneal dialysis patients. Perit Dial Int 2003;23:184–190.

19 Piccoli A, Rossi B, Pillon L, et al: A new method for monitoring body fluid variation by bioimpedance analysis: the RXc graph. Kidney Int 1994;46:534–539.

20 Piccoli A, Italian CAPD-BIA Study Group: Bioelectric impedance vector distribution in peritoneal dialysis patients with different hydration status. Kidney Int 2004;65:1050–1063.

21 van de Kerkhof J, Konings CJ, van Kreel B, et al: Bioimpedance analysis and assessment of intracellular water in peritoneal dialysis patients. Perit Dial Int 2003;23:591–593.

22 Crepaldi C, Soni S, Chionh CY, et al: Application of body composition monitoring to peritoneal dialysis patients. Contrib Nephrol. Basel, Karger, 2009, vol 163, pp 1–6.

23 Papakrivopoulou E, Lillywhite S, Davenport A: Is N-terminal probrain-type natriuretic peptide a clinically useful biomarker of volume overload in peritoneal dialysis patients? Nephrol Dial Transplant 2012;27:396–401.

24 Twardowski ZJ: Clinical value of standardized equilibration tests in CAPD patients. Blood Purif 1989;7:95–108.

25 Ates K: Salt and water in PD: the Turkish contribution. Perit Dial Int 2008;28:224–228.

26 Kuhlmann MK, Zhu F, Seibert E, et al: Bioimpedance, dry weight and blood pressure control: new methods and consequences. Curr Opin Nephrol Hypertens 2005;14:543–549.

27 Khandelwal M, Oreopoulos DG: Is there a need for low sodium dialysis solution for peritoneal dialysis patients? Adv Perit Dial 2004;20:156–162.

28 Mitch WE, Wilcox CS: Disorders of body fluids, sodium and potassium in chronic renal failure. Am J Med 1982;72:536–550.

29 Wang AY: The 'heart' of peritoneal dialysis. Perit Dial Int 2007;27(suppl 2):S228–S232.

30 Van Biesen W, Lameire N, Verbeke F, et al: Residual renal function and volume status in peritoneal dialysis patients: a conflict of interest? J Nephrol 2008;21:299–304.

31 Dell'Aquila R, Berlingò G, Pellanda MV, et al: Continuous ambulatory peritoneal dialysis and automated peritoneal dialysis: are there differences in outcome? Contrib Nephrol 2009;163:292–299.

32 Liao CT, Chen YM, Shiao CC, et al: Rate of decline of residual renal function is associated with all-cause mortality and technique failure in patients on long-term peritoneal dialysis. Nephrol Dial Transplant 2009;24:2909–2914.

33 Tzamaloukas AH: Risk of extracellular volume expansion in long-term peritoneal dialysis. Adv Perit Dial 2005;21:106–111.

34 Wang AY: Cardiovascular risk factors in peritoneal dialysis patients revisited. Perit Dial Int 2007;27(suppl 2):S223–S227.
35 Paniaqua R, Amato D, Mujais S, et al: Predictive value of brain natriuretic peptides in patients on peritoneal dialysis: results from the ADEMEX Trial. Clin J Am Soc Nephrol 2008;3:407–415.
36 Moon J, Tobkin SE, Roberts MD, et al: Total body water estimations in healthy men and women using bioimpedance spectroscopy: a deuterium oxide comparison. Nutr Metab 2008;5:7.
37 Mattsson S, Thomas BJ: Development of methods for body composition studies. Phys Med Biol 2006;51:R203–R228.
38 Chen YC, Lin CJ, Wu CJ, et al: Comparison of extracellular volume and blood pressure in hemodialysis and peritoneal dialysis patients. Nephron Clin Pract 2009;113:c112–c116.
39 Bavbek N, Akay H, Altay M, et al: Serum BNP concentration and left ventricular mass in CAPD and automated peritoneal dialysis patients. Perit Dial Int 2007;27:663–668.
40 Kotanko P, Levin NW, Zhu F: Current state of bioimpedance technologies in dialysis. Nephrol Dial Transplant 2008;23:808–812.
41 Song JH, Lee SW, Kim GA, et al: Measurement of fluid shift in CAPD patients using segmental bioelectrical impedance analysis. Perit Dial Int 1999;19:386–390.
42 Fuller NJ, Elia M: Potential use of bioelectrical impedance of the 'whole body' and of body segments for the assessment of body composition: comparison with densitometry and anthropometry. Eur J Clin Nutr 1989;43:779–791.
43 Roos AN, Westendorop RG, Frölich M, et al: Tetrapolar body impedance is influenced by body posture and plasma sodium concentration. Eur J Clin Nutr 1992;46:53–60.
44 McCullough AJ, Mullen KD, Kalhan SC: Measurement of total body and extracellular water in cirrhotic patients with and without ascites. Hepatology 1991;14:1102–1111.
45 Rallison LR, Kushner RF, Penn D, et al: Errors in estimating peritoneal fluid by bioelectrical impedance analysis and total body electrical conductivity. J Am Coll Nutr 1993;12:66–72.
46 Caillette A, Labeeuw M, Zech P: Total body water determination using tetrapolar impedancemetry in CAPD patients. Nephrol Dial Transplant 1994;9:585.

Mikko Haapio
Consultant Nephrologist
Helsinki University Central Hospital, Division of Nephrology
PO Box 340
FI–00029 HUS (Finland)
Tel. +358 9 4711, E-Mail mikko.haapio@hus.fi

Ronco C, Rosner MH, Crepaldi C (eds): Peritoneal Dialysis – State-of-the-Art 2012.
Contrib Nephrol. Basel, Karger, 2012, vol 178, pp 246–250

Today's Approaches to Prevent Peritonitis

Beth Piraino

Renal Electrolyte Division, Department of Medicine, Pittsburgh, Pa., USA

Abstract

Peritonitis continues to be a significant problem in patients on peritoneal dialysis. There is a striking variability of peritonitis rates from one center to another. These results suggest that all centers can strive for the low levels of peritonitis that are seen at some centers of excellence (0.3 episodes per year at risk or lower). Routine monitoring of PD related infections as organism specific rates (rather than proportions) is critical to achieving lower rates. Training and retraining of PD patients may be key to lowering peritonitis rates, particularly from organisms that commonly come from contamination such as coagulase-negative staphylococcus (CNS). Rates of CNS peritonitis may be used as a hallmark of adequate patient training, with a goal of a CNS peritonitis rate of 0.03 episodes per year at risk or less. New technology in connectology would be helpful to lower peritonitis related to contamination. Protocols to prevent peritonitis related to exit site infection include exit site mupirocin or exit site gentamicin as part of routine care. A randomized control trial (RCT) comparing exit site medi-honey to intranasal mupirocin is nearing completion and may prove to be an attractive alternative. Enteric peritonitis may be due to a bowel source; there are limited data on approaches to prevention. Procedures such as colonoscopy are clearly a risk for peritonitis and prophylaxis is recommended. Bowel approaches such as the prescription of a probiotic should be tested in a multicenter RCT to see if such approaches may lower enteric peritonitis. Hypokalemia is a known risk factor for peritonitis from *Enterobacteriacea* and should be prevented/treated. More research is needed to test various approaches to reduce peritonitis. Until more RCTs have been done, best demonstrated practices (as outlined in the recent ISPD position paper) should be utilized to lower peritonitis rates.

Peritonitis continues to remain a major problem in patients on peritoneal dialysis (PD). It not only can lead to technique failure and hospitalizations, but may also be associated with an increased risk of death [1]. Peritonitis-associated death, defined as death due to sepsis from peritonitis, death with a positive effluent culture, death within 14 days of the onset of peritonitis, or death during a hospital admissions with peritonitis, occurs in 5% of all PD patients [1]. An increased frequency of peritonitis is associated with an increased risk of dying, especially in older patients [1]. The cause of death is often cardiovascular. Risk factors for death-associated with peritonitis include fast peritoneal transport, poor nutritional status, particularly lower normalized protein catabolic rate, and non-Gram-positive bacteria [2]. A lot of attention has been focused in recent years on approaches to decrease peritonitis risk [3–5]. The 2005 ISPD Guidelines on Peritoneal Dialysis Infections included portions on prevention, which in 2010 and 2011 were further expanded and updated [4, 5]. Unfortunately, the data on how to prevent infections are rather limited.

There is a striking variation in peritonitis rates from one center to another (table 1). Recent published registries from Scotland and Australia confirm the markedly wide range in rates of peritonitis from one program to another [6, 7]. Interestingly, the overall rate of peritonitis was the same in the two countries, 0.6 episodes per year at risk. Within the two countries some programs had much lower rates than the national average, others quite a bit higher

Table 1. Total and organism-specific peritonitis rates given as episodes per year at risk by countries or registries

	Australia (7)	Scotland[1] (6)	Japan (8)
Number of centers	72	10	13
Total peritonitis	0.60	0.60	0.28
Range rates by center	0.13–2.0	0.40–0.78	0.09–0.42
CN *Staphylococcus*	0.15	0.18	0.03
S. aureus	0.07	0.09	0.03
Pseudomonas	0.02	0.01	0.01
Other GNR	0.11	0.05	0.03
Other	0.17	0.15	0.08
Culture negative	0.08	0.12	0.09
Fungus	0.02	0.02	0.01

[1]Does not add to 0.60 due to rounding.

[6, 7]. This variation is unexplained, although the Australian authors pointed out that many programs in their country were not following current guidelines. A recent report from the Tokai area of Japan had considerably lower rates, approximately one half the rates for Scotland and Australia [8]. Of note, the rates in Japan were strikingly lower for coagulase-negative *Staphylococcus*, Gram-negative rod and 'other' peritonitis, all of which might relate to adequacy of patient training in the procedure and particularly hand washing technique.

Measuring a Center's Peritonitis Rates

The first step to improving outcomes in a program is to determine the peritonitis rate of the center. This should be calculated frequently, but at least yearly. The program should calculate not only the overall rate (number of peritonitis episodes in the program for a period of time divided by dialysis years at risk for the program for the same period), but also the episodes as organism-specific rates (episodes by each micro-organism divided by dialysis years at risk). The organism-specific rates for Scotland, Australia and part of Japan are shown in table 1. Such information permits comparison of the organism specific rates to those published in the literature, and to previous years so that trends can be determined. This provides an absolute risk of infection by organism rather than a percentage, which is much less useful, as the overall rate may vary from year to year. As an example, in a recently published paper on peritonitis from a single Brazilian center, the overall rate was 0.65 episodes per year at risk, very similar to both Australia and Scotland [9]. The rate of coagulase-negative *Staphylococcus* peritonitis was 0.18 episodes per year at risk, also similar to the rate reported in Australia and Scotland, but the *Staphylococcus aureus* peritonitis rate was 0.05 (better) and the rate of *Pseudomonas* peritonitis 0.03 (a bit worse). This gives comparative data that percentages do not provide.

Organism specific rates give important clues to causality (table 2). Coagulase-negative *Staphylococcus*, for example, is widely accepted as primarily being due to contamination during the procedure. A high absolute rate of coagulase negative staphylococcus peritonitis (any rate above 0.04 episodes per year at risk) strongly indicates a problem with patient training, hand hygiene and possibly the dialysis equipment, particularly the connectology, used. Rates of coagulase negative staphylococcus of 0.03 episodes per year at risk are achievable (as shown by the rate in the Japanese registry in table 1 and the rate in our own program). If the rates of coagulase-negative *Staphylococcus* peritonitis are high in a program, the training program should be re-examined.

Interventions to Lower Peritonitis Due to Contamination: Training Methods

Training of PD patients to prevent peritonitis is not particularly well studied. Most experts in the field believe that one-on-one training by a well-trained PD nurse is best, and that adult learning approach combining theory and practice with repetition of the procedure under close supervision is a good approach [5]. The length of training is best

Table 2. Causes of peritonitis and commonly associated organisms

Causes	Predominant organisms
Contamination	coagulase-negative *Staphylococcus*, GNR, *S. aureus*
Enteric source	*Enterobacteraciae*, *Candida*, anaerobes, *Enterococcus*
Exit site, tunnel infections	*S. aureus*, *P. aeruginosa*, diphtheroids, GNR
Bacteremia	*Streptococcus*, *S. aureus*
Gynecologic	*Streptococcus*, fungus, GNR

tailored to the patient but should never be rushed or fit into a rigid time line. It is important to test the patient at the end of training to ensure mastery of information. A recent study from China showed that more experienced nurses had patients with the longest period to first Gram positive peritonitis [10]. Peritonitis rates were very good at this center: 0.17, 0.23 and 0.26 episodes per year at risk in patients trained by the most experienced to least experienced nurses. Training was one-on-one.

Recognizing contamination and the correct approach is critical to preventing peritonitis. While it is impossible to cover every possible type of contamination during training it is possible to teach the theory so that the patient can translate this information. Everyone in the program needs to understand the seriousness of contamination and the appropriate corrective action to prevent peritonitis from developing. If potentially contaminated fluid has been infused into the abdominal space, then prophylactic antibiotics are required, and I believe a culture of the effluent is helpful as well. If no fluid has been infused, then a simple tubing exchange may be done.

Re-training is also not well studied but current information suggests that many patients slip away from the correct procedure once home. Reinforcing the training at regular intervals may well be beneficial. A multicenter randomized trial on 'Prevention of Peritonitis in Peritoneal Dialysis' was started on January 2010 to test retraining as a method to prevent peritonitis (ClinicaTrials.gov). Until the results of this study are available, it might be prudent to consider retraining/reinforcing at the time of the home visit which ideally should be within the first month of PD to assess the environment, then again at 3 months and 6 months.

Connectology to Prevent Peritonitis

Connectology has long been known to markedly impact infection risk. Spike technology is associated with an increased risk of infection, and is fortunately being eliminated from the market. Flush of effluent through the tubing after connection, prior to fill, is also been clearly shown to decrease risk of peritonitis. Di Bonaventura et al, have tested in vitro the effect of a new PD connector on heavy contamination with both *Staphylococcus epidermidis* and *Pseudomonas aeruginosa*, and found that the new connector completely eliminated the entrance of bacteria into the bag [11]. Further studies will be needed.

Protocols to Prevent Peritonitis due to Catheter Exit Site and Tunnel Infections

There is a large body of evidence showing that *S. aureus* carriage is a risk factor for both *S. aureus* exit site infection and peritonitis in PD patients [3–5]. There is also considerable evidence to indicate that use of an antibiotic such as mupirocin or gentamicin at the exit site as part of daily care is useful to decrease the risk of exit site infections, and therefore *S. aureus* peritonitis and possibly peritonitis due to Gram negative organisms [12]. This approach has been opposed on the grounds of enhancing resistance to mupirocin, but mupirocin is rarely used as a treatment, so the gains from preventing serious infections (and thus the morbidity and mortality associated) seem to outweigh the potential of resistance to this antibiotic. Furthermore, use of mupirocin decreases the use of other much more important antibiotics by decreasing infection risk. Gentamicin at the exit site has been shown in one multicenter randomized control trial to out-perform mupirocin in preventing both exit site infections and peritonitis, with some slight increase in risk of fungal exit site infections [12]. A recent comparison of two periods at a single center, first period using mupirocin for exit site care, and the second period using gentamicin for exit site care, found that Gram-negative peritonitis fell from 0.10 versus 0.06 episodes per year at risk ($p = 0.07$), and fungal peritonitis increased slightly (0.01 vs. 0.04 episodes per year at risk [$p = 0.067$]) [13]. The gentamicin cream was less effective in preventing *S. aureus* exit site infection (0.022 vs. 0.055 episodes per year at risk, $p = 0.03$) although both rates are low, as can be seen by the *S. aureus* rates of 0.07 and 0.09 episodes per year at risk in Australia and Scotland as shown in table 1, and similar to the rate of 0.03 episodes per year at risk seen in Japan. Each center will need to decide whether mupirocin or gentamicin is preferable at the exit site. Currently, a randomized control trial of medi-honey applied to the exit site versus intranasal mupirocin application is nearing completion and may allow another choice.

Preventing Peritonitis from Gastrointestinal Sources

Other protocols are directed at preventing gastrointestinal sources of peritonitis, an area rather poorly understood or studied. Many episodes of single organism Gram negative peritonitis may well relate to contamination and possibly can be decreased by better techniques and in particular hand washing. However, some Gram-negative peritonitis is likely from transmural migration. It may be that bowel pathology such as diverticulitis, ischemic bowel, constipation, and colitis are all potential sources of peritonitis. Yip et al. [14] found that in the 104 Chinese PD patients who underwent either barium enema or colonoscopy, that diverticulosis, especially of the ascending colon, was an independent risk factor for enteric peritonitis (HR 6.89, 95% CI of 1.43 to 33.3, $p = 0.016$). Colonoscopy without antibiotic prophylaxis also poses a risk of serious peritonitis and can mostly be prevented by providing antibiotic prophylaxis and keeping the abdomen empty of effluent during the procedure [15].

It has been shown that hypokalemia is a risk factor for *Enterobacteriacea* peritonitis [16]. The exact mechanism has not been determined, but may relate to slower bowel motility which perhaps enhances transmural migration of organisms. While prevention and treatment of hypokalemia have not been studied n a prospective fashion to decrease such risk, it seems reasonable to prevent and treat hypokalemia in PD patients, especially since low potassium levels have also been shown to increase the risk of dying in PD patients. Intestinal microbial imbalance with decreased *Bifidobacterium* species in nondiabetic PD patients is common, and may result in impaired intestinal barrier function and increase vulnerability to transmural migration of pathogenic bacteria [17]. Wang et al. [17] suggest a clinical trial testing the efficacy of oral probiotics in PD patients.

Preventing Relapsing and Repeat Peritonitis

Repeat peritonitis defined as peritonitis with the same organism more than 4 weeks after the initial episode is most often due to *Staphylococcus* [18]. A first episode of coagulase-negative *Staphylococcus* peritonitis is associated with an increased risk of subsequent peritonitis from the same organism (OR 2.1, CI 1.5–2.8, $p < 0.001$) compared to other organisms [19]. The highest risk period is the first 6 months after the peritonitis episode. Whether this is due to repeat contamination or to involvement of the biofilm of the catheter with recrudescence is unclear. A decrease in the albumin level is a risk factor for subsequent peritonitis [20]. Whether a longer course of antibiotic therapy, the addition of rifampin to the therapy, or nutritional intervention might prevent relapsing and repeat peritonitis is poorly studied.

Conclusion

There is marked variation in peritonitis rates from one center to another. Many centers do not follow the ISPD guidelines. High-quality research is lacking on approaches to prevent peritonitis. Further research is very much needed in this area. The recently published ISPD position paper on Prevention of PD-Related Infections is intended to present the best demonstrated practices to lower peritonitis risk, and it is recommended that all centers familiarize themselves with this paper and apply the suggestions as appropriate [5]. Following a center's organism-specific rates is critical to identifying problematic areas to guide programmatic changes in an iterative fashion to reduce infection rates.

References

1 Fried LF, Bernardini J, Johnston JR, Piraino B: Peritonitis influences mortality in peritoneal dialysis patients. J Am Soc Nephrol 1006;7:2176–2182.
2 Pajek J, Gucek A, Kloberne A, Pintar T: Severe peritonitis in patients treated with peritoneal dialysis: a case series study. Ther Apheresis Dial 2011;15:250–256.
3 Piraino B, Bailie GR, Bernardini J, et al: ISPD Ad Hoc Advisory Committee. Peritoneal dialysis-related infections recommendations: 2005 update. Perit Dial Int 2005;25:107–131.
4 Li PK, Szeto CC, Piraino B, Bernardini J, Figueiredo AE, Gupta A, Johsnon DW, Kuijper EJ, Lye WC, Salzer W, Schaefer F, Struijk DG: Peritoneal dialysis-related infections recommendations: 2010 Update. Perit Dial Int 2010;30:393–423.
5 Piraino B, Bernardini J, Brown E, Figueiredo A, Johnson DW, Lye WC, Price V, Ramalakshmi S, Szeto CC: ISPD position statement on reducing the risks of peritoneal dialysis-related infections. Perit Dial Int 2011;31:614–630.
6 Brown MC, Simpson K, Kerssens JJ, Mactier RA, Scottish Renal Registry: Peritoneal dialysis-associated peritonitis rates and outcomes in a national cohort are not improving in the post-millennium (200–2007). Perit Dial Int 2011;31:639–650
7 Ghali J, Bannister KM Brown FG, Rosman JB, Wiggins KJ, Johnson DW, McDonald SP: Microbiology and outcomes of peritonitis in Australian peritoneal dialysis patients. Perit Dial Int 2011;31:651–662.
8 Mizuno M, Ito Y, Tanaka A, et al: Peritonitis is still an important factor for withdrawal from peritoneal dialysis therapy in the Tokai area of Japan. Clin Exp Nephrol 2011;5:727–737.
9 Oliveira LG, Luengo J, Caramori CT, Montelii AC, Cunha M, Barretti P: Peritonitis in recent years: clinical findings and predictors of treatment response of 170 episodes at a single Brazilian center. Int Urol Nephrol 2012 Feb 3 [Epub ahead of print].
10 Yang Z, Xu R, Zhuo M, Dong J: Advanced nursing experience is beneficial for lowering the peritonitis rate in patients on peritoneal dialysis. Perit Dial Int 2012;32:60–66.
11 Di Bonaventura G, Cerasoli P, Pompillo Arrizza F, Liberator L, Stingone A, Sirolli V, Arduini A, Bonomini M: In vitro microbiology studies on a new peritoneal dialysis connector. Perit Dial Intern 2012 Feb 1 [Epub ahead of print].
12 Bernardini J, Bender F, Florio T, Sloand J, PalmMonatalbano L, Fried L, Piraino B: Randomized double-blind trial of antibiotic exit site cream for prevention of exit site infection in peritoneal dialysis patients. J Am Soc Nephrol 2005;16:539–545.
13 Pierce DA, Williamson JC, Mauck VS, Russell GB, Palavecino E, Burkart JM: The effect on peritoneal dialysis pathogens of changing topical antibiotic prophylaxis. Perit Dial Int 2012 Feb 1 [Epub ahead of print]
14 Yip T, Tse KC, Lam MF, Cheng SW, Lui SL, Tang S, Ng M, Chan TM, Lai KN, Lo WK: Colonic diverticulosis as a risk factor for peritonitis in Chinese peritoneal dialysis patients. Perit Dial Int 2010;30:187–191.
15 Yip T, Tse KC, Lam MF, Cheng SW, Lui SL, Tang S, Ng M, Chan TM, Lai KN, Lo WK: Risks and outcomes of peritonitis after flexible colonoscopy in CAPD patients. Perit Dial Int 2007;27:560–564.
16 Chuang YW, Shu KH, Yu TM, Cheng CH, Chen CH: Hypokalaemia: an independent risk factor of *Eneterobacteriaceae* peritonitis in CAPD patients. Nephrol Dial Transplant 2009;24:1603–1608.
17 Wang IK, Lai HC, Yu CJ, Liang CC, Chang CT, Kuo HL, Yang YF, Lin CC, Lin HH, Liu YL, Chang YC, Wu YY, Chen CH, Li CY, Chuang FR, Huang CC, Lin CH, Lin HC: Real-time PCR analysis of the intestinal microbiotas in peritoneal dialysis patients. Appl Environ Microbiol 2012;78:1107–1112.
18 Burke M, Hawley CM, Badve S, McDonald SP, Brown FG, Boudvilee N, Wiggins KJ, Bannister KM, Johnson DW: Relapsing and recurrent peritoneal dialysis-associated peritonitis: a multicenter registry study. Am J Kidney Dis 2011;58:429–436.
19 Nessim SJ, Nisenbaum R, Bargman JM, Jassal V: Microbiology of peritonitis in peritoneal dialysis patients with multiple episodes. Perit Dial Int 2012 Feb [Epub ahead of print].
20 Ozturk S, Soyluk O, Karakaya D, Yazici H, Caliskan YK, Yildiz A, Bozfakioglu S: Is decline in serum albumin an ominous sign for subsequent peritonitis in peritoneal dialysis patients? Adv Perit Dial 2009;25:172–177.

Prof. Beth Piraino
Renal Electrolyte Division, Department of Medicine, Suite 200
3504 Fifth Avenue
Pittsburgh, PA 15213 (USA)
Tel. +1 412 383 4899, E-Mail Piraino@pitt.edu

Ronco C, Rosner MH, Crepaldi C (eds): Peritoneal Dialysis – State-of-the-Art 2012.
Contrib Nephrol. Basel, Karger, 2012, vol 178, pp 251–257

Transplant Outcomes and Dialysis Modality

Richard Fuquay · Isaac Teitelbaum

Division of Renal Diseases and Hypertension, University of Colorado School of Medicine, Aurora, Colo., USA

Abstract

The prevalence of end-stage renal disease continues to rise, and patients are treated for increasing periods of time with hemodialysis, peritoneal dialysis, and transplantation. Transition from one treatment modality to another is common, and the astute clinician should be aware of a wide array of observational data regarding the advantages and disadvantages of certain modalities around these transition points. In this paper, we explore data that informs lifelong care of the ESRD patient. The discussion focuses on the impact of dialysis modality on the likelihood of transplantation, and then moves to short-term and long-term outcomes after transplantation. Large observational studies indicate that peritoneal dialysis patients may experience increased rates of graft thrombosis and early (3-month) graft failure. Importantly, however, compared to their HD counterparts PD patients enjoy advantages in shorter time to transplantation, decreased rates of delayed graft function (DGF), and enhanced long-term transplant survival.

'Integrated care' is a concept introduced by Davies et al. [1] which conceptualizes hemodialysis (HD), peritoneal dialysis (PD), and transplantation as three complementary treatment modalities, each with advantages and disadvantages for an individual patient. The typical end-stage renal disease (ESRD) patient will evolve though different stages of a chronic illness with myriad treatment options. In this paradigm, rather than viewing modality change as a negative event described as 'technique failure', changes should be anticipated as usual events for patients living with a chronic disease. Nephrology centers' ability to offer individualized counseling and a full array of therapeutic options are necessary for the 'integrated care' concept to function.

Dialysis technology and immunosuppressive strategies are improving, and accordingly patients can be expected to live longer and undergo more transitions of care, starting with the transition from chronic kidney disease (CKD) to renal replacement therapy (RRT). Subsequent to starting RRT, clinical circumstances may dictate changes from HD to PD, or vice versa, based upon clinical circumstances. The number of incident US ESRD patients may have reached a plateau in 2006 at slightly over 100,000 per year, while the number of prevalent dialysis patients is still slowly rising [2], as is the number of patients undergoing kidney transplantation. Guiding patients toward optimal management of this complicated and chronic disease will require knowledge of the benefits and pitfalls of RRT modality changes. This paper will aim to summarize and assess existing data to assist nephrologists as they counsel patients on the impact of PD versus HD as a dialysis modality before transplantation. We will first discuss likelihood of transplantation and survival on the wait-list, then turn to short-term transplant outcomes in relation to dialysis modality, and finally examine long-term transplant outcomes.

Does Dialysis Modality Influence the Likelihood of Transplantation or Mortality While on the Wait-List?

There are three reasons to study a patient's waiting time to transplantation. The first is the cumulative mortality disadvantage that accrues to patients undergoing dialysis as opposed to transplantation [3]. The second is the inconvenience and psychological burden the patient bears as he or she waits for transplant. Finally, there is data indicating that increasing dialysis vintage is associated with increased likelihood of adverse immunologic and nonimmunologic outcomes after transplantation [4–7]. Therefore, when choosing a dialysis modality, it is of potential interest for the patient – and his or her nephrologist – to know whether the likelihood of either transplantation (i.e. length of time on the waiting list), or death while awaiting transplantation, will be impacted by the initial choice of dialysis modality.

The most robust data, and that which is most relevant to the US, is derived from a retrospective US Renal Data System (USRDS) database study published by Snyder et al. [8] in 2002. This study was an analysis of CMS data on over 250,000 dialysis patients that received 22,776 renal transplants in the US between 1995 and 1998. The proportion of HD and PD patients in this study was 87 and 13%, respectively. The authors found that patients treated with PD had roughly twice the unadjusted transplantation rate of their HD-treated counterparts at 1, 3 and 5 years after listing. After adjustment for demographics and comorbidities, transplantation was 1.39 times more likely in PD-treated patients than HD-treated patients (CI 1.35–1.43, $p < 0.0001$). HD- and PD-treated patients were listed 87 and 86% of the time, respectively, and there was no difference in listing rates for cadaveric or living donation. Though one cannot infer causality from these data, they indicate that in the US, PD-treated patients are waiting less time for transplantation.

Data from French dialysis centers also demonstrates that the waiting time to transplantation is shorter for PD-treated patients than HD-treated patients [9]. This retrospective study detailed 6,420 wait-listed and 3,464 transplanted adult patients in French centers between 1997 and 2000. Compared to the US, this is a smaller overall dialysis population, with a greater proportion undergoing transplantation. The proportion of patients receiving PD, HD, and preemptive transplantation was 10, 80 and 10%, respectively; this proportion is similar to the overall US ESRD population. PD patients' waiting time to transplantation was 0.71 ($p < 0.0001$) that of HD patients' waiting time. However, this statistical advantage disappeared when the investigators controlled for the referring dialysis center, as PD-treated patients were disproportionately cared for by nephrology units with low mean wait-times for transplantation. These data involve adequate numbers and directly answer the question of which modality is associated with faster transplantation, but they are quite specific for the French nephrology system. One can only speculate whether such confounding associations are present in the US with a fundamentally different care delivery system.

Additionally, there are data from a single Japanese center involving 1,573 total patients, showing that the overall transplantation rate is higher among PD patients [10]. In contrast, a small Chinese study involving just 402 dialysis patients found that PD patients waited longer before transplantation [5].

What about mortality while awaiting transplantation? Data suggests that there is no difference in survival between wait-listed PD- and HD-treated patients who have not previously received a transplant. A historical prospective cohort study of 12,568 adult patients who were wait-listed for transplantation, before initiating either PD or HD, found 2-year mortality rates of 6.6 and 6.9%, respectively [11]. These mortality rates are statistically equal. It should be noted that these mortality rates are much lower than that of the overall dialysis populations. Statistical adjustment for a number of baseline and laboratory values did not reveal a mortality difference, except for patients with a baseline BMI ≥26 who had increased mortality on PD compared to HD. Notwithstanding this caveat regarding overweight patients, these data indicate that survival on the transplant wait-list is probably equal between PD- and HD-treated patients. This finding was replicated in a 2011 study of Scottish patients with ESRD not due to diabetic nephropathy who were wait-listed for transplantation [12].

Does dialysis modality affect the likelihood of transplantation, or mortality while on the wait-list? In summary, PD patients probably wait less time before undergoing transplantation, based on association data that precludes causal inferences. As pertains to mortality, all dialysis patients, regardless of modality, appear to fare equally well on the wait-list.

Are Short-Term Transplant Outcomes Affected by Previous Dialysis Modality?

Delayed graft function (DGF) is one of the most clinically important short-term outcomes of renal transplantation. It is associated with increased rates of acute rejection, worse allograft survival, and higher risk of patient death [8, 13]. Study of this outcome is hampered by the varying definitions thereof utilized in the transplantation literature. DGF is most commonly defined as failure of allograft function in the first seven days after transplantation, as manifested by the need for dialysis. The decision to dialyze is subjective, however, and practices vary among centers. Alternative definitions based on urine output or the rate of reduction rate of serum creatinine exist, but there is no consensus [14]. We will discuss DGF using the most common definition – need for dialysis – with the limitations included in this definition.

Numerous studies of varying size and methodology have investigated DGF rates and have found either lower rates in PD patients compared to HD patients [8, 15–17], or no difference between PD- and HD-treated patients [18, 19]. Below is a discussion of some of the notable publications examining this important short-term transplantation outcome.

A two-center, case-control study of 234 patients found that PD patients undergoing transplantation had a lower incidence of DGF (defined as need for dialysis after surgery) and a faster decline in serum creatinine compared to their HD-treated counterparts [20]. The authors did not report a difference in the incidence of infection or surgical complication. There was, however, a statistically significant increase in the number of acute rejection episodes in the PD group compared to the HD group. Nevertheless, overall short-term outcomes were identical with similar levels of serum creatinine and percentage of grafts functioning at 6 months after transplantation.

These data were echoed in a larger retrospective study [21] of 10,584 patients in the United Network for Organ Sharing (UNOS) database, in which anuria occurred in 11.9% of HD patients vs. 8.3% of PD patients (RR 1.49, 95% CI 1.28 to 1.74, $p < 0.001$). DGF occurred in 28.6% of HD patients versus 20.0% of PD patients (RR 1.60, 95% CI 1.44 to 1.78, $p < 0.001$). Both of these associations were further strengthened when analysis was restricted to African-American patients. As the authors indicate in their discussion, clinicians' perception of less hemodynamic insult from PD may have biased clinicians to more readily perform dialysis in PD patients, and thus raise the apparent rate of DGF (due to the shortcomings of the definition discussed above), but that was not observed.

This study also reported that cold ischemia times were equal for PD- and HD-treated patients undergoing transplantation surgery [21]. This finding differs from the French study cited earlier which reported a different cold ischemia times of 20.5 and 22.4 h for PD and HD patients, respectively ($p < 0.0001$) [9]. One might expect that patients performing a continuous dialysis modality like PD would have lower mean cold ischemia times, as there would be no need to delay certain transplantation surgeries to perform hemodialysis. However, that is not consistently demonstrated by the data, and we should not assume that a difference in cold ischemia time is the cause of the lower DGF rate in PD patients.

Table 1. Studies and their findings regarding graft thrombosis

Author	Year	Setting	n	Major findings
Luna et al. [29]	2010	Spain	577	no difference in thrombosis
Palomar et al. [30]	2007	Spain	197	increased thrombosis in PD
Van der Vliet et al. [31]	1996	The Netherlands	916	increased thrombosis in CAPD
Perez Fontan et al. [32]	1996	Spain	660	no difference in thrombosis
Murphy et al. [33]	1994	Northern Ireland	202	increased thrombosis in CAPD
Ojo et al. [34]	1999	UNOS	84,513	increased thrombosis in PD
Vats et al. [35]	2000	Pittsburgh (pediatrics)	2,495	increased thrombosis in PD
Snyder et al. [8]	2002	USRDS	505	increased thrombosis in PD
McDonald et al. [36]	2003	Seattle (pediatrics)	7,247	increased thrombosis in PD

The best large-scale evidence regarding short-term outcomes after transplantation is from Snyder et al. [8]. This retrospective study of over 22,000 transplanted patients found a lower incidence of DGF among PD patients (RR 0.74, 95% CI 0.67–0.81, $p < 0.0001$) after adjustment for multiple clinical covariates. Analysis of grafts surviving less than three months showed that PD-treated patients had a higher unadjusted risk for both graft failure (OR 1.23, CI 1.09–1.39, $p < 0.001$) and death-censored graft failure (OR 1.33, CI 1.16–1.53, $p < 0.0001$) than did HD-treated patients. It is difficult to reconcile the findings that PD patients have less DGF, yet more early graft failure. In a subset of patients for which data was reported on the cause of early graft failure (which may introduce some confounding due to reporting bias), there was a statistically significant increase in graft thrombosis among PD-treated patients compared to HD-treated patients. None of the other 7 specified causes of early graft failure exhibited statistically significant differences between PD and HD patients. Post-transplant graft thrombosis has been studied in a number of studies, which are summarized in table 1.

Are short-term transplant outcomes affected by previous dialysis modality? In summary, data from Snyder and others report less DGF associated with previous PD treatment. Although there is varying size and methodology of the studies reporting an association between PD and increased graft thrombosis, the association occurs consistently enough to suggest an etiologic link. The frequency of this complication is very low, however, and overall patient and graft outcomes at 6 months are identical for patients previously treated with HD or PD.

Are Long-Term Transplant Outcomes Affected by Previous Dialysis Modality?

Post-transplant mortality has been studied in a number of small studies. Mortality after transplantation has been found to be equal among PD and HD patients in a single-center American study [4], a single-center Tunisian study [22], a single-center Turkish study [23], and three single-center British studies [24–26]. Post-transplant mortality is significantly better among PD patients in the experience of a single European center [27]. These results make it difficult to conclude which patient population – if either – fares better after transplantation. Similarly, data from the larger study by Snyder et al. [8] demonstrate that in patients whose grafts survived for at least three months after transplantation, there were no differences in graft failure, death-censored graft failure, or mortality between patients performing HD or PD prior to transplantation.

The largest study of this issue to date is a USRDS-based analysis of 92,844 patients who underwent kidney or kidney-pancreas transplantation during the 1990s. The authors report

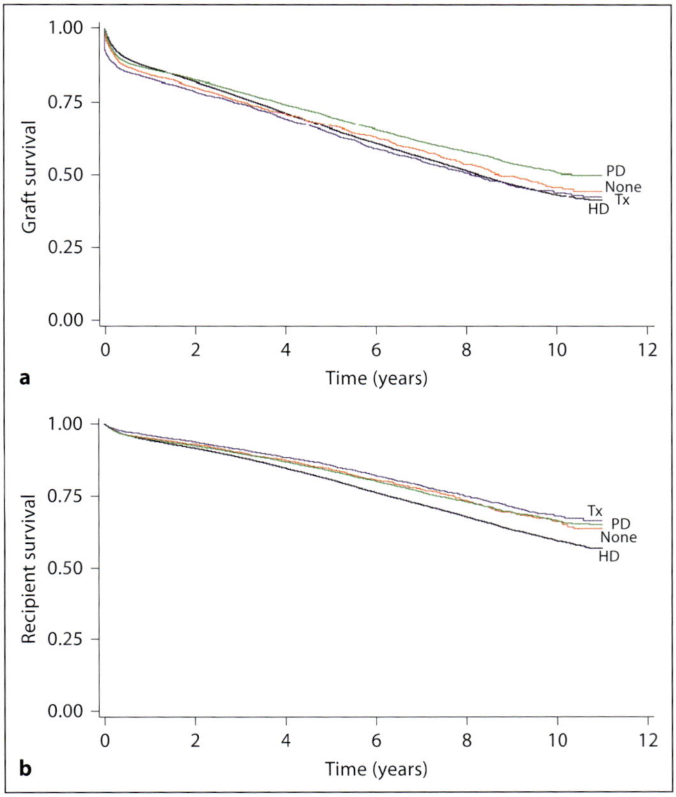

Fig. 1. Graft (**a**) and recipient survival (**b**) according to predominant modality (>50% of time on dialysis). From Goldfarb et al. [28], with permission.

small, but statistically significant, differences in graft failure between PD-treated, HD-treated, and previously transplanted patients [28]. In comparison to HD-treated patients, PD-treated patients had a lower likelihood of graft failure (HR 0.97, 95% CI 0.94–1.0, $p < 0.05$; see fig. 1), while previously transplanted patients had a higher likelihood of graft failure (HR 1.65, 95% CI 1.51–1.8, $p < 0.001$). Even more striking, PD patients had decreased mortality (HR 0.94, 95% CI 0.91–0.97, $p < 0.001$) compared to HD patients. Interestingly, previously transplanted patients had the lowest likelihood of mortality (HR 0.80, 95% CI 0.68–0.93, $p < 0.005$). It should be noted that in this study, survival was defined as total number of grafts functioning or patients alive at the end of the decade of observation, without consideration of when the transplantation surgery occurred.

Are long-term transplant outcomes affected by modality? Viewing these data as a whole, one finds some heterogeneity based on population and era. Furthermore, association studies cannot allow inferences of causality. Yet, the retrospective studies with large patient populations suggest that there may be some differences in recipient and graft survival that are favorable to patients treated with PD before transplantation.

Conclusion

Optimizing therapeutic options for the complex ESRD patient is no easy task. This paper has attempted to synthesize data that will assist nephrologists in counseling their patients on waiting time to transplantation and important short- and long-term outcomes after transplantation.

Complex clinical decisions are rarely addressed in randomized controlled trials; therefore nephrologists frequently must wade into partial and confusing data to counsel ESRD patients on the risks and benefits of different treatment paradigms. This challenging data set will improve only slowly and incrementally. In the meantime, nephrologists must continually study data and apply it to patients in an individualized manner.

References

1 Davies SJ, Van Biesen W, Nicholas J, Lameire N: Integrated care. Perit Dial Int 2001;21(suppl 3):S269–S274.
2 Collins AJ, Foley RN, Herzog C, et al: United States Renal Data System 2008 Annual Data Report. Am J Kidney Dis 2009;53(suppl):S1–S374.
3 Wolfe RA, Ashby VB, Milford EL, Ojo AO, Ettenger RE, Agodoa LY, Held PJ, Port FK: Comparison of mortality in all patients on dialysis, patients on dialysis awaiting transplantation, and recipients of a first cadaveric transplant. N Engl J Med 1999;341:1725–1730.
4 Cosio FG, Alamir A, Yim S, Pesavento TE, Falkenhain ME, Henry ML, Elkhammas EA, Davies EA, Bumgardner GL, Ferguson RM: Patient survival after renal transplantation. I. The impact of dialysis pre-transplant; Kidney Int 1998;53:767–772.
5 Yang Q, Zhao S, Chen W, Mao H, Huang F, Zheng Z, Chen L, Fei J, Yu X: Influence of dialysis modality on renal transplant complications and outcomes. Clin Nephrol 2009;72:62–68.
6 Meier-Kriesche HU, Port FK, Ojo AO, Rudich SM, Hanson JA, Cibrik DM, Leichtman AB, Kaplan B: Effect of waiting time on renal transplant outcome. Kidney Int 2000;58:1311–1317.
7 Goldfarb-Rumyantzev A, Hurdle JF, Scandling J, Wang Z, Baird B, Barenbaum L, Cheung AK: Duration of end-stage renal disease and kidney transplant outcome. Nephrol Dial Transplant 2005;20:167–175.
8 Snyder JJ, Kasiske BL, Gilbertson DT, Collins AJ: A comparison of transplant outcomes in peritoneal and hemodialysis patients. Kidney Int 2002;62:1423–1430.
9 Chalem Y, Ryckelynck JP, Tuppin P, Verger C, Chauve S, Glotz D: Access to, and outcome of, renal transplantation according to treatment modality of end-stage renal disease in France. Kidney Int 2005;67:2448–2453.
10 Mitome J, Yamamoto H, Kato N, Hayakawa H, Ikeda M, Yokoyama K, Nakayama M, Kawaguchi Y, Hosoya T: Dialysis as bridge therapy for renal transplantation: single center experience, a comparison of hemodialysis and continuous ambulatory peritoneal dialysis. Nippon Jinzo Gakkai Shi 2005;47:813–820.
11 Inrig JK, Sun JL, Yang Q, Briley LP, Szczech LA: Mortality by dialysis modality among patients who have end-stage renal disease and are awaiting renal transplantation. Clin J Am Soc Nephrol 2006;1:774–779.
12 Traynor JP, Thomson PC, Simpson K, Ayansina DT, Prescott GJ, Mactier RA: Comparison of patient survival in non-diabetic transplant-listed patients initially treated with haemodialysis or peritoneal dialysis. Nephrol Dial Transplant 2011;26:245–252.
13 Giral-Classe M, Hourmant M, Cantarovich D, Dantal J, Blancho G, Daguin P, Ancelet D, Soulillou JP: Delayed graft function of more than six days strongly decreases long-term survival of transplanted kidneys. Kidney Int 1998;54:972–978.
14 Daly PJ, Power RE, Healy DA, Hickey DP, Fitzpatrick JM, Watson RW: Delayed graft function: a dilemma in renal transplantation. BJU Int 2005;96:498–501.
15 Perez Fontan MP, Rodriguez-Carmona A, Garcia Falcon T, Moncalian J, Oliver J, Valdes F: Renal transplantation in patients undergoing chronic peritoneal dialysis. Perit Dial Int 1996;16:48–51.
16 Van Biesen W, Vanholder R, Van Loo A, Van Der Vennet M, Lameire N: Peritoneal dialysis favorably influences early graft function after renal transplantation compared to hemodialysis. Transplantation 2000;69:508–514.
17 Cacciarelli TV, Sumrani NB, DiBenedetto A, Hong JH, Sommer BG: The influence of mode of dialysis pretransplantation on long-term renal allograft outcome. Ren Fail 1993;15:545–550.
18 Triolo G, Segoloni GP, Salomone M, Piccoli GB, Messina M, Massara C, Bertinet DB, Vercellone A: Comparison between two dialytic populations undergoing renal transplantation. Adv Perit Dial 1990;6:72–75.
19 Cardella CJ, Harding ME, Abraham G, et al: Renal transplantation in older patients on peritoneal dialysis. Transplant Proc 1989;21:2022–2023.
20 Vanholder R, Heering P, Loo AV, Biesen WV, Lambert MC, Hesse U, Vennet MV, Grabensee B, Lameire N: Reduced incidence of acute renal graft failure in patients treated with peritoneal dialysis compared with hemodialysis. Am J Kidney Dis 1999;33:934–940.
21 Bleyer AJ, Burkart JM, Russell GB, Adams PL: Dialysis modality and delayed graft function after cadaveric renal transplantation. J Am Soc Nephrol 1999;10:154–159.
22 Helal I, Abderrahim E, Ben Hamida F, Zouaghi K, Ounissi M, Barbouche S, Hedri H, Ezzine S, Ben Abdallah I, Chrif M, Bardi R, Ayed K, Ben Maiz H, Ben Abdallah T, Kheder A: Impact of dialysis modality on post-transplantation results in kidney transplantation. Transplant Proc 2007;39:2547–2549.

23 Caliskan Y, Yazici H, Gorgulu N, Yelken B, Emre T, Turkmen A, Yildiz A, Aysuna N, Bozfakioglu S, Sever MS: Effect of pre-transplant dialysis modality on kidney transplantation outcome. Perit Dial Int 2009;29(suppl 2):S117–S122.
24 Evangelista JB Jr, Bennett-Jones D, Cameron JS, Ogg C, Williams DG, Taube DH, Neild G, Rudge C: Renal transplantation in patients treated with haemodialysis and short term and long term continuous ambulatory peritoneal dialysis. Br Med J (Clin Res Ed) 1985;291:1004–1007.
25 Joseph JT, Jindal RM: Influence of dialysis on post-transplant events. Clin Transplant 2002;16:18–23.
26 O'Donoghue D, Manos J, Pearson R, Scott P, Bakran A, Johnson R, Dyer P, Martin S, Gokal R: Continuous ambulatory peritoneal dialysis and renal transplantation: a ten-year experience in a single center. Perit Dial Int 1992;12:242, 245–249.
27 Van Biesen W, Veys N, Vanholder R, Lameire N: The impact of the pre-transplant renal replacement modality on outcome after cadaveric kidney transplantation: the Ghent experience. Contrib Nephrol. Basel, Karger, 2006, vol 150, pp 254–258.
28 Goldfarb-Rumyantzev AS, Hurdle JF, Scandling JD, Baird BC, Cheung AK: The role of pretransplantation renal replacement therapy modality in kidney allograft and recipient survival. Am J Kidney Dis 2005;46:537–549.
29 Luna E, Cerezo I, Collado G, Martinez C, Villa J, Macias R, Garcia C, Cubero JJ: Vascular thrombosis after kidney transplantation: predisposing factors and risk index. Transplant Proc 2010;42:2928–2930.
30 Palomar R, Morales P, Rodrigo E, Castaneda O, Fernandez-Fresnedo G, Gomez-Alamillo C, Arias M: Venous graft thrombosis in patients on peritoneal dialysis before transplantation. Transplant Proc 2007;39:2128–2130.
31 Van der Vliet JA, Barendregt WB, Hoitsma AJ, Buskens FG: Increased incidence of renal allograft thrombosis after continuous ambulatory peritoneal dialysis. Clin Transplant 1996;10:51–54.
32 Perez Fontan M, Rodriguez-Carmona A, Garcia Falcon T, Tresancos C, Bouza P, Valdes F: Peritoneal dialysis is not a risk factor for primary vascular graft thrombosis after renal transplantation. Perit Dial Int 1998;18:311–316.
33 Murphy BG, Hill CM, Middleton D, Doherty CC, Brown JH, Nelson WE, Kernohan RM, Keane PK, Douglas JF, McNamee PT: Increased renal allograft thrombosis in CAPD patients. Nephrol Dial Transplant 1994;9:1166–1169.
34 Ojo AO, Hanson JA, Wolfe RA, Agodoa LY, Leavey SF, Leichtman A, Young EW, Port FK: Dialysis modality and the risk of allograft thrombosis in adult renal transplant recipients. Kidney Int 1999;55:1952–1960.
35 Vats AN, Donaldson L, Fine RN, Chavers BM: Pretransplant dialysis status and outcome of renal transplantation in North American children: a NAPRTCS Study. North American Pediatric Renal Transplant Cooperative Study. Transplantation 2000;69:1414–1419.
36 McDonald RA, Smith JM, Stablein D, Harmon WE: Pretransplant peritoneal dialysis and graft thrombosis following pediatric kidney transplantation: a NAPRTCS report. Pediatr Transplant 2003;7:204–208.

Isaac Teitelbaum, MD
Division of Renal Diseases and Hypertension, University of Colorado School of Medicine
12605 E. 16th Avenue, F774
Aurora, CO 80045 (USA)
Tel. +1 720 848 7601, E-Mail isaac.teitelbaum@ucdenver.edu

Ronco C, Rosner MH, Crepaldi C (eds): Peritoneal Dialysis – State-of-the-Art 2012.
Contrib Nephrol. Basel, Karger, 2012, vol 178, pp 258–263

Neutrophil Gelatinase-Associated Lipocalin in the Early Diagnosis of Peritonitis: The Case of Neutrophil Gelatinase-Associated Lipocalin

Francesca Katiana Martino[a] · Ilenia Filippi[b] · Davide Giavarina[c] · Manish Kaushik[b] · Maria Pia Rodighiero[a] · Carlo Crepaldi[a] · Caterina Teixeira[b] · Asunciòn Ferrer Nadal[b] · Mitchell H. Rosner[d] · Claudio Ronco[a,b]

[a]Department of Nephrology Dialysis and Transplantation, [b]International Renal Research Institute (IRRIV) and [c]Clinical Chemistry and Haematology Laboratory, San Bortolo Hospital, Vicenza, Italy; [d]Department of Medicine, University of Virginia Health System, Charlottesville, Va., USA

Abstract

Neutrophil gelatinase-associated lipocalin (NGAL), a protein involved in iron handling, has been recognized as a marker of inflammation. In this regard, serum and urine NGAL levels have proven a useful diagnostic tool for acute kidney injury. Bacterial peritonitis is an all too common complication of peritoneal dialysis (PD) and while diagnosis in most cases is routine, there are times when patients present with typical symptoms but do not have an elevated PD effluent white blood cell count. Furthermore, patients may present with an elevated PD fluid white count, a cloudy effluent and no evidence of active infection. In these cases, a discriminating role for peritoneal fluid NGAL would be useful to distinguish bacterial and nonbacterial PD fluid infection. A small case control study was performed which demonstrated a very high sensitivity and specificity for peritoneal fluid NGAL. These preliminary data show that peritoneal fluid NGAL may be a useful tool for the early and accurate diagnosis of peritonitis.

Neutrophil Gelatinase-Associated Lipocalin and Its Biological Role

Neutrophil gelatinase-associated lipocalin (NGAL) belongs to the lipocalin family of proteins. It consists of a single polypeptide chain with a molecular mass of 25,000 Da and was initially identified in the granules of human granulocytes. The function of NGAL has been extensively evaluated in the last decade. Specifically, NGAL is involved in innate immunity during bacterial infection and it modulates various eukaryotic cellular responses (apoptosis, proliferation and differentiation) [1]. During infection, bacteria acquire much of their iron from the host by synthesizing siderophores that scavenge iron and transport it into the pathogen. NGAL is constitutively synthesized and stored in intracellular granules of human neutrophils and it is secreted into the extracellular compartment, where NGAL binds bacterial siderophores. Finally, the NGAL-siderophore complex blocks iron bacterial traffic and consequently it limits bacterial growth (fig. 1). Moreover, NGAL seems to act as a modulator of cell homeostasis by iron shuttling between the extracellular and intracellular space. These inflammatory properties demonstrate why NGAL secretion has been reported in the setting of some diseases in the absence of bacterial infection, such as inflammatory conditions and kidney injury. Numerous studies have shown its usefulness in the diagnosis of acute kidney disease [2, 3], and currently NGAL concentration in the urine is considered a valid tool to detect renal tubular injury [4].

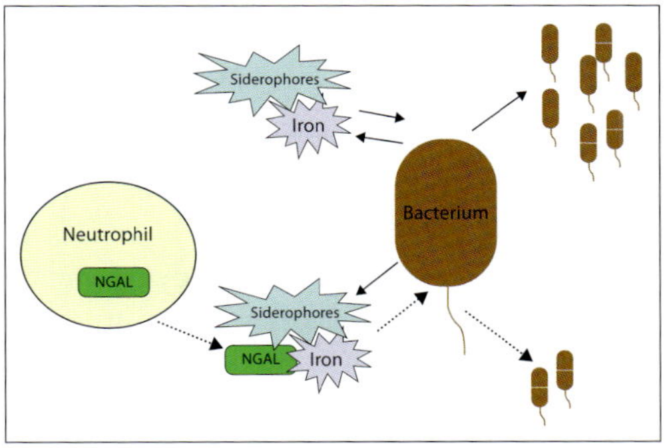

Fig. 1. Role of NGAL during infection. Key events during infection without and with NGAL: In absence of NGAL, the siderophore-iron complex delivers iron into bacterial cell and permits bacterial proliferation. The NGAL secreted from neutrophils in response to infection binds to the siderophore-iron complex. This siderophore-iron-NGAL complex blocks the iron delivery into bacterial cell and limits bacterial proliferation.

Peritoneum during Peritonitis

The peritoneum is a simple structure consisting of a single layer of mesothelial cells (MC) and a connective tissue stratum with fibroblasts, mast cell, macrophages and blood vessels. During bacterial peritonitis, bacterial lipopolysaccharides induce the production of proinflammatory cytokines in MC by the activation of Toll-like receptors, which are constitutively expressed in MC. However, MC undergo epithelial to mesenchymal transdifferentiation, a reversible process where MC change their phenotype losing microvilli, tight-junction and apical-basal polarity; consequently, modifying cytoskeleton organization and increasing migration and invasive capacity [5]. All these changes engender a reparative process with restoration of the peritoneal membrane, but at the same time they contribute to peritoneal fibrosis. Factors, that have a role in this pathway, are transforming growth factor-β_1, interleukin-1β (IL-1β) epidermal growth factor, and hepatocyte growth factor; all of which are increased during peritonitis. The presence of these cytokines in the peritoneal space delays the return of the MC to a normal phenotype and aggravates the fibrotic process of peritoneum membrane.

Why Could NGAL Be a Good Marker in Peritonitis?

We know, as highlighted in the previous paragraph, NGAL is up-regulated during infection. Of note, two studies have shown a significant increase of NGAL during peritonitis. In 1995, Axelsson et al. [6] demonstrated in a general population how severe acute peritonitis was accompanied by an increase of NGAL levels in plasma and in peritoneal exudates. In 2007, Leung et al. [7] confirmed in a small group of PD patients an increase of NGAL value in peritoneal dialysis (PD) effluent during peritonitis. Moreover, the latter study proved the ability of human peritoneal MC to secret NGAL under inflammatory conditions in vitro. The presence of IL-1β up-regulated the synthesis and secretion of NGAL from MC within the first few hours of exposure [7]. As discussed above, MC and IL-1β are also pivotal elements during peritonitis to restore peritoneal homeostasis. Therefore, all these aspects make NGAL a potential marker of peritonitis, because this molecule is secreted by MC in peritoneal space when there is an inflammatory insult.

NGAL in Peritoneal Dialysis Effluent and Systemic Condition

In patients with chronic kidney disease who need renal replacement therapy, the expression of NGAL in PD effluent (*peritoneal-NGAL*) could be influenced by the underlying clinical co-morbidities, inflammatory status or hydration status and also by dialysis modality. Specifically, a high value of plasma NGAL could result in high value of *peritoneal-NGAL* and consequently *peritoneal-NGAL* could lose its meaning as marker of peritoneal inflammation or peritoneal infection. In our previous study [8], we demonstrated that *peritoneal-NGAL* in the basal condition was poorly represented in peritoneal effluent and its value was minimally influenced by plasma NGAL levels and by dialytic creatinine clearance. In fact, these issues explained only 9.5% of total variance model, likely because local factors most strongly affect the concentration of *peritoneal-NGAL*.

This behavior of NGAL is not surprising because NGAL is a protein with a relatively high molecular weight (25,000 Da) and this can strongly influence its transport through the peritoneal membrane [9]. Indeed, proteins with similar molecular weight, such as cystatin C [10], have low peritoneal diffusive capacity.

Why Could NGAL Be Useful in Peritonitis Management?

Peritonitis is the most serious infectious complication in PD. Though in the last few years the number of peritonitis episodes has declined with improved technique and with patient education, this complication remains an important issue in the treatment of PD patients. Currently, two of the following features are essential for the clinical diagnosis of peritonitis:

1 clinical signs and symptoms of peritoneal inflammation: pain, discomfort, nausea/vomiting, diarrhea or constipation,
2 cloudy drainage with WBC > 100 cells/mm^3 and with at least 50% polymorphonuclear cells,
3 positive culture or Gram stain.

As reported in the Guidelines of the International Society of Peritoneal Dialysis 2010 [11], antibiotic therapy should be initiated as soon as possible, when drainage appears cloudy, without waiting for laboratory confirmation. On the other hand, cloudy effluent can be related to different problems such as chemical peritonitis, eosinophilia in the effluent, hemoperitoneum, chylous effluent, and treatment with a dihydropyridine calcium channel antagonist; all these conditions are not related to peritoneal infection and do not require antibiotic therapy. Moreover, in a small percentage of patients the presence of clear drainage is not enough to exclude peritonitis and in a limited number of cases the WBC count can be unclear to elucidate the presence of infective process. Consequently, in these indeterminate scenarios, where the decision to start treatment is guided by clinical judgment, another diagnostic tool could be useful to assist the physician to take the correct treatment decision.

NGAL as Marker of Peritonitis: Preliminary Results

On the basis of previous observations regarding NGAL and peritonitis, we designed a study to evaluate NGAL in PD effluent as a specific and early diagnostic marker of peritonitis. We also studied the reliability of NGAL for the prediction of peritonitis compared to the current laboratory markers of peritonitis.

Material and Methods

A case-control study was carried out at the Peritoneal Dialysis Center in San Bortolo Hospital, Vicenza, Italy, in the period from January 1st, 2011 to June 30th, 2011. All patients on PD who were cared for at our center for more than 3 months were eligible for the study. The case group was composed of all patients who arrived at our center with signs and symptoms suggestive of peritonitis, while patients who came to our center for a routine visit (without any sign or symptom of peritonitis) immediately after a patient with suspected peritonitis formed the control group. All patients provided informed consent before study enrollment. All the patients underwent blood and peritoneal dialysate effluent examination. Peritonitis was defined by the standard criteria as discussed above.

Clinical Data Collection
Baseline demographic data were recorded at the time of enrollment. The following clinical features were collected: age, etiology of CKD, dialysis vintage, kind of PD therapy.

Laboratory Measurements
Venous blood samples were drawn from all patients during visits and the following biochemical parameters were specifically evaluated: C-reactive protein (CRP), procalcitonin, WBC count in peritoneal effluent, *peritoneal-NGAL* and microbiological examination. *Peritoneal-NGAL* and WBC count in peritoneal effluent were evaluated by overnight collection of dialysate in control group, while in case group peritoneal effluent analysis was evaluated in any suspicious drainage. Samples were aliquotted and stored at –80°C before assay, and subsequently measured by the Archictect platform (Abbott Diagnostics, Abbott Park, Ill., USA). This is a two-step (sandwich) assay using chemiluminescent microparticle immunoassay technology.

Statistical Analysis
All continuous variables were reported as median values and interquartile range (IQR), while categorical variables were described by percentage. Mann-Whitney U and Pearson χ^2 tests were used to compare continuous and categorical variables, as appropriate. The predictive efficacy of a variable for predicting peritonitis was evaluated using ROC curve analysis, with the area under the ROC curve (AUC). All reported p values were two sided, and statistical significance was set at $p < 0.05$. Statistical analysis was performed with SPSS version 17.0 (SPSS Inc., Chicago, Ill., USA).

Results

56.5% of patients were male, 26.1% were diabetic, 84.1% had hypertension. Median patient age was 61 years (IQR 46.5–71) and median duration of PD was 30 months (IQR 11–51). The characteristics of cases and controls are reported in table 1. During the study period, we had 30 episodes of peritonitis.

Between cases and controls there were significant differences for the following parameters: CRP ($p < 0.001$), procalcitonin ($p = 0.038$), *peritoneal-NGAL* ($p < 0.001$), and WBC in peritoneal effluent ($p < 0.001$).

The AUCs for the prediction of bacterial peritonitis for serum CRP, serum procalcitonin, WBC count in peritoneal effluent and *peritoneal-NGAL* were 0.81 ($p = 0.001$), 0.70 ($p = 0.039$), 1 ($p < 0.001$), and 0.99 ($p < 0.001$), respectively (fig. 2). In 4 cases (6.6%) the WBC count was more than 100/mm^3 without a clinical diagnosis of peritonitis. In these 4 cases, *peritoneal-NGAL* was not increased (the values were comparable with control group, $p = 0.09$). There was no case of peritonitis when the WBC count was less than 100/mm^3.

Discussion

To our knowledge, the present study is the first one evaluating the reliability of *peritoneal-NGAL* as a diagnostic marker to predict peritonitis episodes. In our series, *peritoneal-NGAL* turned out to be strongly correlated with peritonitis and the test performance of *peritoneal-NGAL* was comparable with that of WBC count in peritoneal effluent.

Moreover, although *peritoneal-NGAL* correlated strongly with WBC count in peritoneal effluent, occasionally it seemed to have a different behavior. In 6.6% of patients (all in the control group) the WBC count was elevated (>100 cells/mm^3) but these patients had no clinical or microbiological evidence of peritonitis. Interestingly, these patients did not demonstrate a rise of *peritoneal-NGAL*. This preliminary observation, despite the paucity of the case number and the

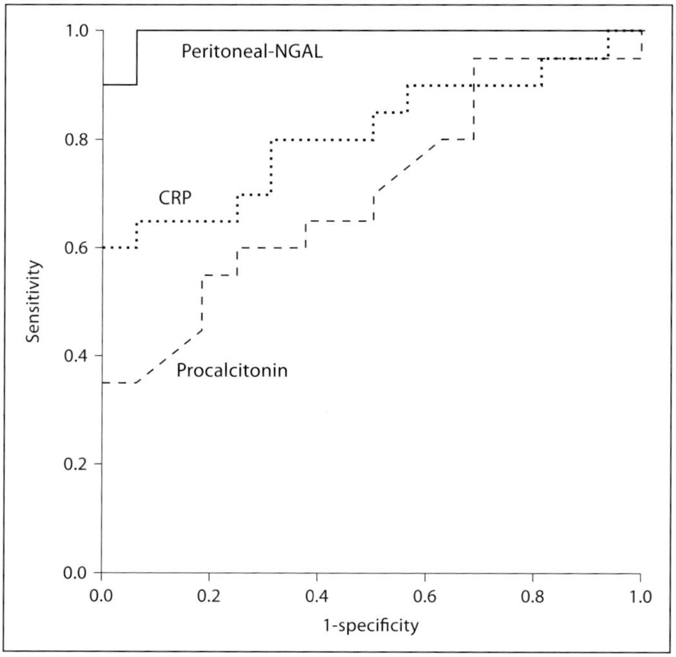

Fig. 2. ROC curve. Diagonal segments are produced by ties.

Table 1. Characteristics of enrolled patients according to the presence of an episode of peritonitis

	Cases median (IQR)	Controls median (IQR)
Age, years	66.5 (52.2–73)	70 (59.7–73.2)
Male, %	73.3	73.3
CAPD, %	70	76.7
C-reactive protein, mg/dl	4.9 (1.18–9.8)	0.57 (0.15–0.86)
Procalcitonin, ng/ml	0.73 (0.36–2.77)	0.44 (0.28–0.64)
Peritoneal-NGAL, ng/ml	327 (187.5–829.7)	57.5 (34.5–92)
WBC count in peritoneal effluent, n/mm^3	3,400 (1,680–7,460)	20 (10–45)

CAPD = Continuous ambulatory peritoneal dialysis; *peritoneal-NGAL* = NGAL in peritoneal dialysis effluent; WBC = white blood cell; IQR = interquartile range.

need of confirmation with lager series, seems to suggest a specific role of *peritoneal-NGAL* in its ability to exclude peritonitis independently from WBC count in peritoneal effluent.

Although we have shown its potential usefulness in the diagnosis of peritonitis, we should not forget its biological role during inflammation: *peritoneal-NGAL* could also be used as marker of peritoneal inflammation, as suggested by demonstration of its up-regulation during inflammation [12] and its secretion by MC [7]. This makes the role of NGAL in peritoneal inflammation very interesting, but could be a confounding factor in the diagnosis of peritonitis. In any case, more studies are needed to evaluate the role of *peritoneal-NGAL* in PD as a marker of inflammation. We therefore plan to evaluate in a different series the value of *peritoneal-NGAL* as marker of peritoneal inflammation compared to IL-6, IL-8, CA125, and hyaluronan.

The present study suffers from some limitations. First, the number of cases and controls are limited to express consistent evidence about peritoneal-NGAL during peritonitis, but we plan to collect a larger series to support our results. Second, the assay used to measure *peritoneal-NGAL* was not specifically created for peritoneal dialysate effluent assay, but currently there is no specific kit for *peritoneal-NGAL*.

In conclusion, in our study *peritoneal-NGAL* was evaluated for the first time as marker of peritonitis and the preliminary results have shown its reliability to diagnose a peritonitis episode.

Disclosure Statement

All authors have made a substantial contribution to the information or material submitted for publication. All have read and approved the final manuscript. The study did not receive any kind of funding. Manuscript or portions thereof are not under consideration by another journal or electronic publication and have not been previously published. Professor C. Ronco has received speaking honoraria from Abbott, Alere, and Gambro. All other authors have no competing interests.

References

1 Schmidt-Ott KM, Mori K, Li JY, et al: Dual action of neutrophil gelatinase-associated lipocalin. J Am Soc Nephrol 2007;18:407–413.
2 Soni SS, Ronco C, Katz N, Cruz DN: Early diagnosis of acute kidney injury: the promise of novel biomarkers. Blood Purif 2009;28:165–174.
3 Bolignano D, Donato V, Coppolino G, et al: Neutrophil gelatinase-associated lipocalin (NGAL) as a marker of kidney damage. Am J Kidney Dis 2008;52:595–605.
4 Devarajan P: Biomarkers for the early detection of acute kidney injury. Curr Opin Pediatr 2011;23:194–200.
5 Aroeira LS, Aguilera A, Sanchez-Tomero JA, et al: Epithelial to mesenchymal transition and peritoneal membrane failure in peritoneal dialysis patients: pathologic significance and potential therapeutic intervention. J Am Soc Nephrol 2007;18:2004–2013.
6 Axelsson L, Bergenfeldt M, Ohlsson K: Studies of the release and turnover of a human neutrophil lipocalin. Scand J Clin Lab Invest 1995;55:577–588.
7 Leung JC, Lam MF, Tang SC, Chan LY, Tam KY, Yip TP, et al: Roles of neutrophil gelatinase-associated lipocalin in continuous ambulatory peritoneal dialysis-related peritonitis. J Clin Immunol 2009;29:365–378.
8 Martino F, Filippi I, Giavarina D, et al: Neutrophil gelatinase-associated lipocalin (NGAL) in peritoneal dialysate effluent: evaluation in peritoneal dialysis patients in basal condition. Perit Dial Int. Submitted.
9 Kabanda A, Goffin E, Bernard A, Lauwerys R, Van Ypersele De Strihou C: Factors influencing serum level and peritoneal clearances of low molecular weight proteins in continuous ambulatory peritoneal dialysis. Kidney Int 1995;48:1946–1952.
10 Montini G, Amici G, Milan S, et al: Middle molecule and small protein removal in children on peritoneal dialysis. Kidney Int 2002;61:1153–1159.
11 Li PK, Szeto CC, Piraino B, Bernardini J, et al: Peritoneal dialysis-related infections recommendations: 2010 update. Perit Dial Int 2010:30:393–423.
12 Karlsen JR, Borregaard N, Cowland JB: Induction of neutrophil gelatinase-associated lipocalin expression by co-stimulation with interleukin-17 and tumor necrosis factor-α is controlled by IkB-ζ but neither by C/EBP-ß nor C/EBP-δ. J Biol Chem 2010;285:14088–14100.

Dr. Francesca Katiana Martino
Nephrology, Dialysis and Transplantation, San Bortolo Hospital
Viale Rodolfi 37
IT–36100 Vicenza (Italy)
Tel. +39.0444.753650, E-Mail francesca.martino.k@hotmail.it

Ronco C, Rosner MH, Crepaldi C (eds): Peritoneal Dialysis – State-of-the-Art 2012.
Contrib Nephrol. Basel, Karger, 2012, vol 178, pp 264–270

Prognostic Factors for Peritonitis Outcome

Sadie van Esch · Raymond T. Krediet · Dirk G. Struijk

Division of Nephrology, Academic Medical Centre, University Hospital and Dianet, Amsterdam, The Netherlands

Abstract

Despite advances in treatment and prevention, peritonitis remains a major problem in peritoneal dialysis (PD) patients with often technique failure as a consequence. The last decades the focus of PD peritonitis has changed from lowering peritonitis incidence to improvement of peritonitis outcome. Prognostic factors for peritonitis outcome can influence decision making during the treatment of peritonitis, for example to take out the PD catheter early in the time course of peritonitis and prevent further damage to the peritoneal membrane. In this paper, we give a review of the literature about prognostic factors for peritonitis outcome. In most studies, age, gender, diabetes, time on PD, a precursor of calcitonin:procalcitonin, IL-6 and albumin did not show a significant effect on peritonitis outcome. The following factors have been associated with poor outcome of peritonitis: Gram-negative organisms, *Mycobacterium* species, fungal peritonitis, polymicrobial peritonitis, concurrent exit site or tunnel infection, Caucasian race, low residual GFR, persistently elevated peritoneal dialysate white cell count, CRP, and low levels of sICAM-1 and hyaluronan at the end of peritonitis treatment. In fungal peritonitis, abdominal pain, bowel obstruction, the catheter remaining in situ and *Candida parapsilosis* are factors associated with higher mortality rate and a greater risk of technique failure. Recent antibiotic therapy and peritonitis are associated with poor treatment response in culture-negative peritonitis. Recurrent peritonitis episodes have a poor therapeutic response and high mortality and have a worse prognosis than relapsing ones. Older age, long PD duration and continuous elevated serum CRP levels are predictors of adverse outcomes in PD patients after peritonitis-related catheter removal. Peritonitis remains a serious complication of PD with marked morbidity. It is a common cause of technique failure. The rate of PD-related peritonitis has decreased over the last decades due to advances in treatment and prevention. Nowadays, the focus moved from lowering peritonitis incidence towards improving peritonitis outcome. It is useful to have prognostic factors for peritonitis outcome, because they can influence decision-making during the treatment of peritonitis, for example to take out the PD catheter early in the time course of peritonitis and prevent further damage to the peritoneal membrane. In the last decades, many publications appeared about prognostic factors for peritonitis outcome. This article summarizes those prognostic factors, based on an extensive review of the literature.

Age at Onset of Peritonitis and Age at Start of Peritoneal Dialysis

The influence of age as a prognostic factor for outcome of peritonitis is controversial. In many studies age at the onset of peritonitis did not have an independent effect on outcome nor did patient age at the start of peritoneal dialysis (PD) [1–3].

However, one study showed that older PD patients experienced a higher risk of severe peritonitis and peritonitis-related mortality [4].

Gender

Several studies did not find an effect of gender on peritonitis outcome [1, 2, 5].

Race

In Caucasians peritonitis more often leads to hospital admission and more often results in death than in Blacks and this effect was age independent [5]. This is consistent with other data demonstrating a significant difference in the rate of treatment failure: in Blacks 11.1% vs. 22.5% in Caucasians [1].

Diabetes, History of Steroid Use, Previous Renal Transplantation, Malignancy

Because these factors interfere with the host immune defenses, it seems apparent that they adversely affect outcome. It is not clear if diabetes has a negative impact on peritonitis outcome: in the literature conflicting results are reported. For example, patients with treatment failure of peritonitis were more likely to have diabetes in the study of Chow et al. [6], but others could not identify diabetes as a predictor of outcome [1, 4, 5]. Several studies could not find an impact of history of steroid use, previous renal transplantation or malignancy on peritonitis outcome [1, 4].

Residual Renal Function

Perez et al. [4] were the first to demonstrate that baseline GFR has a specific and consistent inverse correlation with the later incidence of peritonitis and peritonitis-related mortality. They postulate that PD patients with good residual renal function need a lower number of bag exchanges which may reduce the chances for contamination and infection. In addition, residual renal function may predict the risk of peritonitis by performing as a marker of poor condition of PD patients, because low or absent GFR can point to late referral or secondary selection of PD, after chronic hemodialysis, which is associated with inadequacy of dialysis, malnutrition, inflammation and volume overload.

Time on Peritoneal Dialysis

Conflicting results are reported in the literature. One study found that a longer PD duration had a significant negative effect on outcome; patients who had been on PD for more than 2.4 years had a 24.4% rate of treatment failure of peritonitis, compared to 16.5% for patients less than 2.4 years on PD [1]. In contrast, Troitle et al. [7] found just the opposite: patients on PD for more than 37 months had a better outcome than those on PD for 12 months or less, but the groups differed in race and comorbidity, in favor of the group on PD for longer than 37 months. Yang et al. [3] found duration of PD was only of borderline significance. Others reported that PD duration was not predictive of outcome, including mortality, and that time on PD was not related with the length of hospital stay [8, 9]. The authors of the first paper postulate that PD duration is of importance for outcome of peritonitis, because the peritoneal membrane characteristics and peritoneal macrophages change over time in PD which may contribute to decreased peritoneal host defense [1].

Number of Peritonitis Episodes Previously Experienced

Some studies found that the number of peritonitis episodes a patient experienced, had no influence on the outcome of the present peritonitis [1], others found that the incidence of peritonitis was a strong independent predictor of peritonitis-related mortality [4].

Concurrent Exit Site Infection

Concurrent exit site infection or tunnel infection has been shown to have an adverse outcome [3, 5]. However, in one study the presence of a purulent exit site was associated with a significantly higher rate of treatment failure of peritonitis (35.2 vs. 18.3%, $p = 0.004$), but in a regression analysis it did not independently effect outcome [1].

Peritoneal Dialysis Fluid Cell Count

In several studies peritoneal dialysate white cell count (PDE WBC) is found to have prognostic meaning in outcome of peritonitis. For PDE WBC $\geq$1,090/mm^3 on day 3, the sensitivity was 75% and the specificity was 74% for the prediction of treatment failure, defined as catheter loss or peritonitis-related death. In a multiple logistic regression analysis, peritoneal white cell count of $\geq$1,090/mm^3 on day 3 was an independent risk factor for prediction of treatment failure after adjustment for conventional risk factors; a more than 9-fold increased risk existed for catheter loss and death. Peritoneal white cell count >100/mm^3 for more than 5 days was associated with treatment failure (OR 7.38; 95% CI 3.38–16.1; $p < 0.0001$) [6]. Similar findings are obtained by others [1, 10]. In a study by Martikainen et al. [11], dialysate leukocytes >500/mm^3 on day 4 indicated poor outcome. Others looked at the influence of peritoneal cell count at admission to the hospital: it was positively correlated with the length of hospital stay. If it took more than 24 h from the onset of symptoms to hospital admission, PD effluent leucocyte percentage was higher and PD effluent lymphomononuclear cell percentage was lower, which was associated with a longer length of hospital stay [8].

Growth Factors, Cytokines, Adhesion Molecules, Inflammatory Markers

Procalcitonin, one of the calcitonin precursors, has been suggested as a marker for infection and low-grade inflammation. However, in a prospective study on PD patients that developed peritonitis, procalcitonin failed to predict outcome of peritonitis [12].

IL-6 is known to stimulate adhesion molecules like intercellular adhesion molecule-1 (ICAM-1). ICAM-1 plays an important role in the inflammatory response and host defense. It stimulates hyaluronan (HA) which is an important component of the extracellular matrix. In 36 patients with peritonitis the above-mentioned parameters were measured at the onset, on day 4, at the end of treatment and 2 months after the onset of peritonitis. Concentrations of sICAM-1 in patients completing the antibiotic therapy were higher at the onset and on day 4 of peritonitis than at the end of the treatment with antibiotics. Concentrations of sICAM-1 at the end of the treatment with antibiotics in patients with a relapse/re-infection were significantly lower than in patients with no relapse/re-infection. The same findings were found for HA. The authors hypothesize that lower levels of sICAM-1 and HA at the end of treatment in patients with a relapse/re-infection may be a sign of reduced immune defense of the peritoneum which may be due to destruction of peritoneal cells during a severe episode of peritonitis or a reduced immune defense capacity of the peritoneal membrane. Or it may be that during severe infections activated leukocytes bind more ICAM-1 which in turn binds HA. For Il-6, the highest concentrations were seen at onset and on day 4 of peritonitis in patients completing the treatment with antibiotics. IL-6 failed to differentiate between a good or poor outcome of peritonitis [11].

There are conflicting results for CRP as a marker of peritonitis outcome. In one study, the mortality rate was significantly higher in patients with CRP >3.0 mg/l than in patients with CRP <3.0 mg/l on day 42 after the onset of peritonitis [12]. In a prospective cohort study of PD patients with incident peritonitis, higher baseline levels of CRP were associated with an increased risk of short-term adverse outcomes, including death, switch to hemodialysis, persistent infection and relapse of peritonitis. After recovering from peritonitis, higher CRP levels were associated with an increased risk of long-term events: a second peritonitis or death [9]. Elsurer et al. [8] found that CRP was independently associated with the length of hospital stay because of peritonitis. Some researchers found a relationship between CRP >100 mg/l on day 4 of peritonitis and poor outcome [11]. However, others were not able to find a relationship between CRP and outcome [3].

Several studies showed that a low albumin level is associated with technique failure and death [3]. The suggested reasons for this relationship are: the fact that albumin is an inverse acute-phase reactant, low albumin, and possibly hypoglobulinemia, predisposes to recurrent infections [13], and low albumin may reflect the underlying problem of malnutrition [14]. On the other hand, some investigators did not find a relationship between low albumin and peritonitis outcome [1].

Causative Organism

Peritonitis caused by Gram-negative organisms has a worse outcome than peritonitis due to Gram-positive organisms. Krishnan et al. [1] reported about 399 episodes of bacterial peritonitis between 1996 and 2000. They found a resolution rate for single Gram-positive peritonitis of 87.3%, compared to 63.6% for single Gram-negative peritonitis episodes, p = 0.001. *Staphyococcus aureus* resulted in significantly lower resolution rates than other Gram-positive organisms, 68.6% for *S. aureus* versus 94.2% for other Gram-positive organisms. More than half of the PD catheter losses (57%) among single Gram-positive organism-induced peritonitis were attributed to *S. aureus* infections [3, 15]. Of the Gram-negative organisms, *Serratia marcescens* had the highest rate of treatment failure (85.7%), followed by *Pseudomonas aeruginosa* peritonitis (78.6%) [1]. Chow et al. [6] found that Gram-negative organisms, *Pseudomonas*, fungal and *Mycobacterium* species were independent risk factors for treatment failure.

The number of organisms cultured is another risk factor for catheter loss. Micro-organisms of the Enterobacteriaceae family are the major pathogens responsible for catheter loss in polymicrobial peritonitis [3].

Fungal Peritonitis

Many studies have found that the use of antibiotics and bacterial peritonitis within the previous 3 months are predisposing factors for the development of fungal peritonitis [16–18]. Antibiotics, by killing the bowel flora, promote fungal colonization of the intestinal or genitourinary tract, with subsequent invasion across the mucosal barrier to the peritoneal cavity. *Candida parapsilosis* has been shown to be an independent risk factor associated with mortality [17]. Abdominal pain, bowel obstruction, and the catheter remaining in situ are other factors associated with higher mortality rate and a greater risk of technique failure [10, 19, 20].

Culture-Negative Peritonitis

Szeto et al. [2] analyzed 212 episodes of culture-negative peritonitis from 1995 to 2001. Primary response was defined as resolution of abdominal pain, clearing of the dialysate, PDE WBC <100/ml on day 10 with antibiotics alone. If the PDE was still cloudy at day 10, the Tenckhoff catheter was removed or the antibiotics were changed. Complete cure was defined as resolution of peritonitis without the need for catheter removal, antibiotic switch or relapse within 120 days. Recent antibiotic therapy (within 30 days of onset of peritonitis) was associated with a lower primary response rate (31 of 56 versus 113 of 156 episodes; p = 0.019) and lower complete cure rate (12 of 56 vs. 68 of 156 episodes; p = 0.003). A history of peritonitis from 31 to 120 days before the onset also resulted in a lower complete cure rate (p = 0.001). Multivariate logistic regression analysis showed that only recent antibiotic therapy was an independent predictor of poor primary response rate, odds ratio 2.12 (95% CI 1.12–3.98; p = 0.02). The authors speculate that the use of antibiotics alters body flora and provokes peritonitis by fastidious organisms; conversely, there might be an accumulation of antibiotics that might hinder PDE culture. Only recent peritonitis was an independent predictor of poor complete cure rate, odds ratio 2.87 (95% CI 1.56–5.29; p = 0.001). They argue that antibiotics probably alter local bacterial flora and provoke the development of resistant bacterial strains.

Recurrent and Relapsing Peritonitis

Recently, an article has been published about the characteristics of recurrent and relapsing peritonitis in a retrospective study over 14 years. According to the ISPD guidelines relapsing peritonitis is defined as a peritonitis that appears within 4 weeks after a prior peritonitis with the same organism or a sterile peritonitis. A recurrent peritonitis occurs within 4 weeks of a prior episode but with a different organism. The authors report that relapsing peritonitis most often is caused by coagulase-negative *Staphylococcus* and *Pseudomonas* species. Recurrent peritonitis is often caused by non-*Pseudomonas* Gram-negative organisms and polymicrobial growth. They suggest that this can point to an underlying pathological state of the bowel; or that recent antibiotic use disturbs the gastrointestinal flora and provokes transmural migration of bowel organisms to the peritoneal cavity. In their study the recurrent group had a significant lower primary response rate (71.2 vs. 86.4%), lower complete cure rate (42.4 vs. 72.3%), and higher mortality rate (20.8 vs. 7.7%) than the control group; as well as a lower primary response rate (71.2 vs. 88.5%), lower complete cure rate (42.4 vs. 62.4%) and higher mortality rate (20.8 vs. 7.0%) than the relapsing group. The control group consisted of first peritonitis episodes without relapse or recurrence. In conclusion, recurrent peritonitis has a poor therapeutic response and high mortality. Recurrent peritonitis has a worse prognosis than relapsing peritonitis. The authors discuss that recurrent peritonitis deserves an equal and perhaps a more aggressive treatment as for relapsing episodes [21].

Risk Factors for Adverse Outcomes after Peritonitis-Related Technique Failure

Moon et al. [22] investigated the risk factors for developing short-term complications after peritonitis-related technique failure. Patients were divided into four groups according to adverse outcomes that developed within 90 days after PD catheter removal: no complications, recurrent ascites, encapsulating peritoneal sclerosis (EPS) and death directly related to peritonitis. They performed a multivariate analysis of risk factors for adverse outcomes. Serum CRP level at 72 h of peritonitis and PD duration were significant predictors for the development of EPS. For peritonitis-related death, CRP level at 72 h and age at PD catheter removal (per 1 year increase: OR 1.11) were identified as significant determinants. Only effluent WBC at 72 h was associated with the development of ascites. The authors conclude that persistently elevated serum CRP level, older age, and long PD duration are significant predictors of adverse outcomes in PD patients after peritonitis-related catheter removal.

In summary, many prognostic factors for peritonitis outcome are investigated and contradictory results are reported in the literature (table 1). Gram-negative organisms, *Mycobacterium* species, fungal peritonitis, polymicrobial peritonitis, concurrent exit site or tunnel infection: all these factors have been found to result in a poor outcome of peritonitis. In addition, it seems that Caucasians have a worse outcome compared to Blacks. PDE WBC $\geq$1,090/mm^3 on day 3 is an independent risk factor for prediction of treatment failure as well a PDE WBC >100/mm^3 for more than 5 days. Furthermore, low levels of sICAM-1 and HA at the end of treatment are negative prognostic indicators. Most data reveal CRP as a marker of peritonitis outcome. At present, only one study looked at the GFR and found an inverse correlation with peritonitis-related mortality. Recent antibiotic therapy and peritonitis are associated with poor treatment response in culture-negative peritonitis. In fungal peritonitis, abdominal pain, bowel obstruction, the catheter remaining in situ and *C. parapsilosis* are factors associated with higher mortality rate and a greater risk of technique failure. Recurrent peritonitis episodes have a poor therapeutic response and high mortality and have a worse prognosis than relapsing ones. Continuous elevated serum CRP level, older age, and long PD duration are significant predictors of adverse outcomes in PD patients after peritonitis-related catheter removal. The following parameters have not shown a clear effect on peritonitis outcome: age, gender, diabetes, time on PD, procalcitonin, IL-6 and albumin.

Table 1. Prognostic factors for peritonitis outcome

Factor	Prognostic value	References
Age	no	Krishnan et al. [1], Szeto et al. [2], Yang et al. [3]
	yes	Perez et al. [4]
Gender	no	Krishnan et al. [1], Szeto et al. [2], Golper et al. [5]
Race: caucasians have a worse outcome compared to Blacks	yes	Krishnan et al. [1], Golper et al. [5]
Diabetes, history of steroid use, previous renal transplantation, malignancy	no	Krishnan et al. [1], Perez et al. [4] Golper et al. [5]
	yes	Chow et al. [6]
Residual renal function	yes	Perez et al. [4]
Time on PD	no	Elsurer et al. [8], Zalunardo et al. [9]
	yes	Krishnan et al. [1], Troidle et al. [7]
Number of peritonitis episodes previously experienced	no	Krishnan et al. [1]
	yes	Pérez et al. [4]
	no	Krishnan et al. [1]
Concurrent exit site infection	yes	Yang et al. [3], Golper et al. [5]
PD fluid cell count: PDE WBC $\geq$1,090/mm^3 on day 3, PDE WBC $\geq$100/mm^3 for >5 days	yes	Krishnan et al. [1], Chow et al. [6], Elsurer et al. [8], Wang et al. [10], Martikainen et al. [11]
Growth factors, cytokines, adhesion molecules, inflammatory markers		
Procalcitonin	no	Lam et al. [12]
sICAM-1 and hyaluronan	yes	Martikainen et al. [11]
IL-6	no	Martikainen et al. [11]
CRP	no	Yang et al. [3]
	yes	Elsurer et al. [8], Zalunardo et al. [9],
Albumin	no	Martikainen et al. [11], Lam et al. [12]
	yes	Krishnan et al. [1]
		Blake et al. [14]
Causative organism	yes	
Risk factors for poor outcome: Gram-negative organisms, Pseudomonas, fungal and *Mycobacterium* sp.		Krishnan et al. [1], Chow et al. [6]
Among Gram-positive organisms, *S. aureus* has a worse outcome		Krishnan et al. [1], Yang et al. [3], Choi et al. [15]
Polymicrobial peritonitis as risk factor for catheter loss		Yang et al. [3]
Culture-negative peritonitis: recent peritonitis or recent antibiotic therapy	yes	Szeto et al. [2]
Fungal peritonitis: abdominal pain, bowel obstruction, catheter remaining in situ, *C. parapsilosis*	yes	Wang et al. [10], Lo et al. [17], Goldie et al. [19], Prasad et al. [20]
Recurrent and relapsing peritonitis: recurrent peritonitis has a poor therapeutic response and high mortality; recurrent peritonitis has a worse prognosis than relapsing peritonitis	yes	Szeto et al. [21]

Table 1. Continued

Factor	Prognostic value	References
Risk factors for adverse outcomes (ascites, EPS, death) after peritonitis-related technique failure: persistently elevated CRP level, older age, long PD duration	yes	Moon et al. [22]

References

1 Krishnan M, Thodis E, Ikonomopoulos D, et al: Predictors of outcome following bacterial peritonitis in peritoneal dialysis. Perit Dial Int 2002;22:573–581.
2 Szeto CC, Wong TY-H, Chow KM, Leung CB, Li PK-T: The clinical course of culture-negative peritonitis complicating peritoneal dialysis. Am J Kid Dis 2003;42:567–574.
3 Yang CY, Chen TW, Lin YP, et al: Determinants of catheter loss following continuous ambulatory peritoneal dialysis peritonitis. Perit Dial Int 2008;28:361–370.
4 Perez Fontan M, Rodriguez-Carmona A, Garcia-Naveiro R, Rosales M, Villaverde P, Valdes F: Peritonitis-related mortality in patients undergoing chronic peritoneal dialysis. Perit Dial Int 2005;25:274–284.
5 Golper TA, Brier ME, Bunke M, et al: Risk factors for peritonitis in long-term peritoneal dialysis: the Network 9 peritonitis and catheter survival studies. Am J Kid Dis 1996;28:428–436.
6 Chow KM, Szeto CC, Cheung KK-T, et al: Predictive value of dialysate cell counts in peritonitis complicating peritoneal dialysis. Clin J Am Soc Nephrol 2006;1:768–773.
7 Troidle L, Gorban-Brennan N, Kliger AS, Finkelstein FO: Effect of duration of chronic peritoneal dialysis therapy on the development of peritonitis. Perit Dial Int 1999;19:376–379.
8 Elsurer R, Afsar B, Sezer S, Ozdemir FN: Peritoneal cells at admission: do they have prognostic significance in peritonitis? Ren Fail 2010;32:335–342.
9 Zalunardo NY, Rose CL, Ma IWY, Altmann P: Higher serum C-reactive protein predicts short and long-term outcomes in peritoneal dialysis-associated peritonitis. Kidney Int 2007;71:687–692.
10 Wang AYM, Yu AWY, Li PKT, et al: Factors predicting outcome of fungal peritonitis in peritoneal dialysis: analysis of a 9-year experience of fungal peritonitis in a single center. Am J Kid Dis 2000;36:1183–1192.
11 Martikainen TA, Ekstrand AV, Honkanen EO, Teppo AM, Gr+Ânhagen-Riska C: Dialysate leukocytes, sICAM-1, hyaluronan and IL-6: predictors of outcome of peritonitis? Blood Purif 2004;22:360–366.
12 Lam MF, Leung JCK, Lam CWK, et al: Procalcitonin fails to differentiate inflammatory status or predict long-term outcomes in peritoneal dialysis-associated peritonitis. Perit Dial Int 2008;28:377–384.
13 Gulati S, Stephens D, Balfe JA, Secker D, Harvey E, Balfe JW: Children with hypoalbuminemia on continuous peritoneal dialysis are at risk for technique failure. Kidney Int 2001;59:2361–2367.
14 Blake PG, Flowerdew G, Blake RM, Oreopoulos DG: Serum albumin in patients on continuous ambulatory peritoneal dialysis – predictors and correlations with outcomes. J Am Soc Nephrol 1993;3:1501–1507.
15 Choi P, Nemati E, Banerjee A, Preston E, Levy J, Brown E: Peritoneal dialysis catheter removal for acute peritonitis: a retrospective analysis of factors associated with catheter removal and prolonged postoperative hospitalization. Am J Kid Dis 2004;43:103–111.
16 Bordes A, Campos-Herrero MI, Fernandez A, Vega N, Rodriguez JC, Palop L: Predisposing and prognostic factors of fungal peritonitis in peritoneal dialysis. Perit Dial Int 1995;15:275–276.
17 Lo SHK, Chan CK, Shum HP, Chow VCC, Mo Kl, Wong KS: Risk factors for poor outcome of fungal peritonitis in Chinese patients on continuous ambulatory peritoneal dialysis. Perit Dial Int 2003;23:S123–S126.
18 Matuszkiewicz-Rowinska J: Update on fungal peritonitis and its treatment. Perit Dial Int 2009;29:S161–S165.
19 Goldie SJ, Kiernan-Troidle L, Torres C, et al: Fungal peritonitis in a large chronic peritoneal dialysis population: a report of 55 episodes. Am J Kid Dis 1996;28:86–91.
20 Prasad KN, Prasad N, Gupta A, Sharma RK, Verma AK, Ayyagari A: Fungal peritonitis in patients on continuous ambulatory peritoneal dialysis: a single centre Indian experience. J Infect 2004;48:96–101.
21 Szeto CC, Kwan BC-H, Chow KM, et al: Recurrent and relapsing peritonitis: causative organisms and response to treatment. Am J Kid Dis 2009;54:702–710.
22 Moon SJ, Han SH, Kim DK, et al: Risk factors for adverse outcomes after peritonitis-related technique failure. Perit Dial Int 2008;28:352–360.

Dr. Dirk G. Struijk
Division of Nephrology, Department of Medicine, Academic Medical Centre, Amsterdam and Dianet
Meibergdreef 9
NL–1105 AZ Amsterdam (The Netherlands)
Tel. +31 20 5669 111, E-Mail d.g.struijk@amc.uva.nl

Ronco C, Rosner MH, Crepaldi C (eds): Peritoneal Dialysis – State-of-the-Art 2012.
Contrib Nephrol. Basel, Karger, 2012, vol 178, pp 271–277

Improving the Care of Diabetic Patients on Peritoneal Dialysis

Pranav Dalal · Madhukar Misra

Division of Nephrology, University of Missouri, Columbia, Mo., USA

Abstract

An overwhelming majority of patients on dialysis reach end-stage renal disease (ESRD) secondary to diabetes mellitus (DM). Although renal transplantation offers the best option for these patients, shortage of available kidneys becomes a major impediment. Besides hemodialysis (HD), peritoneal dialysis (PD) is also a commonly offered dialysis modality to these patients. However, PD in diabetics poses unique challenges. A constant exposure to glucose in the dialysate may further worsen the internal milieu of hyperglycemic diabetic individuals. A number of factors may help improve outcomes in such patients. Protection of the peritoneal membrane and residual renal function (RRF) are extremely important in this regard. Close monitoring of blood glucose levels and prompt management of peritoneal and exit site infections can prevent long term complications. This brief review addresses some important measures that can help improve outcomes of such patients on PD.

Diabetes mellitus (DM) has become the leading cause of end-stage renal disease (ESRD) worldwide. According to United States Renal Data System (USRDS) report, diabetic nephropathy was responsible for 44% of patients starting on dialysis in 2009 compared to 28% in 1984. Nearly ten times more patients are being treated for ESRD in 2009 than in 1980 [1]. Despite significant improvement in the survival of diabetic patient on hemidialysis (HD) and peritoneal dialysis (PD), it remains lower compared to renal transplantation and dialysis in nondiabetics. Renal transplantation is the preferred treatment for ESRD as it leads to better quality of life and improved survival. However, only a limited number of patients receive renal transplantation due to short supply of donor kidneys. It is therefore vitally important to critically appraise the dialysis modalities available to diabetic patients for maximizing outcomes. In this brief review we will examine the current status of PD together with ways to enhance various outcomes in diabetic patients on PD.

In general, the outcomes of patients on PD can be viewed as being dependent on several nonmodifiable and modifiable risk factors. While demographics and genetics largely determine the former, the latter include the residual renal function (RRF), infections, volume status and the functional and structural integrity of the peritoneal membrane.

Patient and Technique Survival in Diabetes

Studies comparing survival between HD and PD have yielded conflicting results. The five year mortality is higher in diabetic ESRD patients compared to their nondiabetic counterparts, mainly related to the co-existing cardiovascular disease. Between 1993–1997 and 1998–2002, the 5-year survival improved significantly for diabetic patients on dialysis. The improvement was more significant for patients on PD than patients on HD [2]. Vonesh et al. [3] compared the mortality amongst ESRD patients on HD versus PD from six large-scale registries and three cohort studies conducted in the US, Canada, Denmark and Netherlands. PD was associated with equal or better survival among nondiabetic patients and younger diabetic patients in all four countries. Among older diabetic patients, the Canadian and Danish registries data showed similar survival between HD and PD. In the US, HD was associated with better survival in diabetics aged 45 and older. A more recent analysis of 16,643 patients from the Dutch End-Stage Renal Disease Registry (RENINE) showed that the survival advantage of PD over HD decreases over time, with age and in the presence of diabetes as primary disease [4].

Serkes et al. [5] reported similar survival between patients on CAPD and HD. However, the CAPD patients had significantly higher treatment change over rate than HD patients. Also, the relative risk of modality change was significantly higher in diabetic CAPD patients compared to diabetic HD patients. Van Biesen et al. [6] showed the technique success rate was significantly higher in HD patients compared to PD patients at 3 years of follow-up. Again, the risk of technique failure was significantly higher in diabetics compared to nondiabetic patients. A matched-pairs analysis showed survival advantage for patients who started on PD and who were transferred to HD later compared to patients who were started and remained on HD.

Key Factors that Determine Outcomes in the Diabetic PD Patient

Residual Renal Function

RRF contributes to solute clearance and fluid removal. It contributes to adequacy of dialysis in PD patients and improves the quality of life. RRF is directly correlated with patient survival in both HD and PD patients [7]. The reanalysis of data from CANUSA study showed that each 5 liters/week increase in renal glomerular filtration rate (GFR) was associated with 12% decrease in the relative risk of death. Each 250-ml increment in urine volume was associated with a 36% decrease in overall mortality [8]. In a prospective observational study involving 231 PD patients, Wang et al. [9] reported a 50% reduction in all-cause mortality and cardiovascular death for every 1 ml/min increase in residual GFR. Moist et al. [10] showed that the patients treated with peritoneal dialysis had a 65% lower risk of RRF loss than those on hemodialysis during the first year of dialysis. Also, in this study, diabetes was an independent predictor of rapid decline in RRF. In a study by Liao et al. [11], the rate of decline of RRF was a more powerful prognostic factor than baseline RRF associated with all-cause mortality and technique failure in long-term PD patients.

Loss of RRF is associated with fluid overload, reduced erythropoiesis, retention of uremic toxins, malnutrition, congestive heart failure, cardiac hypertrophy, atherosclerosis, vascular, and valvular calcification and an overall increase in cardiovascular morbidity and mortality. It is therefore imperative to preserve RRF in diabetic dialysis patients. In two different, prospective, randomized, open-label studies, the use of Ramipril and Valsartan was associated with a slower decline in RRF compared to placebo in patients on PD [12, 13]. High-dose diuretics use was associated with increase urine volume, greater sodium removal and less weight gain without compromising RRF in CAPD patients [14]. The use of neutral pH, low glucose degradation product (GDP) lactate in the Euro-balance trial (retrospective registry data) showed better preservation of RRF compared to a traditional PD solution [15]. However, when tested in a well-powered randomized trial, Fan et al. [16] failed to show the benefits of using a biocompatible solution in the preservation of RRF in 93 PD patients.

Infection

Diabetes impairs antibacterial defenses and increases the risk of infection. Peritonitis is one of the major causes of morbidity in PD patients. High GDPs in PD solutions accelerate leukocyte apoptosis and adversely affect peritoneal defense [17]. However, analysis of large population-based studies reveals a similar incidence of PD peritonitis and PD catheter-related infections in diabetic and nondiabetic patients [18, 19]. In a recent retrospective analysis of observational data on more than 200 PD patients, Han et al. [20] found DM as an independent risk factor for PD peritonitis. The time to first episode of PD peritonitis was significantly longer in nondiabetic patients. On the other hand, this was not the case when larger North American data bases were analyzed. Mujais et al. [21] evaluated data on the microbiology and outcomes of peritonitis in USA and Canada involving about 10,000 PD patients. The rate of exit site infection was 0.184 and 0.193 infections per patient-year at risk in the USA and Canada, respectively. The rate of PD peritonitis was one infection every 32.7 patient-months at risk in the USA and one infection every 27.6 patient-months at risk in the Canada. They also evaluated the outcome of peritonitis episode according to diabetes status. The rates of resolution of peritonitis were similar in diabetic and nondiabetic groups. Diabetes did not affect the incidence of PD catheter removal and risk of death and outcomes were comparable in both countries – the USA and the Canada. It is therefore apparent that the theoretical concerns about the enhanced rates of peritoneal infections in diabetic patients may not be borne out by available evidence.

Volume Management

Fluid overload is an important contributor for the high technique failure rate in peritoneal dialysis patients. Diabetic patients tend to be more fluid overloaded compared to nondiabetic patients [22]. Restriction of salt and water intake may limit weight gain and help reduce the use of hypertonic glucose solutions for ultrafiltration. Patient education is of upmost importance. In a study from China, intensive patient education by a nurse, focusing on the importance of dietary salt and fluid restriction, the detrimental effects of using more hypertonic glucose solution, and the consequences of fluid overload was helpful in achieving dietary compliance with salt and fluid restriction, improving fluid status and minimizing the use of hypertonic glucose solution [23].

A recently published randomized control trial compared the effects of Icodextrin (ICO) and glucose-based solutions (GLU) in 41 Japanese patients with ESRD from DM nephropathy. The technique survival rate was 71.4% in ICO and 45.0% in GLU, with most of the technique failure due to volume overload. Net ultrafiltration volume was significantly higher in ICO throughout the study period. There were no apparent benefits of icodextrin use on residual renal and peritoneal functions, hemoglobin A1c, glycoalbumin, and lipid profile at 24 months [24].

Peritoneal Membrane Integrity

Long-term PD patients develop progressive increase in peritoneal membrane permeability, decrease in ultrafiltration capacity and peritoneal fibrosis [25]. In a study of peritoneal membrane morphology in patients before the start of PD, the uremic diabetic patients had higher average peritoneal thickness compared to nondiabetic patients. The hyalinizing vasculopathy was more frequent in uremic patients with diabetes than uremic patients without diabetes [26]. Conventional PD solutions contain glucose as the main osmotic agent and lactate as the buffering agent. Persistent exposure to high glucose and GDPs lead to ultrastructural changes in the peritoneal membrane including neoangiogenesis, mesothelial damage and fibrosis. While the pathophysiologic mechanisms underlying these changes are not fully understood, the activation of the local renin-angiotensin-aldosterone system (RAAS) is thought to play an important role. The peritoneal mesothelial cells constitutively express angiotensinogen, angiotensin-converting enzyme (ACE), angiotensin II type 1 and type 2 receptors, as well as transforming growth factor-β (TGF-β) and fibronectin [27]. The high glucose concentration, hyperosmolality, low pH, high lactate concentration, and the presence of glucose degradation products in the peritoneal dialysate is related to activation of local RAAS.

The activation of RAAS and production of TGF-β, contributes to epithelial-to-mesenchymal transformation of mesothelial cells, resulting in progressive fibrosis of the peritoneal membrane [28].

Therapeutic measures targeting inhibition of systemic RAAS as well as reducing the activation of peritoneal RAAS can be helpful in protecting the peritoneal membrane. Use of both Losartan and Captopril has been shown to inhibit glucose-induced TGF-β and fibronectin expression in cultured human peritoneal mesothelial cells [27]. Furthermore, Sauter et al. shown that the ACE inhibitors and Losartan are capable of attenuating the inflammation mediated overproduction of mesothelial vascular endothelial growth factor (VEGF) [29]. In a retrospective analysis of data from the Netherlands Cooperative Study on Adequacy of Dialysis (NECOSAD) on 217 long-term CAPD patients, the use of ACE inhibitors or angiotensin receptor blockers (ARBs) was associated with a beneficial effect on small solute transport status as well as better technique survival [30]. In another retrospective analysis, the use of ACE inhibitors or ARB was associated with a reduction in mortality in patients on peritoneal dialysis independent of blood pressure control and other clinical variables. No association with peritoneal membrane function was reported [31]. Although these studies are helpful, no long-term data assessing the effect of ACE inhibitor/ARBs on the human peritoneal membrane in PD patients are currently available.

Use of a glucose-sparing regimen like icodextrin or amino acid-based PD solutions could minimize the glucose exposure to peritoneal membrane, limit local RAAS activation and may help preserve the integrity of the peritoneal membrane. A subgroup analysis evaluated the effect of glucose exposure and icodextrin use on the longitudinal membrane function in anuric automated peritoneal dialysis patients from European Automated Peritoneal Dialysis Outcomes Study (EAPOS). Patients using icodextrin at baseline were more likely to be diabetic and had worse membrane function. At the end of 24 months, patients using icodextrin at the start of the study had no change in the ultrafiltration capacity and smaller increase in the solute transport [32]. Nakao et al. [33] reported slower deterioration of peritoneal membrane function with icodextrin compared to high-glucose-based PD dialysate in diabetic rats with chronic kidney disease. In vivo, the administration of rosiglitazone (peroxisome proliferator-activated receptor-γ (PPAR-γ) agonists) has been shown to diminish the accumulation of advanced glycation end products (AGEs), preserve the mesothelial monolayer, decrease the number of invading mesothelial cells, reduce fibrosis and angiogenesis, and improve peritoneal function. Rosiglitazone appears to produce pleiotropic protective effects on the peritoneal membrane by reducing the accumulation of AGEs and inflammation, and by preserving the mesothelial cells monolayer, highlighting the potential of PPAR-γ activation to ameliorate peritoneal deterioration in PD patients [34].

Blood Sugar Control in the Diabetic Patient on Peritoneal Dialysis

Marked hyperglycemia is associated with increased mortality in diabetic patients on PD [35]. The majority of endogenous insulin is cleared by the kidneys. Uremia alters the insulin metabolism, responsiveness and excretion, making it difficult to control blood sugar in the PD patients. A genuine fasting level is not possible and good glycemic control is difficult to achieve due to continuous glucose exposure. No studies have specifically addressed glycemic control criteria in diabetic PD patients. About 60–80% of instilled glucose in PD solution is absorbed in a 4-hour dwell, corresponding to daily intake of 100–300 g glucose. This is equivalent to 20–30% of daily caloric intake [36]. Diabetic patients have a slight increase in insulin need after being started on PD, but the insulin requirements markedly increase after exposure to hypertonic glucose solutions [37]. Use of one bag of icodextrin or amino acid-containing solution reduces the glucose load by 15–30%.

Metabolites of icodextrin are known to cause an overestimation of blood glucose in glucose meters using glucose dehydrogenase/pyrroloquinoline quinone systems. This can lead to the administration of a high insulin dose and hypoglycemia. Specialized methods for glucose monitoring should be used in diabetic PD patients on icodextrin-based therapy. Intraperitoneal (IP) insulin administration allows quick and consistent absorption. Insulin enters the portal venous circulation and reduces hepatic glucose output which more physiological route than peripheral insulin administration. IP insulin was associated with less fluctuations in blood sugar and lower low-density lipoprotein level compared to subcutaneous insulin [38]. IP insulin eliminates the need for several daily injections and prevents insulin antibody formation. Although IP insulin administration on empty abdomen was observed to require 26% less insulin, the risk of peritonitis was higher. Other potential disadvantages of IP insulin therapy include peritoneal fibroblast proliferation and hepatic subcapsular steatosis [36].

Other Possible Benefits of Peritoneal Dialysis in the Diabetic Patient

Besides other putative general benefits of PD (better hemodynamic tolerance, lack of need for vascular access with its complications, home-based therapy, etc.), PD may be associated with less circulatory stress and myocardial stunning. Progression of diabetic retinopathy and episodes of hemorrhagic retinopathy are less common in PD patients compared to HD patients. Stabilization or improvement in diabetic retinopathy had been reported in patients maintained on CAPD [39, 40]. PD patients have a lower risk of contracting blood-borne diseases like hepatitis C. Patients on PD able to maintain better hemoglobin level at lower erythropoietin doses [41]. Outcome of renal transplants are similar in diabetic and nondiabetic patients [42]. Studies have reported better recipient and graft survival when the patient received at least 50% of their pretransplant dialysis time as PD [43].

In summary, the outcomes in diabetic patients are not different than diabetic patients on PD. However, management of PD in diabetes poses special challenges. An understanding of the changes in the diabetic peritoneum and strategies for peritoneo- protection are vital to preserve membrane function. Use of icodextrin is associated with reduced glucose load, better ultrafiltration and technique survival rate as well as possible preservation of peritoneal membrane integrity and residual renal function. Physician knowledge and patient compliance are important in maintaining diabetic patient on peritoneal dialysis for the long-term. A multipronged approach, as outlined above, is essential in improving the prognosis of diabetic patients on PD.

References

1 US Renal Data System UADR: Atlas of Chronic Kidney Disease and End-Stage Renal Disease in United States. Bethesda, National Institutes of Health, National Institute of Diabetes and Digestive and Kidney Diseases, 2011.

2 US Renal Data System UADR: Atlas of Chronic Kidney Disease and End-Stage Renal Disease in United States. Bethesda, National Institutes of Health, National Institute of Diabetes and Digestive and Kidney Diseases, 2009.

3 Vonesh EF, Snyder JJ, Foley RN, Collins AJ: Mortality studies comparing peritoneal dialysis and hemodialysis: what do they tell us? Kidney Int Suppl 2006;103:S3–S11.

4 Liem YS, Wong JB, Hunink MG, de Charro FT, Winkelmayer WC: Comparison of hemodialysis and peritoneal dialysis survival in The Netherlands. Kidney Int 2007;71:153–158.

5 Serkes KD, Blagg CR, Nolph KD, Vonesh EF, Shapiro F: Comparison of patient and technique survival in continuous ambulatory peritoneal dialysis (CAPD) and hemodialysis: a multicenter study. Perit Dial Int 1990;10:15–19.

6 Van Biesen W, Vanholder RC, Veys N, Dhondt A, Lameire NH: An evaluation of an integrative care approach for end-stage renal disease patients. J Am Soc Nephrol 2000;11:116–125.
7 van der Wal WM, Noordzij M, Dekker FW, et al: Full loss of residual renal function causes higher mortality in dialysis patients; findings from a marginal structural model. Nephrol Dial Transplant Sep 2011;26:2978–2983.
8 Bargman JM, Thorpe KE, Churchill DN: Relative contribution of residual renal function and peritoneal clearance to adequacy of dialysis: a reanalysis of the CANUSA study. J Am Soc Nephrol 2001;12:2158–2162.
9 Wang AY, Wang M, Woo J, et al: Inflammation, residual kidney function, and cardiac hypertrophy are interrelated and combine adversely to enhance mortality and cardiovascular death risk of peritoneal dialysis patients. J Am Soc Nephrol Aug 2004;15:2186–2194.
10 Moist LM, Port FK, Orzol SM, et al: Predictors of loss of residual renal function among new dialysis patients. J Am Soc Nephrol Mar 2000;11:556–564.
11 Liao CT, Chen YM, Shiao CC, et al: Rate of decline of residual renal function is associated with all-cause mortality and technique failure in patients on long-term peritoneal dialysis. Nephrol Dial Transplant Sep 2009;24:2909–2914.
12 Li PK, Chow KM, Wong TY, Leung CB, Szeto CC: Effects of an angiotensin-converting enzyme inhibitor on residual renal function in patients receiving peritoneal dialysis. A randomized, controlled study. Ann Intern Med 2003;139:105–112.
13 Suzuki H, Kanno Y, Sugahara S, Okada H, Nakamoto H: Effects of an angiotensin II receptor blocker, valsartan, on residual renal function in patients on CAPD. Am J Kidney Dis 2004;43:1056–1064.
14 Medcalf JF, Harris KP, Walls J: Role of diuretics in the preservation of residual renal function in patients on continuous ambulatory peritoneal dialysis. Kidney Int Mar 2001;59:1128–1133.
15 Williams JD, Topley N, Craig KJ, et al: The Euro-Balance Trial: the effect of a new biocompatible peritoneal dialysis fluid (balance) on the peritoneal membrane. Kidney Int 2004;66:408–418.
16 Fan SL, Pile T, Punzalan S, Raftery MJ, Yaqoob MM: Randomized controlled study of biocompatible peritoneal dialysis solutions: effect on residual renal function. Kidney Int 2008;73:200–206.
17 Santamaria B, Sanz A, Justo P, et al: Peritoneal defence – lessons learned which apply to diabetes complications. Nephrol Dial Transplant Jul 2006;21(suppl 2):ii12–ii15.
18 Holley J, Bernardini J, Piraino B: Catheter infections in insulin-dependent diabetics on continuous ambulatory peritoneal dialysis. Perit Dial Int 1991;11:347–350.
19 Digenis GE, Abraham G, Savin E, et al: Peritonitis-related deaths in continuous ambulatory peritoneal dialysis (CAPD) patients. Perit Dial Int 1990;10:45–47.
20 Han SH, Lee SC, Ahn SV, et al: Reduced residual renal function is a risk of peritonitis in continuous ambulatory peritoneal dialysis patients. Nephrol Dial Transplant Sep 2007;22:2653–2658.
21 Mujais S: Microbiology and outcomes of peritonitis in North America. Kidney Int Suppl 2006;103:S55–S62.
22 Gan HB, Chen MH, Lindholm B, Wang T: Volume control in diabetic and nondiabetic peritoneal dialysis patients. Int Urol Nephrol 2005;37:575–579.
23 Quan L, Xu Y, Luo SP, Wang L, LeBlanc D, Wang T: Negotiated care improves fluid status in diabetic peritoneal dialysis patients. Perit Dial Int 2006;26:95–100.
24 Takatori Y, Akagi S, Sugiyama H, et al: Icodextrin increases technique survival rate in peritoneal dialysis patients with diabetic nephropathy by improving body fluid management: a randomized controlled trial. Clin J Am Soc Nephrol 2011;6:1337–1344.
25 Heimburger O, Waniewski J, Werynski A, Tranaeus A, Lindholm B: Peritoneal transport in CAPD patients with permanent loss of ultrafiltration capacity. Kidney Int 1990;38:495–506.
26 Honda K, Hamada C, Nakayama M, et al: Impact of uremia, diabetes, and peritoneal dialysis itself on the pathogenesis of peritoneal sclerosis: a quantitative study of peritoneal membrane morphology. Clin J Am Soc Nephrol 2008;3:720–728.
27 Noh H, Ha H, Yu MR, Kim YO, Kim JH, Lee HB: Angiotensin II mediates high glucose-induced TGF-beta1 and fibronectin upregulation in HPMC through reactive oxygen species. Perit Dial Int 2005;25:38–47.
28 Nessim SJ, Perl J, Bargman JM: The renin-angiotensin-aldosterone system in peritoneal dialysis: is what is good for the kidney also good for the peritoneum? Kidney Int 2010;78:23–28.
29 Sauter M, Cohen CD, Wornle M, Mussack T, Ladurner R, Sitter T: ACE inhibitor and AT1-receptor blocker attenuate the production of VEGF in mesothelial cells. Perit Dial Int 2007;27:167–172.
30 Kolesnyk I, Noordzij M, Dekker FW, Boeschoten EW, Krediet RT: A positive effect of AII inhibitors on peritoneal membrane function in long-term PD patients. Nephrol Dial Transplant 2009;24:272–277.
31 Fang W, Oreopoulos DG, Bargman JM: Use of ACE inhibitors or angiotensin receptor blockers and survival in patients on peritoneal dialysis. Nephrol Dial Transplant Nov 2008;23:3704–3710.
32 Davies SJ, Brown EA, Frandsen NE, et al: Longitudinal membrane function in functionally anuric patients treated with APD: data from EAPOS on the effects of glucose and icodextrin prescription. Kidney Int Apr 2005;67:1609–1615.
33 Nakao A, Nakao K, Takatori Y, et al: Effects of icodextrin peritoneal dialysis solution on the peritoneal membrane in the STZ-induced diabetic rat model with partial nephrectomy. Nephrol Dial Transplant 2010;25:1479–1488.
34 Sandoval P, Loureiro J, Gonzalez-Mateo G, et al: PPAR-gamma agonist rosiglitazone protects peritoneal membrane from dialysis fluid-induced damage. Lab Invest 2010;90:1517–1532.
35 Duong U, Mehrotra R, Molnar MZ, et al: Glycemic control and survival in peritoneal dialysis patients with diabetes mellitus. Clin J Am Soc Nephrol 2011;6:1041–1048.

36 Huang CC: Treatment targets for diabetic patients on peritoneal dialysis: any evidence? Perit Dial Int 2007;27(suppl 2):S176–S179.
37 Szeto CC, Chow KM, Leung CB, et al: Increased subcutaneous insulin requirements in diabetic patients recently commenced on peritoneal dialysis. Nephrol Dial Transplant 2007;22:1697–1702.
38 Quellhorst E: Insulin therapy during peritoneal dialysis: pros and cons of various forms of administration. J Am Soc Nephrol 2002;13(suppl 1): S92–S96.
39 Diaz-Buxo JA, Burgess WP, Greenman M, Chandler JT, Farmer CD, Walker PJ: Visual function in diabetic patients undergoing dialysis: comparison of peritoneal and hemodialysis. Int J Artif Organs Sep 1984;7:257–262.
40 Rottembourg J, Bellio P, Maiga K, Remaoun M, Rousselie F, Legrain M: Visual function, blood pressure and blood glucose in diabetic patients undergoing continuous ambulatory peritoneal dialysis. Proc Eur Dial Transplant Assoc Eur Ren Assoc 1985;21:330–334.
41 Richardson D, Ford D, Gilg J, Williams AJ: UK Renal Registry 11th Annual Report (December 2008). Chapter 9: Haemoglobin, ferritin and erythropoietin amongst patients receiving dialysis in the UK in 2007: national and centre-specific analyses. Nephron Clin Pract 2009;111(suppl 1):c149–c183.
42 Tokodai K, Amada N, Kikuchi H, Haga I, Takayama T, Nakamura A: Outcomes of renal transplantation after end-stage renal disease due to diabetic nephropathy: a single-center experience. Transplant Proc 2012;44:77–79.
43 Goldfarb-Rumyantzev AS, Hurdle JF, Scandling JD, Baird BC, Cheung AK: The role of pretransplantation renal replacement therapy modality in kidney allograft and recipient survival. Am J Kidney Dis Sep 2005;46:537–549.

Madhukar Misra, MD
Division of Nephrology, University of Missouri Columbia, C420 CSE Building
5 Hospital Drive
Columbia, MO 65212 (USA)
Tel. +1 573 882 7992, E-Mail misram@health.missouri.edu

Ronco C, Rosner MH, Crepaldi C (eds): Peritoneal Dialysis – State-of-the-Art 2012.
Contrib Nephrol. Basel, Karger, 2012, vol 178, pp 278–283

How to Select among Dialysis Options

Andrew Mooney

Leeds Teaching Hospitals NHS Trust, Leeds, UK

Abstract

End-stage renal disease is an almost unique disease area in which patients not only choose their treatment modality but can also change their mind and their treatment as time goes by. The way that information about treatment options is presented to patients is critical in influencing how they process this information, and it is possible to present information to patients in different ways so that patients can make better decisions about the treatment they receive. It is important to recognize that simply giving more information to patients does not necessarily improve their ability to make decisions. Instead, a series of simple principles should be used when giving information to help patients to choose between dialysis options, and it is possible to put this together into 'patient decision aid' which will reduce bias and increase the likelihood of a patient choosing the treatment which is right for them. If a patient does do this, it is more likely that they will comply with the treatment better, tolerate complications of the treatment better, and experience better outcomes.

Dialysis can be delivered by various modalities, but rates of uptake of different modalities vary widely [1]. Analysis of different national registry data shows that there is a wide geographical variation in the uptake of the different modalities, but also analysis of registry data from individual countries reveals changes in the uptake of different dialysis modalities with time [2]. Comparing the survival rates on the different modalities does not give an explanation of the change in uptake rates [3], and the changes over time mean that case-mix is unlikely to account for these differences. Furthermore, none of the rates of uptake match those which practicing physicians believe to be the best starting therapy for patients new to dialysis [4]. Therefore, it would appear that there are physician, patient and service factors which influence the uptake rates of dialysis modalities, and it would follow that each of these could be subject to manipulation.

Regarding patient factors, the treatment of end-stage chronic kidney disease is almost unique in that it is a chronic treatment of a long term condition where the patient can choose their treatment modality but also change from one modality to another as time goes by. To try to help patients choose between these technical treatments, multiple agencies have invested considerable resources in trying to produce documents to improve patient choice. However, few if any of these resources have been developed with knowledge of the psychology of patient behavior, processing of information-related to health or decision-making. As a result, review of these information resources designed to support decision-making for patients has revealed that often they are not fit for purpose [5].

In many health care settings, there is active promotion of patient care and patient choice. There is an increasing recognition of the role of patient input to clinical decision making, and there are now a series of guidelines of best practice for how to deliver effective predialysis education, especially regarding modality choice [6]. To understand the basis for these guidelines, it is necessary to have some understanding of the psychological science behind decision making, and these are presented in the next section.

Background to Decision Making

All of us, all the time, have to make decisions. Despite our unique experiences, however, all of us have only two ways of making decisions – these are heuristic and systematic. A heuristic decision is one in which 'an option that will do' is chosen – an example would be choosing what to eat from the menu in a restaurant. It is quick, intuitive and usually associated with a satisfactory outcome, but nevertheless chosen without attention to all the details or consequences of the decision taken. This is the method by which most of us make most of our decisions most of the time. A systematic decision, on the other hand, is one that is taken with greater attention to the pro's and con's of the options; one weighs up what these are in each scenario, matches them with one's own beliefs and values, and then chooses an option. An example of a systematic decision might be whether to apply for a new job. Clearly, taking a systematic decision is more time consuming and requires greater effort; however, it is also established that making systematic decisions is associated with making better decisions, i.e. a decision that fits with one's beliefs and values and one which we are less likely to regret in the future [7].

In a dialysis context, when talking to patients about their treatment options, clearly one would want the patient to make a systematic decision. However patients, just like all of us, are seeking to 'short cut' this process and use a heuristic process instead. The way that patients might try to use heuristic methods would be to ask the doctor 'What do you think is best?'. By doing this, the patient is not judging the options against his or her own values and beliefs, but instead asking the doctor to make the judgment against their beliefs. Similar principles may apply if a patient asks to meet other patients who have chosen a particular dialysis modality [7].

In order to support patients' decision making, it is important that information is presented in a way that engages systematic decision making and reduces the likelihood of using heuristic strategies. The next section describes how this can be achieved.

Designing Effective Patient Information

To make information as useful as possible for patients to choose between treatment options, it is important to consider two factors – the patient and the information.

Patient Factors

Starting with the patient, it is important to consider two factors: firstly, where is the patient in their disease pathway, and, secondly, where is the patient in their readiness to make a decision. The first consideration may seem obvious, but as is often the case in this field, it is often overlooked. During a patient's development of chronic kidney disease, they will pass from stages 1 to 5, and at some point need to make choices between dialysis options. It is very helpful for patients to be provided with a 'map' (fig. 1) to show where they are in the decision-making process. By doing this, one engages the patient, increases their understanding, alerts them to the fact that a decision has to be made (which increases the likelihood of systematic processing), and informs them of their options. Although a great deal of effort has been spent in providing information to help choose between dialysis options, our studies have revealed that for patients a much larger decision that they are more acutely aware of is the decision whether to have renal replacement therapy at all [8] – it seems that patients expend

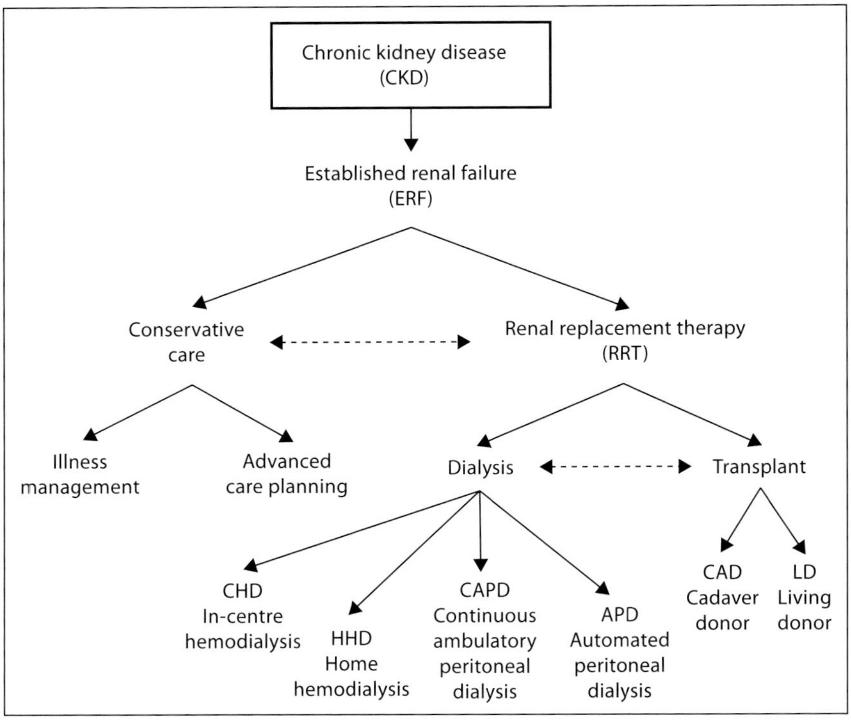

Fig. 1. Schematic diagram to increase patient's understanding of their position in the CKD decision-making process.

a lot of energy on that decision, and then fail to engage as effectively as they could with information about choosing between dialysis options.

The second consideration is where the patient is in their readiness to make a decision. This has parallels with the transtheoretical model of 'readiness to change' which was developed from work with patients who abuse substances and whether they were in a position to effectively try to change their behavior (precontemplation, contemplation, readiness, action, maintenance) [9]. In similar fashion, patients need to be ready to consider future treatment options, and if they are not ready to do so, they do not require decision-making information, but instead require further information about their disease or else further consultations with their doctors or allied professions to come to a position where they can engage with the decision-making information.

Information Factors

Information to help patients make decisions is specific for its purpose, and different from information designed to increase patients knowledge about their illness, or information to improve concordance or compliance with treatment, or information to describe procedures associated with treatment choices (e.g. which ward to report to for fistula formation), etc. It is very important when providing patient literature to be clear what the purpose is of the literature being provided. It should also help the author focus on what information should be included [7].

Readability

However, in keeping with all types of patient information, one of the first principles is that it should be written in simple language – aiming for language that can be understood by a high-school (13–14 years old) student. In English, there are readily available readability scores often now included in word processing software which enable the readability score to be calculated easily [10]. However, in other languages it is recognized that literature read by young children is different to that read by adults and similar principles apply – shorter sentences with shorter words is more easily readable.

Balance

The next and apparently obvious point is that information between the options should be balanced with an equal number of pro's and con's presented for each. By definition, if one is making a decision between options it should be possible to present these data and if there were not an equal number of pro's and con's then there wouldn't be a choice to make. In the case of dialysis modality, there is no convincing evidence that one is superior to the other, so the choice is between lifestyle factors (e.g. treatment in your house vs. treatment at a center) which could be viewed as positive or negative depending on the patient's perspective. Clearly, although this may seem an obvious point, our studies have revealed that patient information is not presented in this way [5]. In addition, our studies have shown that it is more effective to present options side by side, rather than in series – much in the same way that 'price comparison websites' do, so that patients can visualize the options and perform the trade-offs more effectively [11].

Presentation of Risk

The next important thing to consider is the presentation of risk figures. It is essential to avoid using terms such as 'low' or 'high' likelihood of events happening. Such language reflects the values of the author and it is important that patients look at the numbers and make their own value judgments about whether the likelihood is high or low. Therefore, phrases such as 'eight out of ten patients choosing this option experience this outcome' are preferable and more effective at engaging patients and causing them to use systematic decision making processes. All of us would have a different threshold for deciding whether an 80% likelihood of an outcome is acceptable or not [7].

Explaining Medical Terms

Often when writing for patients, professionals are unsure how to use technical terms, as a result of which there is a risk that the text is either unintelligible because too many technical medical terms are used, or else appears patronizing or colloquial as more childish terms are used. It is established that the most effective way to explain these terms to patients are by using the correct term plus an explanation – e.g. 'fistula, which is a surgically created blood vessel especially for use in hemodialysis' is superior to 'fistula' alone or 'special blood vessel' [7].

Avoid Unnecessary Use of Videos, Pictures or Stories

It is often tempting to use videos or other media to provide information to patients. Although such information might be highly memorable to patients and help them to remember key facts, it must be borne in mind that use of such materials can easily tap into patients heuristic processing and prevent the recipient from properly evaluating the information presented. For example, a booklet containing a photograph showing a hemodialysis patient attached to a machine with a nurse in attendance might be contrasted with a photograph of a patient on a fairground ride in the peritoneal dialysis section. Although the intention might be to demonstrate that peritoneal dialysis patients have greater independence, the images might be interpreted that hemodialysis patients receive more care or nurturing; alternatively images of fairground rides might put off patients who have fear of heights or motion sickness from a modality that would otherwise be ideal for them! It has also been demonstrated that videos of different people giving the same information produces different choices among subjects, and it is established in several areas of medical care that patients are more persuasive than doctors over treatment decisions [12].

Avoid Information Leakage

When presenting information, it is easy to surround the facts with other language which reveals the authors attitude to the information. For example, citing an 80% chance of an outcome carries a more positive inference than citing an 80% risk of an outcome. Using the latter phrase might cause the patient to infer that the author did not favor that choice [7]. There are multiple possible examples such as this and it is important that neutral terms are used as much as possible.

Present Information in a Structured Way Matching Patients Beliefs about Illness

All of us when we become ill have a common way of conceptualizing our illness. We all seek information about the illness's identity, natural history, consequences, cause and potential treatments. For example, if you have a sore throat, you might think you have laryngitis (identity), it will last a few days then resolve (natural history), you might need 2–3 days off work (consequences), you got it because you met up with your brother who had something similar and you have been working hard recently (cause) and you might want to take some throat lozenges (treatment). Our response to finding a lump in our supraclavicular fossa might follow a more serious and worrying course, but have similar components. This is a model that has been proposed as a template from which we all respond to illness, which in most cases would be to seek effective intervention [13]. Therefore, if the information we provide for patients can mirror this structure, it might increase the likelihood with which the patient will engage with the information and undertake action to improve their well-being (i.e. make a decision about the treatment they want to receive).

In summary, therefore, there are several components to the structure of information which can help patients make decisions more effectively. Some are simple to activate, e.g. using simple language, others are more complicated and require external expertise, e.g. using illness representation models to structure information. However, all of these can be utilized in patient decision aids, which are described below.

Patient Decision Aids

The summative use of all these techniques is a patient decision aid. This is a complex intervention designed with all the above principles in mind. Its purpose is to enable patients to become involved in decision making by providing information about the options and by clarifying personal values. They are designed to complement, rather than replace, counselling from a health practitioner. However, by using such aids, it should be possible for health services to more easily provide unbiased information to patients to effectively choose treatment options that are right for them.

Conclusions

Including patients in choices about their treatments is important and increasingly so. The principles involved in helping patients make good decisions depend on presenting unbiased balanced information which patients can assimilate with their beliefs and values to come to a decision which suits them. Some principles are relatively easy to include, others are more complex and can all be incorporated into a patient decision aid. The use of such aids, and the support of patients in choosing treatment options that suit them, should result in patients receiving true patient-centered care and also result in patients that are more concordant with treatment regimens and tolerant of treatment complications.

Acknowledgements

The author greatly acknowledges the help of Dr. Hilary Bekker and others in the development of ideas for this manuscript.

References

1 ERA-EDTA Registry Annual Report 2009. Amsterdam, Academic Medical Center, Department of Medical Informatics, 2011.

2 UK Renal Registry Report 2010. Bristol, Southmead Hospital, 2012.

3 Burkart J, Piraino B, Kaldas H, Lee JY, Bender FH, Krediet RT, Boeschoten EW, Dekker FW, Vonesh E, Mujais S: Why is the evidence favouring hemodialysis over peritoneal dialysis misleading? Semin Dial 2007;20:200–202.

4 Ledebo I, Ronco C: The best dialysis therapy? Results from an international survey among nephrology professionals: NDT Plus 2008;1:403–408.

5 Winterbottom A, Conner M, Mooney A, Bekker HL: Evaluating the quality of patient leaflets about renal replacement therapy across UK renal units. Nephrol Dial Transplant 2007;22:2291–2296.

6 Covic A, Bammens B, Lobbedez T, Segall L, Heimburger O, van Biesen W, Fouque D, Vanholder R: Educating end-stage renal disease patients on dialysis modality selection; NDT Plus 2010;3:225–233.

7 Bekker HL, Winterbottom A, Mooney A: Patient information and decision making (editorial). Br J Renal Med 2009;14:28–30.

8 Winterbottom A, Bekker HL, Conner M, Mooney A: Choosing dialysis modality: decision making in a chronic illness context. Health Expectations 2012;under review.

9 Prochaska JO, Butterworth S, Redding CA, Burden V, Perrin N, Leo M, Flaherty-Robb M, Prochaska JM: Initial efficacy of MI, TTM tailoring and HRI's with multiple behaviors for employee health promotion. Prev Med 2008;46:226–231.

10 Flesch R: A new readability yardstick. J Appl Psychol 1948;32:221–233.

11 Mooney A, YoDDA Development Group: Developing a dialysis decision aid: establishing the best way of structuring information. British Renal Society Meeting, Birmingham, 2011, abstr O56.

12 Winterbottom A, Bekker H, Conner M, Mooney A: Patient stories about their dialysis experience biases others' choices regardless of doctor's advice: an experimental study. Nephrol Dial Transplant 2011;6:325–331.

13 Leventhal H, Meyer D, Nerenz D: The common-sense representation of illness danger; in Rachman S (ed): Contributions to Medical Psychology. New York, Pergamon Press, 1980, vol 2, pp 7–30.

Dr. Andrew Mooney
Leeds Teaching Hospitals NHS Trust
Beckett Street
Leeds LS9 7TF (UK)
Tel. +44 113 2066869, E-Mail andrew.mooney@leedsth.nhs.uk

Author Index

Subject Index